A Case-Based Approach to Veterinary Science

A Case-Based Approach to Veterinary Science

Edited by Matthew Benoit

SYRAWOOD
PUBLISHING HOUSE

New York

Published by Syrawood Publishing House,
750 Third Avenue, 9th Floor,
New York, NY 10017, USA
www.syrawoodpublishinghouse.com

A Case-Based Approach to Veterinary Science
Edited by Matthew Benoit

International Standard Book Number: 978-1-68286-624-5 (Hardback)

Cataloging-in-Publication Data

A case-based approach to veterinary science / edited by Matthew Benoit.
    p. cm.
Includes bibliographical references and index.
ISBN 978-1-68286-624-5
1. Veterinary medicine. 2. Veterinary medicine--Case studies. 3. Animals--Diseases.
4. Animal health. I. Benoit, Matthew.
SF745 .C37 2018
636.089--dc23

TABLE OF CONTENTS

PREFACE

Veterinary medicine focuses on the diagnosis, treatment and rehabilitation of unhealthy and sick animals. Veterinary medicine has various branches specializing in particular anatomical systems of animals. Vaccination, treatment as well as surgical procedures are performed on animals for their care and well-being. Detection and prevention of zoonotic diseases is another important part of veterinary medicine. From theories to research to practical applications, case studies related to all contemporary topics of relevance to this field have been included in this book. With state-of-the-art inputs by acclaimed experts of this field, this book targets students and professionals.

After months of intensive research and writing, this book is the end result of all who devoted their time and efforts in the initiation and progress of this book. It will surely be a source of reference in enhancing the required knowledge of the new developments in the area. During the course of developing this book, certain measures such as accuracy, authenticity and research focused analytical studies were given preference in order to produce a comprehensive book in the area of study.

This book would not have been possible without the efforts of the authors and the publisher. I extend my sincere thanks to them. Secondly, I express my gratitude to my family and well-wishers. And most importantly, I thank my students for constantly expressing their willingness and curiosity in enhancing their knowledge in the field, which encourages me to take up further research projects for the advancement of the area.

Editor

Identification of a Novel Enterovirus E Isolates HY12 from Cattle with Severe Respiratory and Enteric Diseases

Lisai Zhu⁹, Zeli Xing⁹, Xiaochun Gai⁹, Sujing Li, Zhihao San, Xinping Wang*

College of Veterinary Medicine, Jilin University, Changchun, Jilin, China

Abstract

In this study, a virus strain designated as HY12 was isolated from cattle with a disease of high morbidity and mortality in Jilin province. Biological and physiochemical properties showed that HY12 isolates is cytopathic with an extremely high infectivity. HY12 is resistant to treatment of organic solvent and acid, and unstable at 60°C for 1 h. Electron microscopy observation revealed the virus is an approximately 22–28 nm in diameter. The complete genome sequence of HY12 consists of 7416 nucleotides, with a typical picornavirus genome organization including a 5′-untranslated region (UTR), a large single ORF encoding a polyprotein of 2176 amino acids, and a 3′-UTR. Phylogenetic analysis clustered HY12 isolates to a new serotype/genotype within the clade of enterovirus E (formerly BEV-A). Alignment analysis revealed a unique insertion of 2 amino acid residues (NF) at the C-terminal of VP1 protein between aa 825 and 826, and several rare mutations in VP1 and VP4 of HY12 isolates in relation to known bovine enterovirus (BEV) strains. This is the first report of an enterovirus E in China, which is potentially associated with an outbreak in cattle with severe respiratory and enteric diseases.

Editor: Lijun Rong, University of Illinois at Chicago, United States of America

Funding: This study is supported by the Key Science and Technology projects from Jilin Province Scientific and Technology Program (20140204064NY); program fund of Jilin province for high-level creative and talented individuals to Xinping Wang. The funders had no role in study design, data collection and analysis, decision to publish, or preparation of the manuscript.

Competing Interests: The authors have declared that no competing interests exist.

* E-mail: wangxp88@hotmail.com

⁹ These authors contributed equally to this work.

Introduction

The genus *enterovirus* within the family *picornaviridae* consists of 9 species of enterovirus (A,B, C, D, E, F, G, H, J) and 3 species of rhinoviruses (A, B, C) based on the latest virus taxonomy[1]. These viruses have many features in common and are the leading etiological agents related to respiratory and digestive diseases in human and animals. Like other species within the genus, bovine enteroviruses (BEVs) are small, non-enveloped viruses with an icosahedral virion and a positive–stranded RNA genome. BEVs have been isolated from cattle with a clinical signs varying from respiratory diseases to enteric, reproductive disease and infertility [2,3,4,5,6,7,8,9,10,11,12,13,14], and even from faeces of the presumably healthy calves[15]. The pathogenicity and virulence of bovine enterovirus is still largely unknown. Failure to experimentally reproduce bovine enterovirus infection in calves showing obvious clinical signs led to the conclusion that BEV is not significant agent in the cattle industry. This argument was seemly further supported by the findings that bovine enterovirus were easily detected in the contaminated waters adjacent to cattle herds; and the discovery that BEV-like sequences are present in shellfish, bottlenose dolphins, and in deer feces from the same geographical area [16,17,18,19,20]. However, with more and more BEV isolates were identified from the fatal enteric and respiratory disease, the pathogenicity and virulence of BEV recurred where its relatedness to the illness be intensively explored [12,21,22,23,24]. Blas-Machdo has showed that calves experimentally infected with

BEV-1 manifested symptoms of respiratory illness similar to those naturally BEV-infected calves; and the BEV-1 was detected to localize mainly in the digestive tract, indicating the potential pathogenicity of BEV [22]. Recently, several strains of BEV were isolated from cattle with a severe diarrhea in China, and genomic sequence analysis indicated that those strains belong to enterovirus F (previously named BEV-B)[12]. Those findings suggest the pathogenicity of BEV as potential causative agents for the respiratory and enteric diseases in cattle.

Classification of bovine enteroviruses undergoes a series of modifications. In the early attempt, BEV were classified into seven serotypes, and later revised to two serotypes [25,26]. Because of the cross-reaction among BEV type-specific sera, it is difficult to type BEV using serological means. With the accumulation of BEV sequence data, classification of BEVs based on virus genetic variability and molecular difference becomes feasible. Based on the generally accepted definition for picornavirus species and serotype, a molecular-based BEV classification by comparing the sequences from 5′-UTR, the capsid protein region were established and used to classify bovine enteroviruses to BEV-A (currently named enterovirus E) and BEV-B (currently named enterovirus F), where different serotypes/genotypes were further divided for either enterovirus E or enterovirus F [27,28,29]. In this study, we reported the identification of a novel enterovirus E isolates HY12 from a cattle herd with an outbreak of a severe respiratory disease and enteritis in Jilin Province.

Table 1. Primers used for differentiation of the potential agents.

virus	Primer sequences (5'-3')	Position
BPV	S GCGCCGCATAAATGTGTCTTGGTG	1326~1349
	AS TGTGGGGCTTTCCGCTTTATCTCA	1738~1715
FMDV	S CGGTGGAAAACTACGGGGGAGAG	40~63
	AS TGCGCCGTAGTTGAAGGAGGTTG	496~473
BEV	S AGGATGATGATTGGCAGATTTTGT	372~395
	AS CATGTGGAAGTGTCTTTTGAGGAA	708~685

BPV: bovine parvovirus; FMDV: foot and mouth disease virus; BEV: bovine enterovirus; S: sense; AS: antisense.

Materials and Methods

The ethics committee in Jilin University has approved this study.

Cell culture and virus isolation

Faecal samples were collected from diarrheic cattle following standard procedures approved by the ethics committee of College of Veterinary Medicine at Jilin University, and processed to inoculate the MDBK cells. Briefly, samples were diluted in a dilution of 1:10 (W/V) with 10 mM phosphate buffered saline (PBS) (pH 7.2). After centrifugation at 8000 r. p. m. for 30 min, the supernatant was filtered with 0.45 nm filter and the flow-through was used to inoculate MDBK cells. The inoculum was discarded after incubation with MDBK cells for 2 h, and the cells were washed with Hank's solution before the addition of Dulbecco's modified eagle's medium (DMEM) (Invitrogen,) supplemented with 2% fetal bovine serum (HyClone), 2 μg/ml gentamycin and 2 mM L-glutamine (Invitrogen). The cells were observed every 4~6 h and cytopathic effects (CPE) were captured using Digital Camera.

Electron microscopy observation

Sample was processed for EM observation by centrifuging at 8000 r. p. m for 30 min at 4°C after virus cultures were frozen and thawed for 3 times. The supernatants were incubated with 1% phosphotungistic acid, and viruses were observed using electron microscopy (JEM-2200FS/CR).

TCID$_{50}$ titration and characterization of isolates HY12

Titration of TCID$_{50}$ for HY12 isolates was performed using 96 well-plates. Briefly, viruses were diluted at a 10×serial dilutions and used to infect the quadruplicate wells for each dilution. 48 h post inoculation, the cytopathic effects were observed and counted, and the TCID$_{50}$ was calculated following a standard procedure[30]. Biological and physiochemical properties of HY12 were characterized according to the standard protocols. HY12 viruses were treated either with organic solvents (chloroform and ether), heated at 50°C, 60°C, 70°C, and 80°C for 1 h, or incubated at pH 3.0 and pH 5.0 before infecting the cells. The stability to heat, acid or organic solvents were determined by comparing the TCID$_{50}$ for treated groups and untreated controls.

RNA isolation, cDNA synthesis and PCR amplification

RNA isolation was performed as previously reported[31]. Briefly, the infected cells were lysed in TRNzol reagent (Tiangen, Beijing), then mixed with 0.2 volume of chloroform and shaken vigorously for 30 sec. After centrifugation at 12,000×g for 20 min at 4°C, the aqueous phase was mixed with equal volume of isopropanol, centrifuged at 12,000×g for 20 min at 4°C. The pellet was washed with 70% ethanol and dissolved in DEPC-

Table 2. Primers used for amplifying the complete genome sequence for HY12.

Fragment	primer sequence (5'-3')	positions
F1	S TTAAAACAGCCTGGGGGTTGTA	1~23
	AS GGTGAAATTTGGTAGCATTGCACT	1379~1356
F2	S CAGTGACACCGACGCAACATC	1150~1170
	AS CTAAAGTACATAAGCCCGAGAAAGT	3159~3135
F3	S TGACGAGAGCATGATCGAGAC	2644~2664
	AS CATCTCAGTGAATTTCTTCATCCA	4011~3988
F4	S AATGGGTTCCGATTCCGTTGTG	3886~3908
	AS AGTCAATTCCAGGGAGGTATCAG	5632~5610
F5	A TCGCTGTCATTCAGAGTGTTTCC	5262~5284
	AS GACGGCTTTTTCCTTTCTTGATCTT	6485~6461
F6	A AATGTGCAAAGAGACATGCCAGAG	6455~6178
	AS ACACCCCATCCGGTGGGTGTAT	7416~7395

S stands for sense; AS refers to antisense.

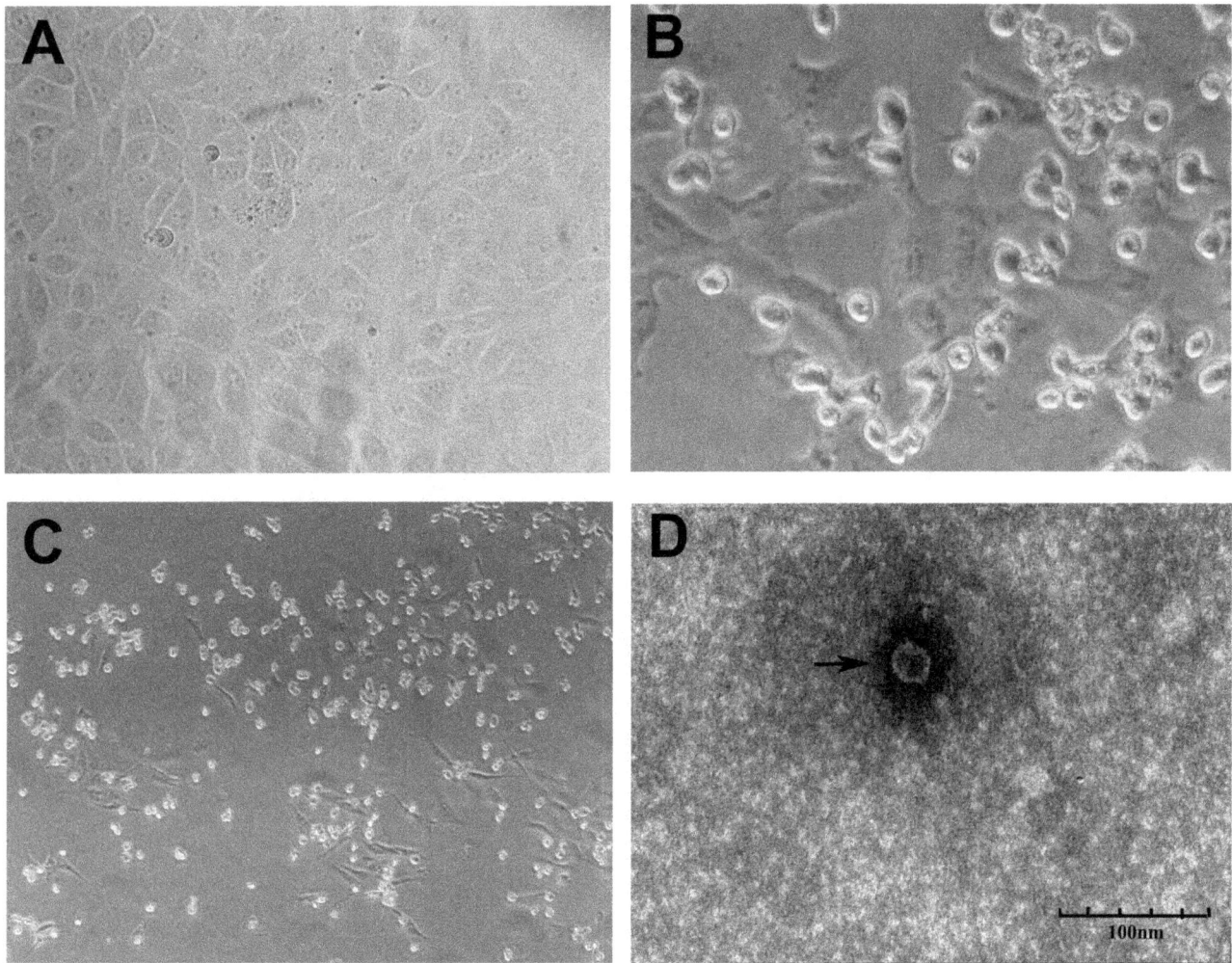

Figure 1. Cytopathic effect of HY12 in cell culture and EM observation. HY12 caused a typical cytopathic effect in MDBK cells after 6–8 h inoculation. Cells became rounded with an increased refraction (B). 24~48 h post infection, majority of the infected cells detached off the flask (C). The normal MDBK cells were used as negative controls (A). HY12 virus particles observed by electron microscopy to be about 22~28 nm in diameter as indicated by arrow (D), the scale bar is 100 nm.

treated H_2O. The resulting RNA was kept at $-80°C$ for further analysis.

The reverse transcriptase reaction was performed using Superscript ^{TM} II Reverse Transcriptase (Invitrogen, Carlsbad,

CA). Briefly, cDNA was synthesized in a volume of 20 μl containing 25 mM Tris-HCI, pH 8.3, 37.5 mM KCI, 1.5 mM MgCI2, 5 mM DTT, 0.25 mM each of dATP, dCTP, dGTP and dTTP, 40 units of RNase inhibitor, 200 units of M-MLV reverse

Table 3. Partial physiochemical properties for HY12 strain.

Treatment		treated groups (TCID50/0.01 ml)	untreated groups (TCID50/0.01 ml)
chloroform		$10^{-10.1}$	$10^{-10.7}$
ether		$10^{-10.0}$	$10^{-10.2}$
Heat-resistant Test(1 h)	50°C	$10^{-8.4}$	$10^{-10.7}$
	60°C	$10^{-0.0}$	$10^{-10.0}$
	70°C	$10^{-0.0}$	$10^{-10.4}$
	80°C	$10^{-0.0}$	$10^{-10.5}$
Acid-resistant(pH)	5.0	$10^{-8.8}$	$10^{-9.6}$
	3.0	$10^{-9.1}$	$10^{-10.4}$

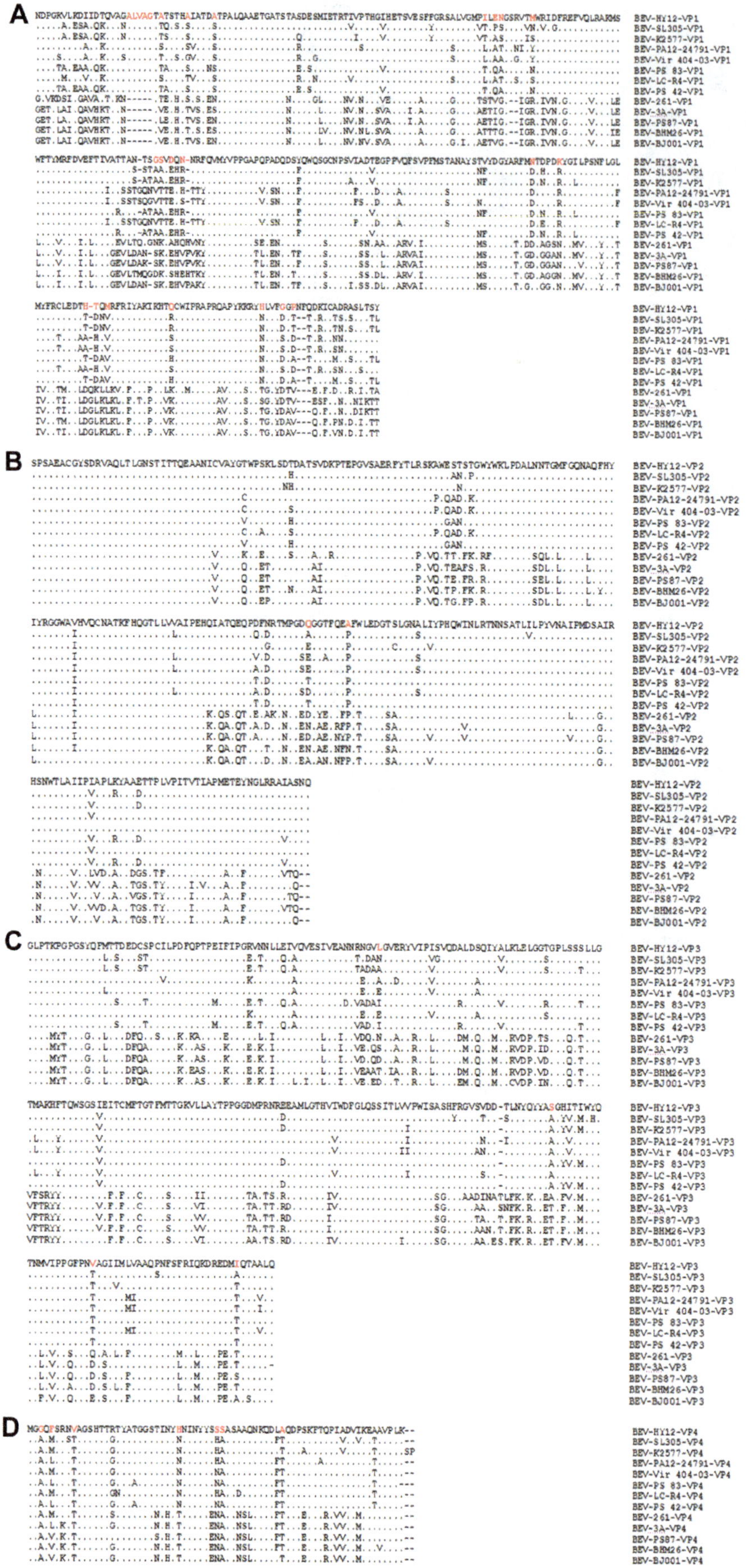

A

```
NDPGRVLKDIIDTQVAGALVAGTATSTHAIATDATPALQAAETGATSTASDESMIETRTIVPTHGIHETSVESFFGRSALVGMPILENGSRVTMWRIDFREFVQLRAARMS   BEV-HY12-VP1
........A.ESA.QK..N.......TQ.S.S...S...............................V.....V....Y......VT.PS...VN.V.G...........   BEV-SL305-VP1
........A.ESA.QK..N.......TS..S...S.............Q........I...V...Y......VT.AS....IS..................          BEV-K2577-VP1
............S....S..SV...S............R..........G.....................S...L.AT..NI.Y..................        BEV-PA12-24791-VP1
......TA.EAA.QK.......TA...S...NS..............R.G......................S...L.AA..G..Y...............          BEV-Vir 404-03-VP1
......M...V..K......S.....TV..S.............R.N...V..............S.....T.QA....N....................            BEV-PS 83-VP1
......TA.EAA.QK.......TA...S...S.........E.S............V..............T.QA...N.....................            BEV-LC-R4-VP1
......TA.EAA.QK.......TA...S...S.........E.S............V..............A.GI..AETVG..T.QA..IP.........           BEV-PS 42-VP1
G.VKDSI.GAVA.T.KN-----.TE.H.S.S.EN.........N..GL..NV.N..SVA....I.A.....G..TSTVG.--IGR.IVN.G...V..LE            BEV-261-VP1
GET.LAI.QAVRKT..N-----.VE.H.TVS.ES.........N.....NV.N..SVA....I.A.....G..AETIG.--IGR.IVN.G...V..LE             BEV-3A-VP1
GET.LAI.QAVRKT..N-----.LE.H.TVS.EN.........N.....NV.N..SVA....I.A.....G..AETIG.--IGR.IVN.G...V..LE             BEV-PS87-VP1
GET.LAI.QAVRKT..N-----.VE.H.T.S.ES.........N..LV..NV.NL.SVA..........G..ATTTG.--IGR.IVN.G...V..LE              BEV-BHM26-VP1
GET.LAI.QAVRKT..N-----.VE.H.TVS.EN.........N..NV.NV.SVA.......A...G.I..AETVG.--IGR.IVN.G...V..LE               BEV-BJ001-VP1

WFTYMRFDVEFTIVATTAN-TSGSVDQN-NRFQVMYVPPGAPQPADQDSYQWQSGCNPSVIADTBGPFVQFSVPFMSTANAYSTVYDGYARFMYTDPDKYGILPSNFLGL   BEV-HY12-VP1
............S-STAA.EHR........F..........V...........NF.....D.H..R.....                                        BEV-SL305-VP1
..........S-ATAA.EHR........................A..V...........NF......D.N..R..L....                              BEV-K2577-VP1
.........I..SSTGQNVTTE.H-TTY...V.SN...F....F...D..A.........S........D...R........F                           BEV-PA12-24791-VP1
.........I..SSTSQGVTTE.S-TTY...V.SN...F....FS..D..A.........S........D...R........F                           BEV-Vir 404-03-VP1
........R....-ATAA.EHR-..........................NF......D.N..R..L....                                         BEV-PS 83-VP1
.........I..SSTGQNVTTE.H-TTY...V.SN...F....P...D..A.........S........D...E..R.....F                           BEV-LC-R4-VP1
........R....-ATAA.EHR-......................A...G.I..AETVG.-...........NF...D.N..R..L....                     BEV-PS 42-VP1
L...V...I.L...EVLTQ.GNK.AHQHVVY.......SE.EN.......S....SN.AA..ARV.I........MS....T.DD.AGSN..MV..Y..T           BEV-261-VP1
L...V...I.L...GEVLDAN-SK.EHVPVKY.......TL.EN..TF.......S.SS..L..ARVAI.......MS....T.GD.GGAN..MV..Y..T          BEV-3A-VP1
L...V...I.L...GEVLDAK-SK.EHVPVKY.......TL.EN..TF.......S.SS..L..ARVAI.......MS....T.GD.GGAN..V..Y..T           BEV-PS87-VP1
L...I...I.L...GEVLTMQGDK.SHEHTKY.......TL.EN...TF.......S...I.SS.DL..ARVAI.......MS....T.GD.AGGN..MV..Y..T      BEV-BHM26-VP1
L...I...I.L...GEVLDAN-SK.EHVPAKY.......TL.EN...TF.......S...I.SS.DL..ARVAI.......MS....T.G..GG.N..MV..Y..T      BEV-BJ001-VP1

MYFRCLEDTH-TQMRFRIYAKIKHTQCWIPRAPRQAPYKKRYHLVFGGPNFQDKICADRASLTSY   BEV-HY12-VP1
.......T-DNV.............R...........N...D.T--T.R..TS.S...TL          BEV-SL305-VP1
.......T-DNV.............R...........N...D.T--T.R..TN.S...TL          BEV-K2577-VP1
....T...AA-H.V.........S.............N...S.D--T.R.SN.....              BEV-PA12-24791-VP1
....T...AA-H.V.........H.............N...D.A--T...M.S...TL            BEV-Vir 404-03-VP1
....T...AA-H.V.........S..............N...S.D--T.R.SN.....             BEV-PS 83-VP1
.......T-DAV.............H.............N...D.A--T...M.S...TL          BEV-LC-R4-VP1
IV..TM..LDQKLLKV.P...P..LK..M......AV...S..TG.YDTV---E.F.D..R.I.TA    BEV-261-VP1
IV..TI..LDGLKLKL.F.T.P..VK......AV...S..SG.YDTV---Q.F..N..NIKTT       BEV-3A-VP1
IV..TI..LDGLKLKL.P...P..VK.......AV...S..TG.YDAV---Q.F..N..DIKTT      BEV-PS87-VP1
IV..TM..LDGLKLKL.P...P..VK.......AV...S..TG.YDAV---Q.F.ND.I.TT        BEV-BHM26-VP1
IV..TI..LDGLKLKL.P...P..VK.......AV...S..TG.YDAV---Q.F.VN.D.I.TT      BEV-BJ001-VP1
```

B

```
SPSAEACGYSDRVAQLTLGNSTITTQEAANICVAYGTWPSKLSDTDATSVDRKPTEPGVSAERFYTLRSKGAWESTSTGWYWKLPDALNNTGMFGQNAQFHY   BEV-HY12-VP2
.........................................H...............................AN.P.....                       BEV-SL305-VP2
.........................................NH..............................................                 BEV-K2577-VP2
.............................C.........................................P.QAD.K....                       BEV-PA12-24791-VP2
.............................C....S.....................................P.QAD.K....                      BEV-Vir 404-03-VP2
..............V.....H.......................................................GAN....                        BEV-PS 83-VP2
.............C..A..S.........................................................P.QAD.K....                  BEV-LC-R4-VP2
..............V.............................................................GAN....                        BEV-PS 42-VP2
.............V...K..E.....S...A...R.............................P.VQ.TT.FK.RF.....SQL.L....L             BEV-261-VP2
..............V...Q...ET.......AI............................P.VQ.TEAFS.R........SDL.L....L              BEV-3A-VP2
..............V...Q.ET........AI............................P.VQ.TP.FK.R.........SBL.L....L             BEV-PS87-VP2
..............V...Q.ET..N...AI............................P.VQ.TP.FK.R.........SDL.L....L.Y             BEV-BHM26-VP2
..............V...Q.EP........AI............................P.VQ.TG.FP.R.........SDL.L....L              BEV-BJ001-VP2

IYRGGWAVHVQCNATKFHQGTLLVVAIPEHQIATQEQPDFNRTMPGDQGGTFQEAFWLEDGTSLGNALIYPHQWINLRTNNSATLILPYVNAIPMDSAIR   BEV-HY12-VP2
...........I......L..............Q.D....A.......P.........S...................V.......                     BEV-SL305-VP2
...........I..............................G.....E.....P.....C....V..........................               BEV-K2577-VP2
...........I.............L....V.D....SE..A.......P..........S...........                                   BEV-PA12-24791-VP2
...........I......L..............A.D....T....T....P........S.......                                        BEV-Vir 404-03-VP2
...........I.............T.D....T....T....P........                                                         BEV-PS 83-VP2
...........I..............A.D....SD.....P.........S.......                                                  BEV-LC-R4-VP2
...........I......L..............T.D....T....T....P.....                                                    BEV-PS 42-VP2
L..........I...........K.QS.QT.E.AK.N..ED.YE...FP.T...SA.................L...G.                            BEV-261-VP2
L..........I...........K.QA.QT.A.D..N..EN.AE.RFP.T...SA.........V...........G.                            BEV-3A-VP2
L..........I...........K.QA.QT.A...N..ED.AE.NYP.T...SA.........V...........V...G.                          BEV-PS87-VP2
L..........I...........K.QA.QT...T..N.EN.AE.NFN.T...SA.........V...........G.                              BEV-BHM26-VP2
L..........I...........K.QA.QT..D..N.EA.AN.NFP.T...SA.........V...........G.                               BEV-BJ001-VP2

HSNWTLAIIPIAPLKYAAETTPLVPITVTIAPMETEYNGLRRAIASNQ   BEV-HY12-VP2
.............V...R...D....                            BEV-SL305-VP2
.............V.......D....                            BEV-K2577-VP2
.............V.........                               BEV-PA12-24791-VP2
.............V...R...D..............V....              BEV-Vir 404-03-VP2
.............V......................                  BEV-PS 83-VP2
.............V...R...D....                            BEV-LC-R4-VP2
.N......V..LVD.A..DGS..TP.........A..F.....VTQ--     BEV-261-VP2
.N......V..V..WW.A..TGS.TY....I.V..A..F......TQ--    BEV-3A-VP2
.N......V..V..A..VGS.TY....I...A..F.......TQ--       BEV-PS87-VP2
.N......V..WD.A..TGS.TY....I...A..F.....VTQ--        BEV-BHM26-VP2
.N......V..V..A..TGS.TY....I...A..F......Q--         BEV-BJ001-VP2
```

C

```
GLPTKPGPGSYQFMYTTDEDCSPCILPDFQPTPEIFIPGRVNNLLEIVQVESIVEANNRNGVLGVERYVIPISVQDALDSQIYALKLELGGTGPLSSSLLG   BEV-HY12-VP3
..............L.S..ST.............E.T..Q.A......T.DAN.......VG.......V.....S.......                        BEV-SL305-VP3
..............L.S..ST.............E.T..Q.A......TADAA.......V.........V.....S.......T...                   BEV-K2577-VP3
.............L..............K........A........E..A.D...A.......A.................                          BEV-PA12-24791-VP3
......................................A........E..E.......V....A.................                          BEV-Vir 404-03-VP3
..........S...T......M...E.T..Q.A......D.VADAI..........R....V....R...T...                                 BEV-PS 83-VP3
..............L..............K........A........E..E.......V....V....R...T...                               BEV-LC-R4-VP3
..............................E.T..Q.A......VAD.I..........R....V....R...T...                             BEV-PS 42-VP3
.MYT..G..L...DFQ..S..K.KA.....E...L.I......L.I..VDQ.N..A.R.L...DM.Q..M..RVDP.TS...Q.T..                    BEV-261-VP3
.MYT..G..L...DFQA.....K.AS...K..E.K.I......L.I..VE.QS..A..R.L...M.Q..M..RVDP.ID...Q.T..                    BEV-3A-VP3
.MYT..G..L...DFQA.....K.AS...K..E.K.I......L.I..VQ.QD..A..R.L...M.Q..M..RVDP.VD...Q.T..                    BEV-PS87-VP3
.MYT..G..L...DFQA.....K.EAS...K..E.K.I......L.I..VEAAT.IA..R.L...DM.Q..M..RVDP.VD...Q.T..                  BEV-BHM26-VP3
.MYT..G..L...DFQA.....K.AS...K..E.K.I...L.I..L..VE.ED..T..R.L...EM.Q..M..CVDP.IN...Q.T..                   BEV-BJ001-VP3

TMAKRHFTQWSGSIEITCMFTGTFMTTGRVLLAYTPPGGDMPRNREEAMLGTHVTWDFGLQSSITLVVPWISASHFRGVSVDD-TLNYQYYASGHITIWYQ   BEV-HY12-VP3
...............................................................Y...T..-S.....A.YV.M.H.                     BEV-SL305-VP3
...............................................D...............I..............A.YV.M.                     BEV-K2577-VP3
..L..Y......V........................................V............I.......N..-I......A.V.M.               BEV-PA12-24791-VP3
..L..Y......V...................................................II............AN....-..A.V.M.             BEV-Vir 404-03-VP3
...............................................D...................................A.YV.M.                BEV-PS 83-VP3
...............................................................I..........S..-I....A.YV.M.                BEV-LC-R4-VP3
VFSRYY.........F.F..C.....S...II........TA.TS.R.........IV.............SG..AADINATLFK.K..EA.FV.M..         BEV-261-VP3
VFTRYY.....V.F.F..C.....S...VI........TA.TT.RD.......IV.............SG..AA..SNFK.R..ET.F.M..               BEV-3A-VP3
VFTRYY.....V.F.F..C.....S...VV........TA.TT.RD........I.............SG..TA..T.FK.R..ET.F.M..               BEV-PS87-VP3
VFTRYY.....V.F.F..C.....S...VI........TA.TT.RD........I.............SG..AAN.T.FK.R..ET.FV.M..              BEV-BHM26-VP3
VFTRYY.........F.F..C.....S...VI......AA.TS.RD.......IV.............SG..AA.ES.FK.R..ET.FV.M..              BEV-BJ001-VP3

TNMVIPPGFPNVAGIIMLVAAQPNFSFRIQRDREDMIQTAALQ   BEV-HY12-VP3
..............T......S.........A.....                 BEV-SL305-VP3
..............T..V.................T....              BEV-K2577-VP3
..............T.....MI.............T....V...          BEV-PA12-24791-VP3
..............T.....MI.............T...I....          BEV-Vir 404-03-VP3
..............T..................T....                BEV-PS 83-VP3
..............T.....MI.............T....V...          BEV-LC-R4-VP3
..L.V..S...Q.A.L.F..........M..L...PE.T....-          BEV-261-VP3
..L.V..Q...D.S..........L..M...PE.S.....              BEV-3A-VP3
..L.V.Q...D.S..F..........L..M...PE.T....              BEV-PS87-VP3
..L.V..A...D.S.L.F..........L..M...PE.T....            BEV-BHM26-VP3
..P.V..Q...E.S..F..........L..M...PE.A.S...            BEV-BJ001-VP3
```

D

```
MGXQFSRNVAGSHTTRTXATGGSTINYHNINYYSSSASAAQNKDDLNQDPSKFTQPIADVIKEAAVPLK--   BEV-HY12-VP4
..A.M..ST.....G...........N...HA......FT.......V..T....--                  BEV-SL305-VP4
..A.M...T.....G...........N...HA......FT.....V..T....SP                    BEV-K2577-VP4
..A.L...T..........G.......N...HA......FT...A....T....--                   BEV-PA12-24791-VP4
..A.M...T.....G...........N...NA......FT.............T....---              BEV-Vir 404-03-VP4
..A.M...T.....G..A.........N...NA......FT.............T....---             BEV-PS 83-VP4
..A.L...T.....GN..........N...NA......FT.............T....--              BEV-LC-R4-VP4
..A.L...T.....G...........N...NA......FT..............T....---            BEV-PS 42-VP4
..A.M...T..........N.H.T...ENA..NSL....FT..E..R.VV..M...---                BEV-261-VP4
..A.L.K.T..........N.H.T...S.H.T...ENA..NSL....FT..E..R.VV..M...           BEV-3A-VP4
..A.V.K.T..........G...N.H.T...ENA..NSL....FT..E..R.VV..M...               BEV-PS87-VP4
..A.V.K.T..........G...N.H.T...ENA..NSL....FT..E..R.VV..M..V....--         BEV-BHM26-VP4
..A.V.K.T..........G...N.H.T...ENA..NSL....T...E..R.VV..M...               BEV-BJ001-VP4
```

Figure 2. Unique amino acid mutations in the capsid proteins encoded by HY12 isolates. The amino acid sequence of HY12 isolates were deduced from the nucleotide sequence, and was aligned with 12 known BEV strains in the GenBank. Alignment analysis was performed using each HY12-encoded structural protein as a template. Results were shown respectively for VP1 (A), VP2 (B), VP3 (C), and VP4 (D). The identical amino acids were marked with symbol "·", and different amino acids to HY12 were presented as individual amino acid symbol. The unique mutation for HY12 was highlighted with red color. Deletion of amino acids were marked as "-".

transcriptase, 2 µg of total RNA, and 2.5 µM random primers. The cDNA synthesis was carried out at 42°C for 1 h.

PCR amplification was done using Taq DNA polymerase (Takara Bio Group). The reaction was performed in a total volume of 50 µl containing 20 mM Tris-HCl, pH 8.4, 50 mM KCl, 3 mM MgCl$_2$, 0.25 mM each of dATP, dCTP, dGTP and dTTP, 5 unit of Taq DNA polymerase, 1 µM of each primer, and 2 µl of cDNA synthesized above. The amplification was done after optimizing the condition. The primers used for amplifying the potential virus sequences were listed in table 1; and primers to amplify the complete genome sequence of HY12 isolates were listed in table 2.

Cloning and sequencing

PCR products were analyzed by electrophoresis using 1% agarose gel and cloned to pGEM-T vector (Promega, Madison, WI). Recombinants were confirmed by sequencing (Sangon Biotech, Shanghai). The resulting sequences were analyzed using DNAstar Lasergene software. The nucleotide sequence served as a template for searching homologous sequences through GenBank (www.ncbi.nlm.nih.gov).

Alignment and phylogenetic analysis

Alignment analysis of multiple sequences was performed using the Clustal W method [32]. The amino acid sequence of HY12 was deduced from the nucleotide sequence. Briefly, the nucleotide sequences of the 5'-UTR, VP1, VP2, VP3 and VP4 were aligned with the corresponding regions of known BEV strains in the GenBank, and phylogenetic analysis was performed by neighbor-joining methods [33].

Results

Virus isolation and EM observation

To isolate the potential etiological agents, the faecal samples were processed and used to inoculate the MDBK cells, and for electron microscopy observation. After incubating with the inoculum, MDBK cells showed a typical cytopathic effect as early as 6–8 h. Initially, cells became rounded with an increasing refraction. 24~48 h post inoculation, majority of the infected cells detached off the flask (Fig 1B–C). To rule out the possibility of toxin effect from the sample, the cultures with inoculum were blindly passaged at least 5 generations, and a similar cytopathic effect was observed for each passage, indicating the CPE is the result of pathogen in the inoculum. To determine the potential viruses, the infected cells were frozen and thawed three times and processed for electron microscopy observation. As shown in Fig 1D, virus particles of 22~28 nm in diameter were observed in infected cells, which was similar to the observation in the faecal sample (not shown). The isolated virus was designated as HY12.

Virus titration and partial physiochemical properties

To determine the infectivity of HY12, TCID$_{50}$ was determined as previously described [30]. Two days post inoculation, wells (cells) with cytopathic effect were counted. Results from three repeats showed the TCID$_{50}$ for HY12 isolates is $10^{-11.68}$/0.1 ml. To further characterize the HY12, partial physico-chemical

properties, heat-resistant, and acid-resistant experiments were performed. As shown in table 3, TCID$_{50}$ for HY12 isolates has no significant change after treating with either chloroform or ether, suggesting it is a non-enveloped virus. The TCID$_{50}$ has no significant change for treatment at 50°C for 1 h; however viruses completely lost infectivity at 60°C for 1 h, indicating it is sensitive to heat treatment at 60°C. As shown in table 3, HY12 isolates is stable to acid treatment at pH 3.0. Taken together, the above results suggest that HY12 is likely a picornavirus.

Molecular characterization and the complete genome sequence of HY12

To characterize the HY12 isolates, the primers for bovine enteroviruses were designed and used to amplify the potential virus genome sequence. Simultaneously, the primers for bovine parvovirus (BPV) and foot and mouth disease virus (FMDV) were used as negative controls. As expected, no fragments for BPV and FMDV were amplified after PCR amplification. However, a fragment with expected size was obtained with the primers for enteroviruses. Further cloning and sequencing this fragment turned out that the fragment consists of a sequence with high homology to a bovine enterovirus strain SL305, confirming HY12's status as an enterovirus.

To further characterize the virus, the complete nucleotide sequence of HY12 isolates was determined using several pair primers (table 2). After sequencing and assembling the PCR-amplified overlapping fragments, the complete genome sequence of HY12 was revealed to consist of 7416 nucleotides, with a typical picornavirus genome organization including a 5'-UTR, a large single ORF, and a 3'-UTR. The ORF is located between nucleotides 818 and 7348, encoding a polyprotein of 2176 amino acids with a predicted molecular weight of 243 kD. Comparison of the nucleotide sequence revealed that HY12 strain has a similar length of nucleotide sequence for 5'-UTR and 3'-UTR to known BEV strains. The complete nucleotide sequence of HY12 isolates was deposited in GenBank (KF748290).

Unique amino acid mutations in the capsid protein encoded by HY12

To analyze the protein encoded by HY12, the deduced amino acid sequence of HY12 was aligned with additional 12 BEV strains. Analysis of deduced amino acid sequence for HY12 revealed a few highly conserved regions including nonstructural proteins 2A, 2B, and P3 in relation to other bovine enterovirus (not shown). Similar to those observed in other enterovirus E, the structural proteins encoded by HY12 contains several relatively conserved regions (Fig. 2). In addition, there are also several variable regions and unique mutations in the capsid proteins, especially in VP1 and VP4. The mutations include an insertion of 5 aa at the N-terminal of VP1; an insertion of 2 aa and a deletion of 1 aa at the middle region of VP1; a unique insertion of 2 aa (NF) at C-terminal region of VP1; and a deletion of 1 aa in the C-terminal for VP3 in relation to the known enterovirus E or F. Furthermore, alignment analysis also revealed rare point mutations within the VP4 for HY12 strain in relation to known enteroviruses E or F (Fig 2).

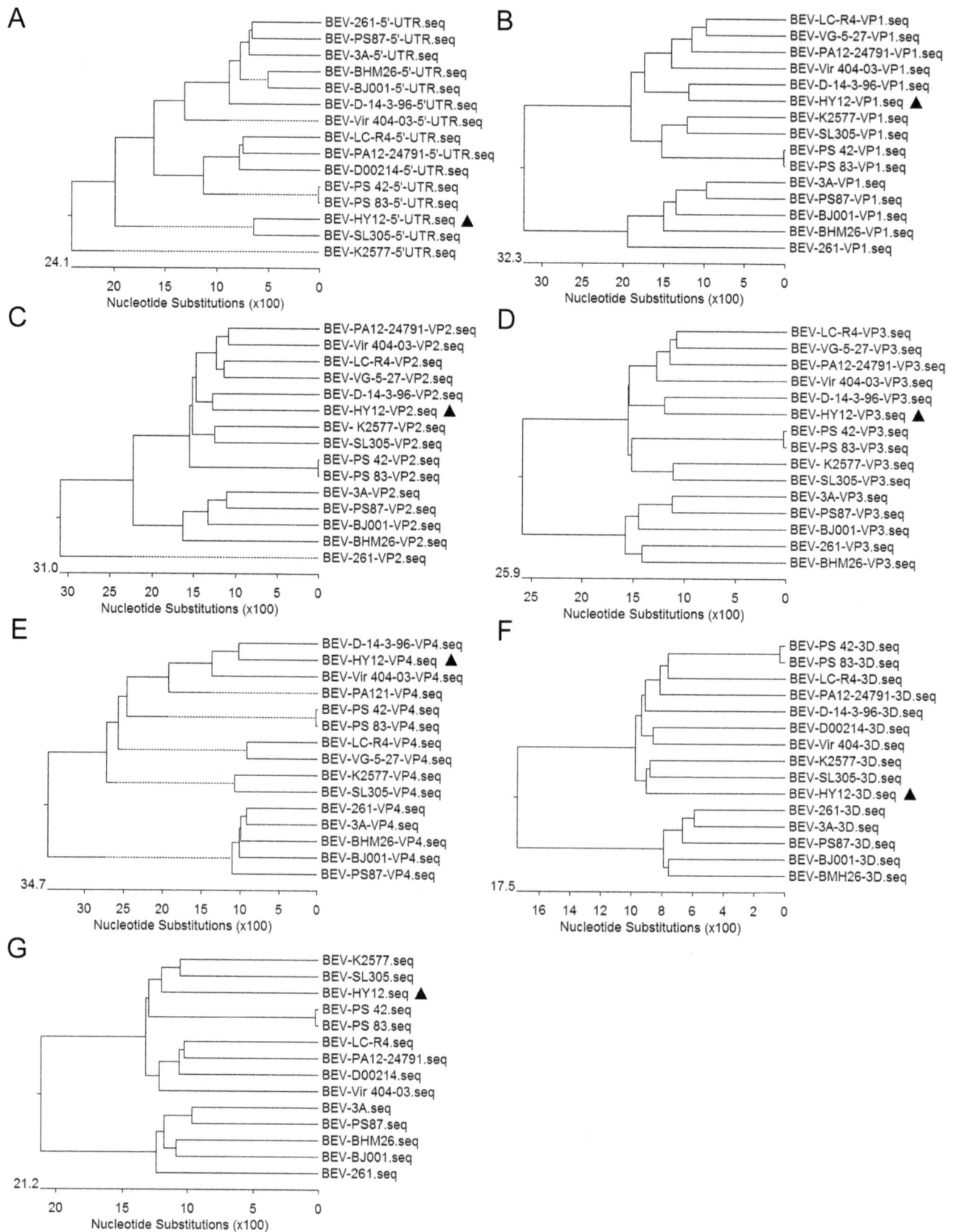

Figure 3. Phylogenetic analysis clustered HY12 strain to a new serotype/genotype within enterovirus E. Phylogenetic tree were generated by neighbor-joining methods by comparing the sequence regions of 5′-UTR, VP1, VP2, VP3, VP4, 3D, and the complete genome sequences for 15 enteroviruses. HY12 strain was placed to the cluster of enteroviruses E after phylogenetic analysis with the all nucleotide sequence regions

except 5′-UTR (B–F). The HY12 strain was revealed as a new serotype/genotype (serotype/genotype 3) that only consists of D14/3/96 and HY12 strains in relation to serotype 1 (LC-R4, VG5-27,Vir 404/03) and serotype 2 (SL305, K2577,PS 42, PS 83) enterovirus strains (B–E). When nucleotide sequences for the non-structural proteins 3D and the complete genome sequence were employed, the HY12 were clustered to the same clade most close to SL305 and K2577 within enteroviruses E (F). However, HY12 strain was clustered to neither clade in enteroviruses E nor enterovirus F using the 5′-UTR sequence (A), suggesting an intraserotypic recombination during HY12 evolution. The position of HY12 was highlighted with a triangle.

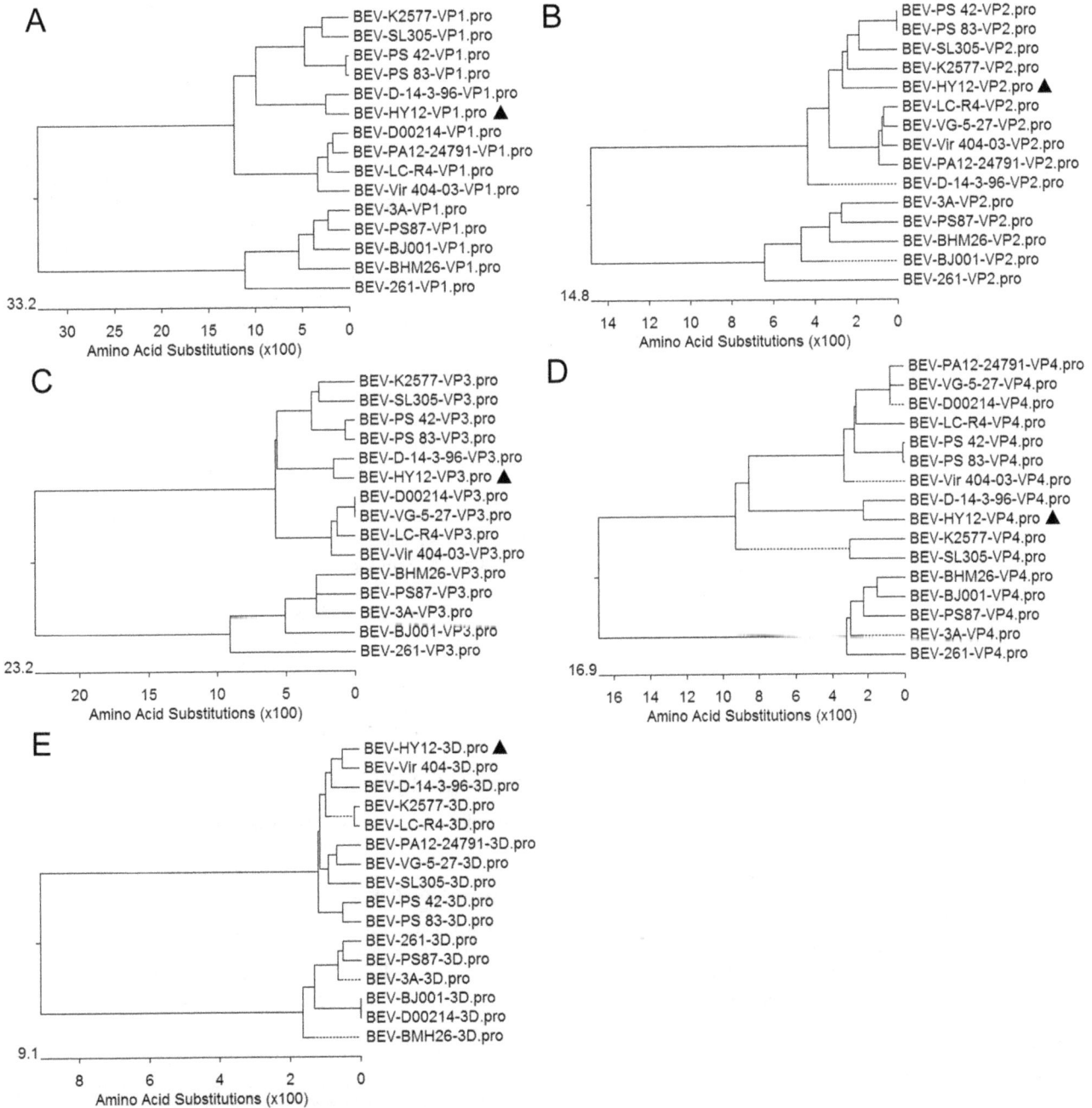

Figure 4. Recombination revealed in the HY12 strain. Neighbor-joining trees of the structural proteins VP1-VP4, and the non-structural protein 3D of 15 enteroviruses were compared. When amino acid sequences for VP1, VP3, and VP4 were used to generate phylogenetic tree, similar patterns were observed as those in Fig 3B, 3D, and 3E, indicating a interserotype recombination for the HY12 strain. Like the observation in Fig 3A, F and G, the HY12 was clustered closely to K2577, SL305, PS 42 and PS 83 strains, an indication of complex interserotypic and intraserotypic recombination in the evolution for HY12. The positions of HY12 were highlighted with a triangle.

HY12 belongs to a novel serotype/genotype in bovine enteroviruses

To define the relationship of HY12 with other enteroviruses, the nucleotide sequences of the 5'-UTR, VP1, VP2, VP3, VP4, 3D, the complete genome sequence of HY12 were aligned with the corresponding regions of known BEV strains, and phylogenetic trees were generated by neighbor-joining methods. As shown in Fig 3, when the nucleotide sequences encoding the structural proteins (VP1,VP2, VP3,VP4) for HY12 were used to generate the phylogenetic tree, the HY12 strain was clustered to enteroviruses E, but was neither in serotype/genotype 1 (LC-R4, VG5-27,Vir 404/03) nor serotype/genotype 2 (SL305, K2577,PS 42, PS 83), it belongs to a new serotype/genotype consisting of the D14/3/96 and HY12 (Fig 3B-E). We named it as serotype/genotype 3. It is interesting to note when nucleotide sequences for the non-structural proteins (3D) and the complete genome sequence were employed, the HY12 were clustered to the same clade most close to SL305 and K2577 within enteroviruses E (Fig 3A, F, and G). However, when the 5'-UTR sequence was aligned with other enteroviruses, the sequence identity of HY12 was 71.7~86.7% with other enteroviruses, and phylogenetic analysis showed the HY12 is neither in the clade for enteroviruses E nor in enterovirus F, it is in a clade with SL305, close to K2577, another separate clade (Fig 3A). As shown in Fig 4, similar expected patterns were revealed when amino acid sequences for VP1, VP3, and VP4 were used to generate phylogenetic tree. Like the observation in Fig 3A, F and G, the HY12 was clustered closely to K2577, SL305, PS 42 and PS 83 (Fig 4B). The above results indicated a complex interserotypic and intraserotypic recombination in the evolution for HY12.

Discussion

In this study, we reported the isolation of an enterovirus HY12 strain from a cattle farm with an unknown disease of high morbidity and mortality. Sequencing results demonstrated that HY12 is a new isolates within enterovirus E. As far as we know, this is the first report of enterovirus E in China. Enteroviruses E and F both belong to the genus *enterovirus* that are etiologically associated with bovine enterovirus infections with clinical signs varying from respiratory diseases to enteritic, reproductive disease and infertility [2,3,4,5,6,7,8,9,10,11,12]. Although there are reports neglecting the pathogenicity of BEVs, increasing reports for isolation of BEVs from respiratory and diarrheic cattle suggest the relatedness of BEV with those diseases. Our detection and isolation of bovine enterovirus HY12 in a cattle farm with severe respiratory and enteric diseases clearly indicate that HY12 might play a critical role in this outbreak as etiological agents.

The classification of bovine enteroviruses undergoes an evolution since their initial discovery. Zell reported a molecular-based BEV classification system based on virus genetic variability and molecular difference, and demonstrated a congruence of this molecular-based classification with previous classification methods [29]. Based on the generally accepted definition for picornavirus

species and serotype, BEVs were classified into enterovirus E (BEV-A) and enterovirus F (BEV-B) by comparing sequences from 5'-UTR, 3'UTR and capsid protein region, where a different serotypes were further divided for either enterovirus E or enterovirus F [27,28,29]. It is generally accepted that picornavirus serotypes are molecularly defined by the diversity of the capsid proteins, while the enterovirus species were determined by the less diverse non-structural protein regions. The percentage of sequence identity was used for species/serotypes definition, where a range from 50% to 55% for heterologous species, 70% to 85 % for heterologous serotypes/homologous species, and greater than 90 % for homologous serotypes [29]. According to this criteria, we defined HY12 enterovirus isolates as enterovirus E since the amino acid sequence identity of VP1 encoded by HY12 is only ranged from 53% to 55% with previously identified BEV-B viruses such as BEV strains PS87, 3A, 261, and two newly strains isolated in China (BHM26, and BJ001). The finding that VP1 of HY12 is about 80-83% with those previously defined BEV-A suggests HY12 is a heterogeneous serotype within enteroviruses E. Moreover, phylogenetic analysis clearly showed that HY12 isolates belongs to neither serotype/genotype 1 (SL305, K2577 PS42, PS83) nor serotype/genotype 2 (LC-R4, Vir 404-03 PA12-24791); it belongs to a new serotype/genotype. The results that HY12 is phylogenetically clustered with D 14/3/96 strain [29], a strain reported to be difficult in serotype/genotype typing further support the classification of HY12 to new serotype/genotype within enterovirus E.

Interserotypic and intraserotypic recombination have been defined previously in poliovirus, echovirus and enteroviruses [1,34,35,36,37]. The incongruence between phylogenies of different genome regions is considered as an indication of recombination events in enteroviruses [29,38]. Phylogenetic analyses of the 5'-UTR, VP1, VP2, VP3, VP4, and 3D of HY12 demonstrated the incongruence between the phylogenies, indicating a complex interserotypic and intraserotypic recombination in the evolution of HY12 isolates.

In conclusion, this study reports the isolation and characterization of a novel enterovirus HY12 strain from a severe outbreak characterized with respiratory and enteric disease in a cattle farm with high mortality and morbidity in China, and provides the molecular evidence for defining HY12 strain as a new serotype/genotype 3 within enterovirus E.

Acknowledgments

The authors thank Professor Shenghua Yang at the Jilin University for his assistance for EM observations.

Author Contributions

Conceived and designed the experiments: XPW. Contributed to the writing of the manuscript: XPW LSZ. Data analysis: ZHS. HY12 characterization: SJL XCG. HY12 genome sequencing: LSZ. HY12 isolation: ZLX.

References

1. King AMQ, Adams MJ, Carsten EB, Lefkowitz E (2012) Virus Taxonomy. Ninth Report of the International Committee for the Taxonomy of Viruses. San Diego: Academic Press. 855–880 p.
2. Moll T, Davis AD (1959) Isolation and characterization of cytopathogenic enterovirus from cattle with respiratory disease. Am J Vet Res 20: 27–32.
3. Straub OC, Boehm HO (1964) Enterovirus as Cause of Bovine Vaginitis. Arch Gesamte Virusforsch 14: 272–275.
4. Buerki F (1962) Studies on bovine Enterovirus. 3. Epizootologic survey. Pathol Microbiol (Basel) 25: 789–795.

5. Straub OC, Kielwein G (1965) Bovine enteroviruses as causative agents of mastitis. Berl Munch Tierarztl Wochenschr 78: 386–389.
6. Rovozzo GC, Luginbuhl RE, Helmboldt CF (1965) Bovine Enteric Cytopathogenic Viruses. I. Characteristics of Three Prototype Strains. Cornell Vet 55: 121–130.
7. Van der Maaten MJ, Packer RA (1967) Isolation and characterization of bovine enteric viruses. Am J Vet Res 28: 677–684.
8. Buczek J (1970) Further characterization of bovine enteroviruses isolated in Poland. Brief report. Arch Gesamte Virusforsch 30: 408–410.

9. Ide PR (1970) Developments in veterinary science. The etiology of enzootic pneumonia of calves. Can Vet J 11: 194–202.

10. Dunne HW, Ajinkya SM, Bubash GR, Griel LC Jr (1973) Parainfluenza-3 and bovine enteroviruses as possible important causative factors in bovine abortion. Am J Vet Res 34: 1121–1126.

11. Weldon SL, Blue JL, Wooley RE, Lukert PD (1979) Isolation of picornavirus from feces and semen from an infertile bull. J Am Vet Med Assoc 174: 168–169.

12. Li Y, Chang J, Wang Q, Yu L (2012) Isolation of two Chinese bovine enteroviruses and sequence analysis of their complete genomes. Arch Virol 157: 2369–2375.

13. Zheng T (2007) Characterisation of two enteroviruses isolated from Australian brushtail possums (Trichosurus vulpecula) in New Zealand. Arch Virol 152: 191–198.

14. McCarthy FM, Smith GA, Mattick JS (1999) Molecular characterisation of Australian bovine enteroviruses. Vet Microbiol 68: 71–81.

15. McFerran JB (1958) ECBO viruses of cattle. Vet Rec 70: 999.

16. Ley V, Higgins J, Fayer R (2002) Bovine enteroviruses as indicators of fecal contamination. Appl Environ Microbiol 68: 3455–3461.

17. Dubois E, Merle G, Roquier C, Trompette AL, Le Guyader F, et al. (2004) Diversity of enterovirus sequences detected in oysters by RT-heminested PCR. Int J Food Microbiol 92: 35–43.

18. Fong TT, Griffin DW, Lipp EK (2005) Molecular assays for targeting human and bovine enteric viruses in coastal waters and their application for library-independent source tracking. Appl Environ Microbiol 71: 2070–2078.

19. Jimenez-Clavero MA, Escribano-Romero E, Mansilla C, Gomez N, Cordoba L, et al. (2005) Survey of bovine enterovirus in biological and environmental samples by a highly sensitive real-time reverse transcription-PCR. Appl Environ Microbiol 71: 3536–3543.

20. Nollens HH, Rivera R, Palacios G, Wellehan JF, Saliki JT, et al. (2009) New recognition of Enterovirus infections in bottlenose dolphins (Tursiops truncatus). Vet Microbiol 139: 170–175.

21. Blas-Machado U, Saliki JT, Boileau MJ, Goens SD, Caseltine SL, et al. (2007) Fatal ulcerative and hemorrhagic typhlocolitis in a pregnant heifer associated with natural bovine enterovirus type-1 infection. Vet Pathol 44: 110–115.

22. Blas-Machado U, Saliki JT, Sanchez S, Brown CC, Zhang J, et al. (2011) Pathogenesis of a bovine enterovirus-1 isolate in experimentally infected calves. Vet Pathol 48: 1075–1084.

23. McClenahan SD, Scherba G, Borst L, Fredrickson RL, Krause PR, et al. (2013) Discovery of a bovine enterovirus in alpaca. PLoS One 8: e68777.

24. Cho YI, Han JI, Wang C, Cooper V, Schwartz K, et al. (2013) Case-control study of microbiological etiology associated with calf diarrhea. Vet Microbiol 166: 375–385.

25. Dunne HW, Huang CM, Lin WJ (1974) Bovine enteroviruses in the calf: an attempt at serologic, biologic, and pathologic classification. J Am Vet Med Assoc 164: 290–294.

26. Knowles NJ, Barnett IT (1985) A serological classification of bovine enteroviruses. Arch Virol 83: 141–155.

27. Zell R, Stelzner A (1997) Application of genome sequence information to the classification of bovine enteroviruses: the importance of 5'- and 3'-nontranslated regions. Virus Res 51: 213–229.

28. Zell R, Sidigi K, Henke A, Schmidt-Brauns J, Hoey E, et al. (1999) Functional features of the bovine enterovirus 5'-non-translated region. J Gen Virol 80 (Pt 9): 2299–2309.

29. Zell R, Krumbholz A, Dauber M, Hoey E, Wutzler P (2006) Molecular-based reclassification of the bovine enteroviruses. J Gen Virol 87: 375–385.

30. Reed LJ, Muench H (1938) A simple method of estimating fifty percent endpoints. Am J Hygiene: 493–497.

31. Wang XP, Zhang YJ, Deng JH, Pan HY, Zhou FC, et al. (2001) Characterization of the promoter region of the viral interferon regulatory factor encoded by Kaposi's sarcoma-associated herpesvirus. Oncogene 20: 523–530.

32. Thompson JD, Higgins DG, Gibson TJ (1994) CLUSTAL W: improving the sensitivity of progressive multiple sequence alignment through sequence weighting, position-specific gap penalties and weight matrix choice. Nucleic Acids Res 22: 4673–4680.

33. Saitou N, Nei M (1987) The neighbor-joining method: a new method for reconstructing phylogenetic trees. Mol Biol Evol: 406–425.

34. Kim H, Kim K, Kim DW, Jung HD, Min Cheong H, et al. (2013) Identification of Recombinant Human Rhinovirus A and C in Circulating Strains from Upper and Lower Respiratory Infections. PLoS One 8: e68081.

35. Yozwiak NL, Skewes-Cox P, Gordon A, Saborio S, Kuan G, et al. (2010) Human enterovirus 109: a novel interspecies recombinant enterovirus isolated from a case of acute pediatric respiratory illness in Nicaragua. J Virol 84: 9047–9058.

36. McIntyre CL, McWilliam Leitch EC, Savolainen-Kopra C, Hovi T, Simmonds P (2010) Analysis of genetic diversity and sites of recombination in human rhinovirus species C. J Virol 84: 10297–10310.

37. Boros A, Pankovics P, Knowles NJ, Reuter G (2012) Natural interspecies recombinant bovine/porcine enterovirus in sheep. J Gen Virol 93: 1941–1951.

38. Smura T, Blomqvist S, Paananen A, Vuorinen T, Sobotova Z, et al. (2007) Enterovirus surveillance reveals proposed new serotypes and provides new insight into enterovirus 5'-untranslated region evolution. J Gen Virol 88: 2520–2526.

2

Asymptomatic Cattle Naturally Infected with *Mycobacterium bovis* Present Exacerbated Tissue Pathology and Bacterial Dissemination

Álvaro Menin[1]*, Renata Fleith[1], Carolina Reck[2], Mariel Marlow[3], Paula Fernandes[1], Célso Pilati[2], André Báfica[1]*

1 Laboratory of Immunobiology, Universidade Federal de Santa Catarina, Florianópolis, Santa Catarina, Brazil, 2 Laboratory of Histology and Immunohistochemistry, Universidade do Estado de Santa Catarina, Lages, Santa Catarina, Brazil, 3 Laboratory of Protozoology, Universidade Federal de Santa Catarina, Florianópolis, Santa Catarina, Brazil

Abstract

Rational discovery of novel immunodiagnostic and vaccine candidate antigens to control bovine tuberculosis (bTB) requires knowledge of disease immunopathogenesis. However, there remains a paucity of information on the *Mycobacterium bovis*-host immune interactions during the natural infection. Analysis of 247 naturally PPD+ *M. bovis*-infected cattle revealed that 92% (n = 228) of these animals were found to display no clinical signs, but presented severe as well as disseminated bTB-lesions at *post-mortem* examination. Moreover, dissemination of bTB-lesions positively correlated with both pathology severity score (Spearman r = 0.48; p<0.0001) and viable tissue bacterial loads (Spearman r = 0.58; p = 0.0001). Additionally, granuloma encapsulation negatively correlated with *M. bovis* growth as well as pathology severity, suggesting that encapsulation is an effective mechanism to control bacterial proliferation during natural infection. Moreover, multinucleated giant cell numbers were found to negatively correlate with bacterial counts (Spearman r = 0.25; p = 0.03) in lung granulomas. In contrast, neutrophil numbers in the granuloma were associated with increased *M. bovis* proliferation (Spearman r = 0.27; p = 0.021). Together, our findings suggest that encapsulation and multinucleated giant cells control *M. bovis* viability, whereas neutrophils may serve as a cellular biomarker of bacterial proliferation during natural infection. These data integrate host granuloma responses with mycobacterial dissemination and could provide useful immunopathological-based biomarkers of disease severity in natural infection with *M. bovis*, an important cattle pathogen.

Editor: Pere-Joan Cardona, Fundació Institut d'Investigació en Ciències de la Salut Germans Trias i Pujol, Universitat Autònoma de Barcelona, CIBERES, Spain

Funding: This work was funded by CAPES (PROCAD), CNPq (INCT/INTEV), National Institutes of Health 394 (GRIP/Fogarty) and the Howard Hughes Medical Institute (ECS Program). AB is a CNPq 395 scientist scholar. The funders had no role in study design, data collection and analysis, decision to publish, or preparation of the manuscript.

Competing Interests: The authors have declared that no competing interests exist.

* E-mail: andre.bafica@ufsc.br (AB); amenin@ccb.ufsc.br (ÁM)

Introduction

Bovine tuberculosis (bTB), caused by infection with the intracellular acid-fast bacilli *Mycobacterium bovis*, is an important neglected zoonosis, which significantly decreases livestock production and economically affects international trade [1–3]. Additionally, *M. bovis* infection is estimated to be responsible for ~10% of human tuberculosis (TB) in Africa [3] and ~2.5% of human cases in Latin America [4], thus underscoring the importance of disease control programs based on the understanding of infection dynamics [5–8].

Currently, no effective vaccine exists for bovine TB. The main procedures to control/eradicate this intractable disease are diagnosis and compulsory slaughter of positive animals [9]. In this context, the most utilized diagnostic tool for *M. bovis* infection in cattle is the single intradermal comparative cervical tuberculin test (SICTT), which measures a delayed type hypersensitivity response to the tuberculin antigen-purified protein derivative (PPD) [10], but may fail to detect specific pathogen infection [11–13]. Indeed, Claridge et al. have recently reported that *Fasciola hepatica* co-infection in bTB diseased cattle significantly decreases

the numbers of PPD-positive animals [11], demonstrating PPD sensitivity could be affected by parasitic co-infections. Together, these data indicate an urgent need for an effective vaccine as well as better diagnostic tests to control bTB. However, there remains a paucity of information on bTB immunopathogenesis, especially during natural infection.

M. bovis primarily infects macrophages, where they can survive, replicate and disseminate into different anatomical sites [14,15]. The risk of transmission as well as the host's survival relies mainly on the ability of well-organized structures called granulomas to contain mycobacterial infection [14–17]. Tuberculous granuloma is a complex host-protective structure generated in response to persistent mycobacterial stimuli with focal accumulation of inflammatory cells, such as multinucleated giant cells and lymphocytes [16,18–21]. In addition, encapsulation, a process involving production of connective tissue around the granuloma, has been shown to be critical for controlling both mycobacterial growth and tissue dissemination [14,15,22].

The pathological outcome of experimental *M. bovis* infection has been associated with diversity and efficiency of host immune response as well as a useful tool for evaluating efficiency of new vaccine antigen candidates and disease severity [23–26]. Furthermore, the presence of cellular populations, such as epithelioid cells, multinucleated giant cells, lymphocytes and neutrophils in the tuberculous granuloma [19,21] during experimental *M. bovis* infection, suggests these cells may play important roles in controlling bTB. Although genetic variability and age-associated factors have been shown to potentially be involved in susceptibility to *M. bovis* infection [2,27–32], fundamental host defense aspects of the natural infection by *M. bovis* have not been fully elucidated. Consistently, cellular immune responses against this major bovine pathogen as well as the tuberculous granulomatous response elicited during natural infection in cattle are poorly understood.

In the present study, we have performed a detailed analysis of several host immune and pathology response parameters in a cohort of 247 naturally *M. bovis*-infected cattle. Our findings reveal that, despite the absence of clinical symptoms, naturally-infected bovines displayed severe lung pathology and bacterial dissemination, which correlate with viable mycobacterial loads within the granuloma. Furthermore, immune-related cells and tissue remodeling of the granuloma were found to correlate with bacterial containment during natural infection. Our results provide useful insights on possible biomarkers of disease severity in natural infection with an important cattle pathogen.

Results

Viable Bacterial Loads Correlate with Tissue Pathology in Naturally *M. bovis*-infected Cattle

Experimental and observational data have demonstrated that bovines display increased resistance to *M. bovis* infection [25,31,33–35]. Such resistance has been thought to impact surveillance programs as well as bacterial dissemination given a possible delay between bTB testing and cattle elimination. To gain insight on the immune-pathological responses induced during the window between infection and appearance of bTB-associated clinical signs, we have studied a cohort of 247 PPD-positive bovines naturally infected with *M. bovis* (**Figs. 1 and 2**). In this cohort, 92.3% of the animals (228 bovines) displayed no clinical signs suggestive of mycobacterial infection (asymptomatic group, AS; **Fig. 2A**). At the post-mortem evaluation, 217 bovines (95.2% of the AS group) presented severe visible bTB-lesions (**Figs. 1A and 2B**) with varying degrees of gross pathology scoring (**Figs. 2C and D**). The majority of animals presented lesions in the lungs, primarily in right cranial lobe and in pulmonary-associated lymph nodes (**Fig. 2E and inset**), suggesting the aerogenous route of transmission was probably the main via of infection in the studied bovine herds. Thus, these findings demonstrate different organs are affected by *M. bovis* and suggest that following primary infection, the bacterium can disseminate to a variety of tissues during natural infection.

To study disease severity and possible immunopathological correlates of *M. bovis* infection, we developed a score system based on anatomical bTB-lesions dissemination (**Fig. 3A**). Using this system, 66.2% (n = 151) of bovines were defined as levels IV and V (**Fig. 3A**), pointing out a possible connection between disseminated infection and disease activity. To validate this hypothesis, we then performed Spearman correlations between viable bacterial loads (CFU counting, **Fig. 1A**), pathology severity (PS score, **Fig. 1C and D**) and bTB lesion dissemination. As demonstrated in **figure 3 (B and C)**, our score system positively correlates with gross pathology severity as well as tissue bacterial loads. These results formally demonstrate that naturally infected cattle with increased pathology severity display higher loads of viable *M. bovis*.

These findings suggest asymptomatic animals could play an important role in bacterial transmission and maintenance of disease before diagnostic and elimination of bovine populations in nature.

Granuloma Encapsulation Negatively Correlates with *M. bovis* Loads in Naturally Infected Cattle

The observed dissemination of *M. bovis* and the presence of severe bTB-lesions in asymptomatic animals suggest the existence of a robust immune response during natural infection [23–25,34]. To investigate bovine-protective factors associated with control of natural infection, which could influence host disease-*M. bovis* interplay and transmission, we have performed a detailed study of the granuloma, a major structure known to be associated with containment of mycobacterial dissemination [14–16,20]. Following analysis of primary lesions from 217 infected AS animals (573 tuberculous granulomas), three major degrees (I-III) of encapsulation intensity were observed, (**Fig. 4A**) in which most of the animals (138; 64%) showed level III (thickly encapsulation), indicating an attempt to limit the infection in such studied cattle. Consistent with these results, a significant negative correlation between encapsulation and viable bacterial loads (Spearman r = −0.61, p = 0.0001) was observed (**Fig. 4B**). Moreover, gross pathology severity (Spearman r = −0.50, p<0.0001) (**Fig. 4C**) and AFB staining (Spearman r = −0.41, p<0.0001) (data not shown) were also found to negatively correlate with encapsulation. Interestingly, AFBs were found to be located mainly within the necrotic caseum centre of granulomas and rarely within macrophages, multinucleated giant cells or mineralized debris (**Fig. 4A, inset**). These data suggest generation of granuloma encapsulation is important to contain *M. bovis* growth in naturally-infected bovine herds.

Analysis of cellular profile of lung granulomatous response from bovines naturally infected with *M. bovis*

We next performed a detailed analysis of the cellular profile of pulmonary granulomas of *M. bovis*-infected asymptomatic animals. As demonstrated in **figure 5A**, histological analysis of the lung tuberculous granulomatous response revealed four major histopathology groups (grades I-IV), which differ on granuloma-associated cell type numbers: Langhans multinucleated giant cells, epithelioid macrophages, neutrophils and lymphocytes (**Fig. 5B**). As expected, multinucleated giant cells displayed a positive correlation with histopathology grades (Spearman r = 0.55, p = <0.0001). In contrast, neutrophil numbers presented a negative correlation with our defined histopathology grades (Spearman r = −2.55, p = <0.0001) (**Fig. 5C**). These data suggest lung granulomas from bovines naturally-infected with *M. bovis*, although chronically infected and encapsulated, are sites of bacterial growth that dynamically recruits neutrophils. In support of this hypothesis, we observed a positive correlation between neutrophil numbers and viable *M. bovis* (Spearman r = 0.27, p = 0.021) (**Fig. 5D**). In addition, *M. bovis* CFU counts negatively correlated with multinucleated giant cell numbers (Spearman r = −0.25, p = 0.03) (**Fig. 5E**) and lung histopathology grades (Spearman r = −0.30, p = 0.009) (**Fig. 5F**). Together, these evidence suggest neutrophils and giant cells may play a role in regulating *M. bovis* growth in the lung during natural infection of bovines.

Discussion

Although bTB is an important neglected zoonosis which significantly decreases livestock production and impacts public

(A)

(B)

(C)

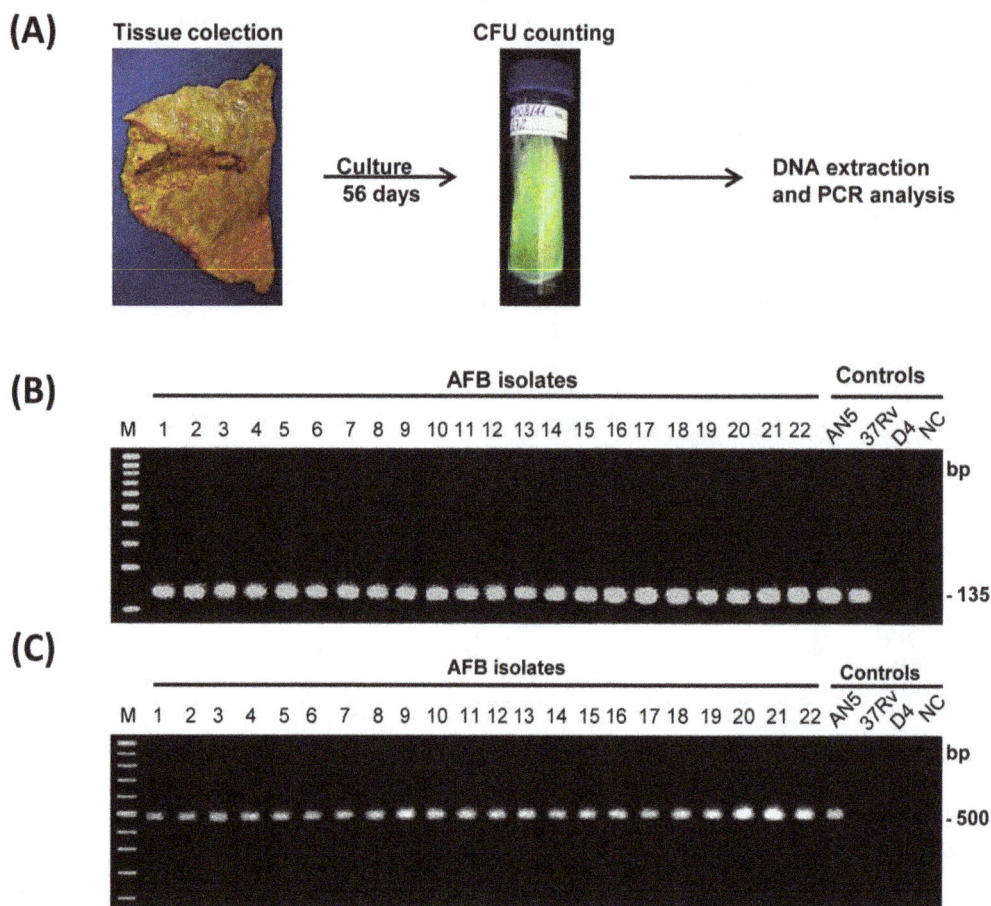

Figure 1. Bacteriology analysis and molecular typing of *M. bovis*. (A) Tissue homogenate obtained from PPD+ asymptomatic animals was inoculated in Ogawa-Kudoh+sodium pyruvate and incubated at 37°C for 8 weeks. After that, colonies were counted and DNA extraction method employed. Purified DNA obtained from **(A)** was used as template for PCR amplification of **(B)** IS1081 (~135 bp) or **(C)** RvD1Rv2031c (~500 bp) gene sequences. Amplification products of single PCR from representative samples are shown. Lane M: 100 bp DNA ladder; lanes 1–22 PCR products of *M. bovis* isolates; AN5 - *Mycobacterium bovis* AN5 strain, standard strain positive control; 37Rv – *Mycobacterium tuberculosis* strain, H37Rv; D4 - *Mycobacterium avium Subsp. avium* D4 strain, non-tuberculosis mycobacteria (NMTBC) member; lane NC, negative control (without DNA).

health, little is known about the dynamics of host-*M. bovis* interactions during natural infection. Moreover, the immunopathological parameters associated with protective host response in cattle during natural *M. bovis* infection remains largely unknown. In this study, we have performed a detailed analysis of important anti-mycobacteria host defense response components in a cohort of 247 naturally *M. bovis*-infected cattle. Despite the absence of clinical signs of bTB, the majority of infected cattle displayed high frequency and severity of the bTB-lesions in the lung (68.6%) (right cranial lobe) as well as pulmonary-associated lymph nodes. In addition, no correlation between the PPD size reactions and pathology severity was observed in our cohort (Spearman r = 0.01 p = 0.85).

Observations obtained from naturally *M. bovis*-infected cattle submitted to low-intensive farming conditions have demonstrated that the majority of lesions were present in mesenteric lymph nodes [32,36]. In contrast, naturally *M. bovis*-infected bovines exposed to intensive husbandry systems display augmented frequency of bTB-lesions in the respiratory tract [31,36,37]. Thus, it is possible that intensive husbandry systems favor *M. bovis* dissemination among dairy herds as a result of increased animal contact [5,38]. Consistent with this hypothesis, we have found that 66% of animals displayed pulmonary and systemic spreading of

bTB infection (levels III/IV) **(Fig. 3A)** suggesting that exposure to the pathogen was first established in the lung tissue. Moreover, the high frequency of lesions observed in the respiratory tract suggests that the major route of *M. bovis* transmission was most likely aerogenous. These evidences are supported by previous studies which demonstrated that bovines infected via the intranasal route by *M. bovis* results in pathology confined to the respiratory tract [39–41]. Involvement of mesenteric lymph nodes was also observed in our cohort, although at a significantly lower frequency (8.8%) **(Fig. 2E)**, suggesting that infection by the oral route may occur simultaneously during natural infection.

It is commonly accepted that *M. bovis* primarily infects macrophages, where they are able to survive, replicate and disseminate into different anatomical sites [14,15,20]. Progression of mycobacterial disease and survival of the host are thought to depend on their ability to limit mycobacterial growth by an effective granulomatous response [14–16,20,42,43]. In the case of experimental *M. bovis* infection in cattle, different stages of granuloma development have been observed to be associated with disease progression [19,21], pointing out a dynamic process of the tuberculous granuloma structure. Our results confirm and extend previous studies [19,21], which suggest an important role for the host granulomatous responses against *M. bovis* during

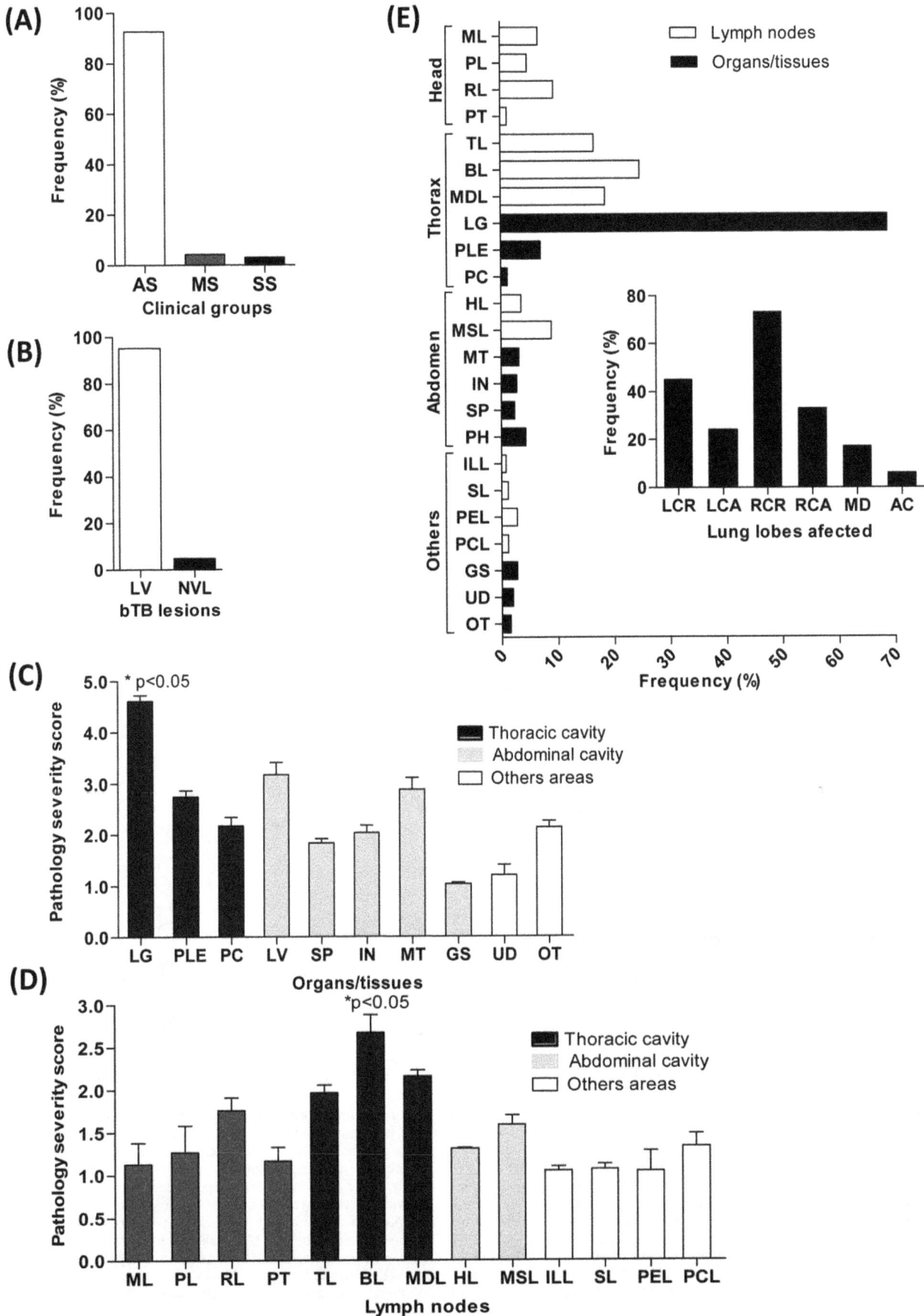

Figure 2. Clinical and gross pathology findings in cattle naturally infected with *M. bovis*. (**A**) Following clinical examination, animals bTB-positive (n = 247) were categorized according to their clinical status into asymptomatic (AS, n = 228), moderate symptoms (MS, n = 11), severe symptoms (SS, n = 8). (**B**) Gross pathology analysis further divided the PPD+ asymptomatic animals into two groups: the presence of visible bTB-lesions (VL) or absence of visible bTB-lesions (NVL). (**C and D**) Severity of tissue gross pathology in asymptomatic bTB bovines was scored by applying a previously described semi-quantitative scoring system (Vordermeier et al, 2002). Results shown are median of scores ± SEM. (**C**) **Organs/Tissues:** thoracic organs and tissues (lung (LG), pleura (PLE), pericardia (PC)); abdominal (liver (LV), spleen (SP), intestine (IN), mesentery (MT), genitor-urinary system (GS), as well as udder (UD), other tissues (OT)); (**D**) **Lymph nodes:** head lymph nodes (mandibular (ML), parotid (PL), retropharyngeal (RL) lymph nodes and palatine tonsil (PT)); thoracic lymph nodes (tracheobronchial (TL), bronchial (BL) and mediastinal (MDL)); abdominal lymph nodes (hepatic (HL), mesenteric (MSL)) as well as Iliac (ILL), Sciatic (SL), pre-scapular (PEL) and pre-crural (PCL) lymph nodes. (**E**) Frequency of bTB-lesions in different organs/lymph nodes affected of asymptomatic bTB bovines. Legends as described in (**C**) and (**D**). (**E, inset**) Frequency of lung lobes affected (left cranial lobe (LCR), left caudal lobe (LCA), right cranial lobe (RCR), right caudal lobe (RCA), middle lobe (MD) and accessory lobe (AC) were determined.

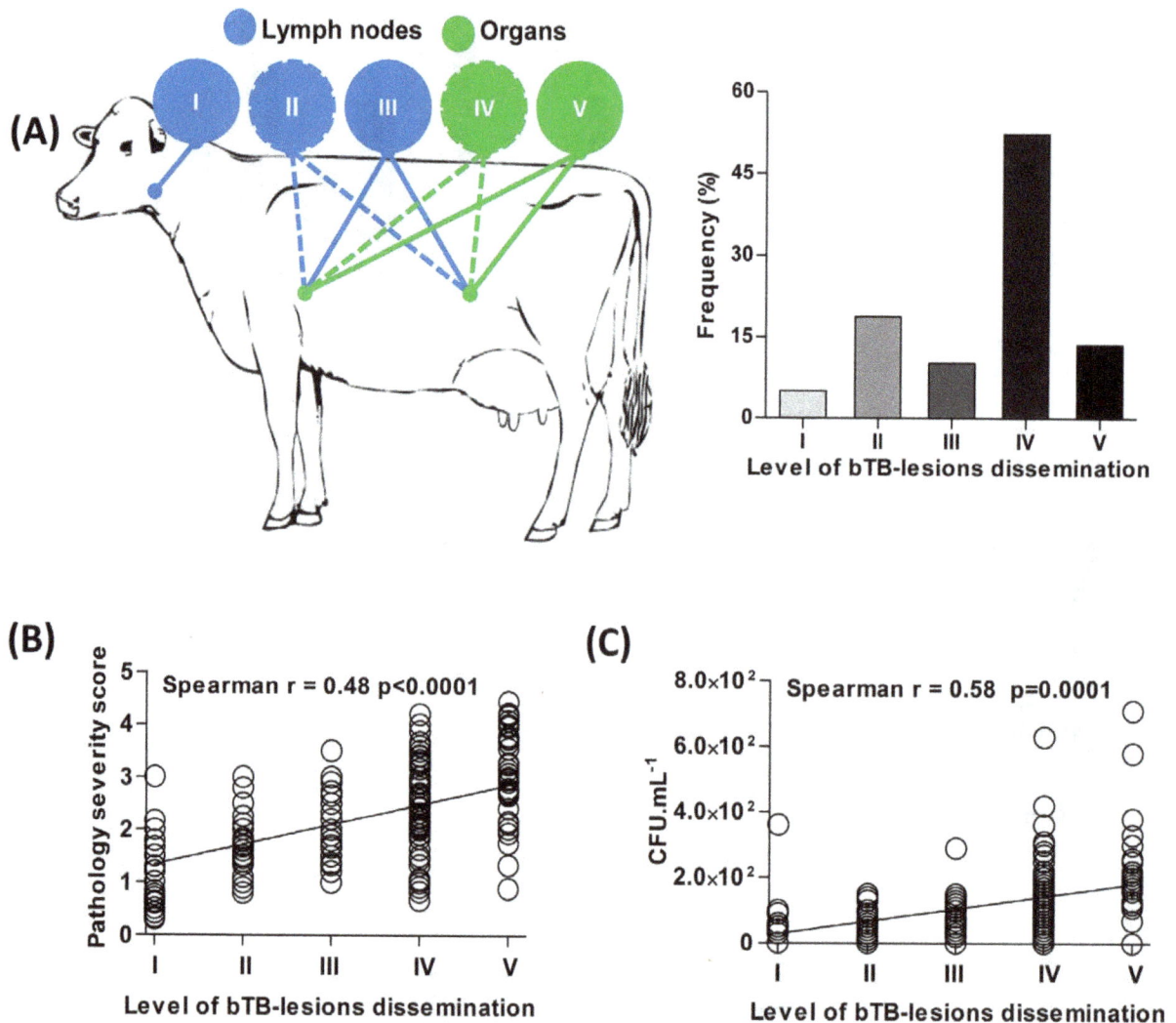

Figure 3. Anatomical dissemination of bTB-lesions and infection burden in asymptomatic cattle naturally infected with *M. bovis*. (**A**) Frequency of animals categorized according to their anatomical dissemination of bTB-lesions into five levels: I, lesions of bTB in the head lymph nodes, including retropharyngeal, mandibular, and parotid lymph nodes; II, presence of lesions of bTB in thoracic lymph nodes, including the mediastinal, bronchial, tracheobronchial lymph nodes, *or* in abdominal lymph nodes, including mesenteric, inguinal, gastric, hepatic, splenic, renal, sub-iliac, medial and lateral iliac lymph nodes; III, simultaneous presence of lesions suggestive of bTB in thoracic *and* abdominal lymph nodes; IV, presence of lesions of bTB in organs of the thoracic *or* abdominal cavity; and V, simultaneous presence of lesions of bTB in organs of thoracic *and* abdominal cavities. Schematic cartoon of the scoring system is represented. Continuous line represents both cavities affected (thoracic and abdominal); dotted line represents only one cavity affected. Green balloons indicate affected organs and blue balloons indicate affected lymph nodes. Correlation between levels of lesion dissemination and pathology severity (**B**) or mycobacterial loads (**C**) in cattle naturally infected with *M. bovis*. In (**B**), the results are expressed applying the gross pathology severity semi-quantitative scoring per animal previously described in [26], and (**C**) as number of CFU.mL^{-1} (colony-forming units per mL of granulomatous tissue homogenate). Spearman's correlation indexes (Spearman's r and p values) are shown in the graphs.

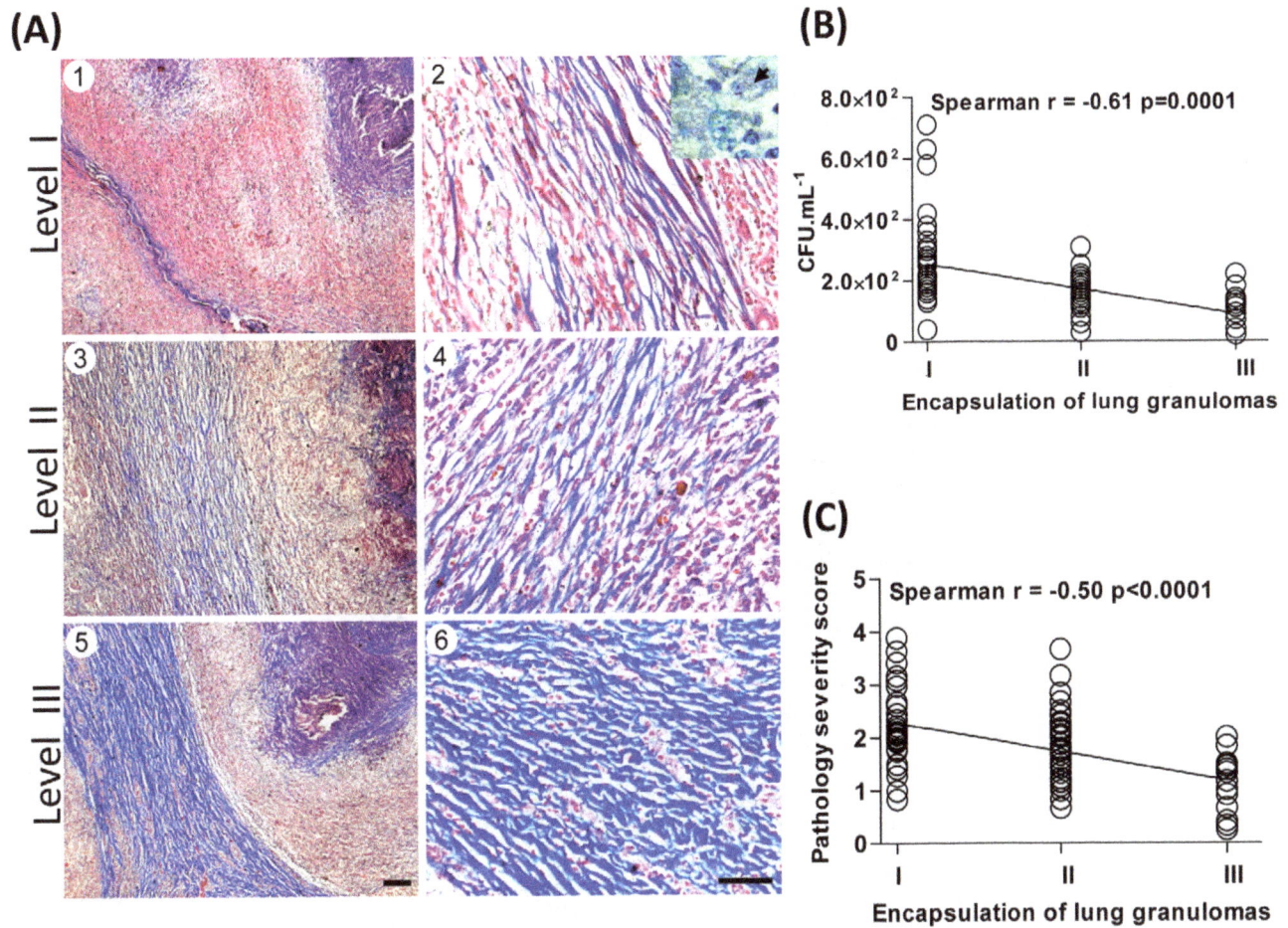

Figure 4. Histopathological analysis of granuloma encapsulation in asymptomatic cattle naturally infected with *M. bovis*. (A) Granulomas were formalin-fixed, paraffin-embedded and 4 μm-sections Massons trichrome stained, categorized and scored according to their intensity of encapsulation of primary granulomas into three levels: (1 and 2) I, thin encapsulation; (3 and 4) II, dense fibrous capsule; and (5 and 6) III, thickly fibrous encapsulation. (A, inset) Acid Fast-Bacilli (AFB). (Left panels, slides shown at 10× magnification; Scale bar = 100 μm. Right panels, slides shown at 40× magnification; Scale bar = 50 μm. Inset, slides shown at 100× magnification. Correlation between intensity of granuloma encapsulation with mycobacterial loads (**B**) or gross pathology severity score (**C**) in cattle naturally infected with *M. bovis* are presented. Spearman's correlation indexes (Spearman's r and p values) are shown in the graphs.

natural infection. We found that anatomical dissemination of bacteria/lesions is associated with tissue mycobacterial loads as well as severity of the gross pathology, suggesting the existence of a dynamic host immune response during natural infection. Although further studies are needed to better characterize the process of *M. bovis* dissemination in naturally-infected bovines, the parameters presented here could be employed as predictive biomarkers of disease progression and utilized in control surveillance programs.

Cattle immune responses against *M. bovis* may be a result of several factors, such as strain resistance, infection route and encapsulation of the tuberculous lesions. Connective tissue deposition (encapsulation) is thought to limit dissemination of bacteria and play a critical role in controlling mycobacterial proliferation by entrapping bacilli inside the lesions [14,20,22,25]. However, Liebana et al. have reported the absence of correlation between AFB numbers and stage of granuloma development during natural infection with *M. bovis* in England and Wales [31]. In our study, histological analysis of granulomatous response and tissue remodeling revealed high frequency of chronic lesions in different tissues, which negatively correlated with viable myco-bacterial counts (**Figs. 4 and 5**).

In order to better investigate the lesion development in cattle naturally infected with *M. bovis*, we first applied the methodology described by Wangoo et al. [21], which performed a descriptive study of the granulomatous responses in lymph nodes from cattle infected with *M. bovis* by the intratracheal route. The employment of such methodology in our samples led us to classify the majority of lesions in different organs/tissues (70–100%) as in the final stage of granuloma development, i.e. stage IV (**Table 1**). Due to increased resistance of cattle to *M. bovis* infection [2,28–30], it is possible that during the natural infection, most of bTB-lesions found in asymptomatic animals are in advanced/chronic stage of development. Interestingly, we found that, despite the observed chronic stage of lesions, thickness of encapsulation could be employed as a marker of lesion development and allowed us to further classify the granulomas into three major groups (I-III) (**Fig. 4**). The amount of connective tissue surrounding the granuloma (thin encapsulation - thickly fibrous encapsulation) negatively correlated with viable *M. bovis* or AFB staining, suggesting a pivotal role of granuloma encapsulation as a host response controlling mycobacterial proliferation during natural infection. In contrast, lymph nodes from experimentally *M. bovis*-

(A)

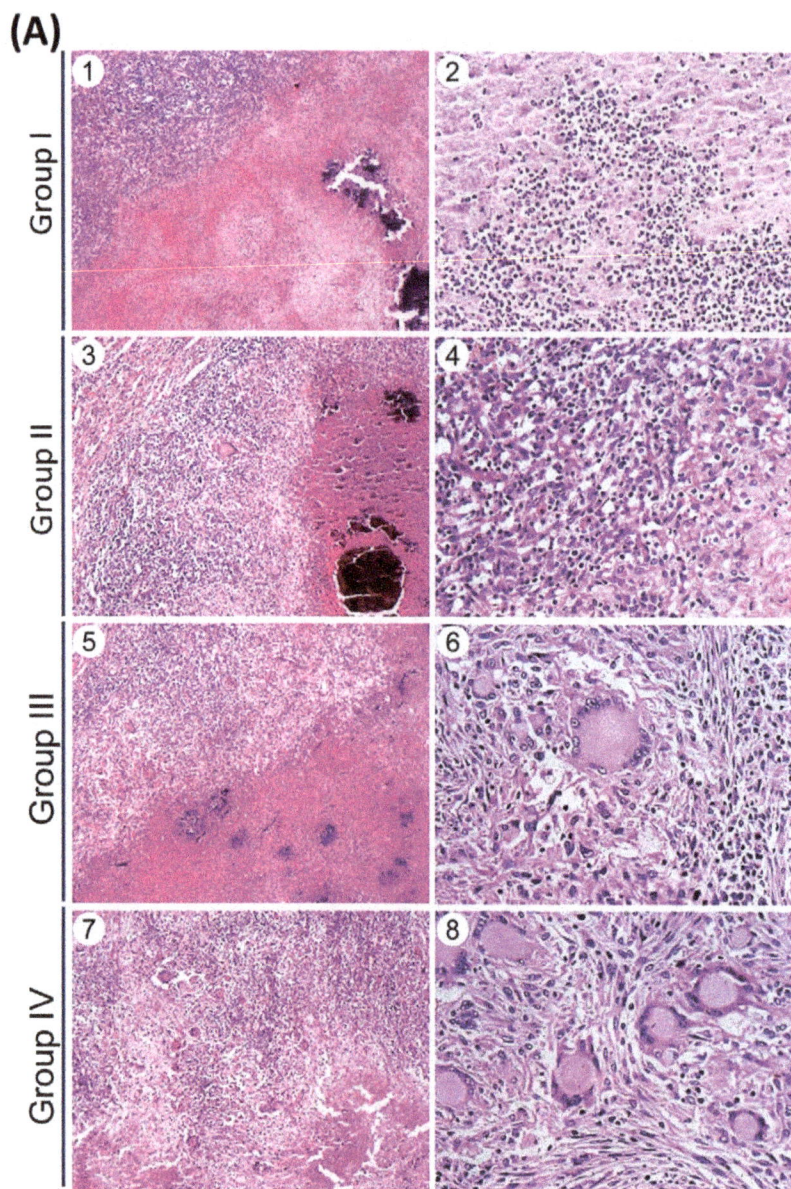

(B)

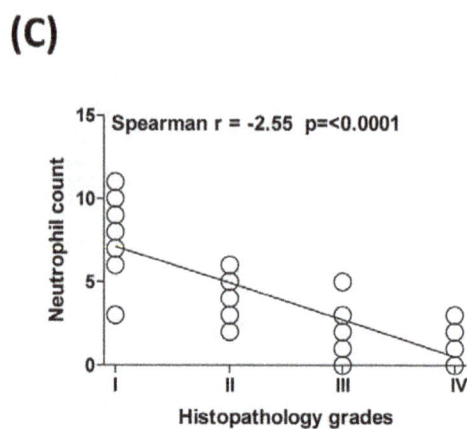

(C)

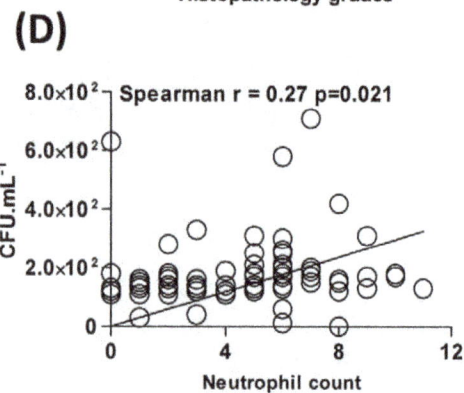

Spearman r = -2.55 p=<0.0001

(D)

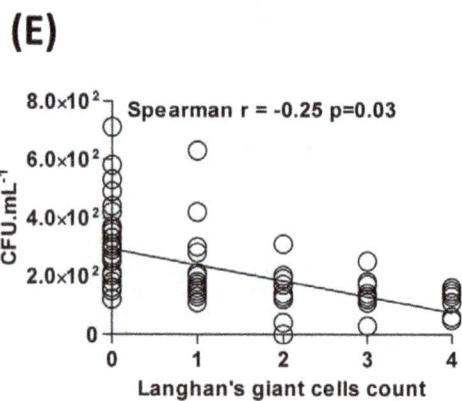

Spearman r = 0.27 p=0.021

(E)

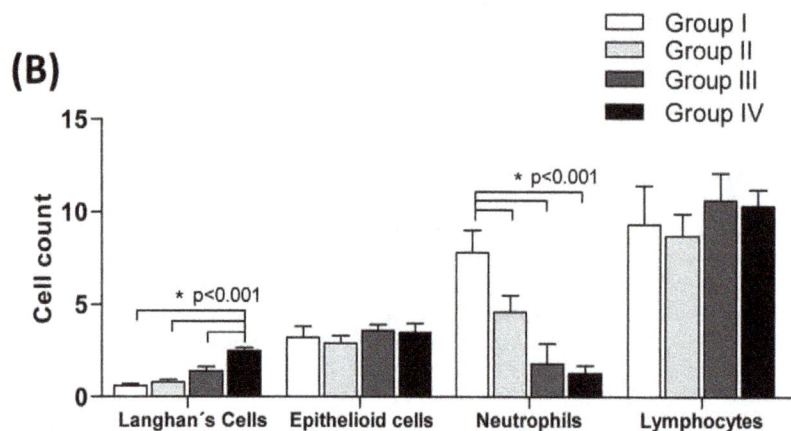

Spearman r = -0.25 p=0.03

(F)

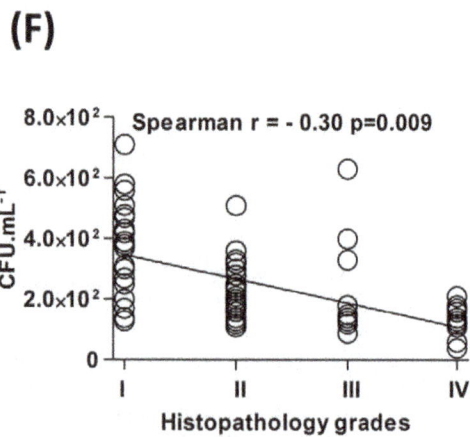

Spearman r = - 0.30 p=0.009

Asymptomatic Cattle Naturally Infected with Mycobacterium bovis Present Exacerbated Tissue...

17

Figure 5. Histopathological analysis of cellular profile of granulomatous response in lung of asymptomatic cattle naturally infected with M. bovis. (A) Lung tissues were categorized according to the granuloma cellular response profile and tissue remodeling into four groups: I-IV. Representative lung-tuberculous granulomatous response patterns are shown: I (1 and 2) encapsulated granulomas with caseous necrosis areas and presence of several scattered lymphocytes and dense clusters of neutrophils near the capsule; II (3 and 4) encapsulated granuloma, with extensive areas of caseous necrosis. Granulomatous cellular response composed primarily of epithelioid macrophages, lymphocytes, multinucleated Langhans giant cells and clusters of neutrophils; III (5 and 6) encapsulated granulomas, with extensive multicentric areas of caseous necrosis and centralized dystrophic mineralization. Granulomatous cellular response composed of epithelioid macrophages and scattered Langhan's giant cells, which surround the necrotic areas with dense clusters of lymphocytes and few neutrophils; III (7 and 8) encapsulated granulomas, with extensive multicentric areas of caseous necrosis and centralized dystrophic mineralization. Granulomatous cellular response composed of epithelioid macrophages admixed with increased numbers of multinucleated Langhan's giant cells, dense clusters lymphocytes and few neutrophils. Left panels, slides shown at 10× magnification; Scale bar = 100 µm. Right panels, slides shown at 40× magnification; Scale bar = 50 µm. **(B)** Results presented are mean ± SEM for each group shown in **(A)**. Correlation between neutrophil counts and histopathology grades **(C)**, Correlation between viable mycobacterial loads and neutrophils **(D)**, multinucleated Langhans giant cells counts **(E)** as well as lung-granulomatous response profile **(F)**. Spearman's correlation indexes (Spearman's r and p values) are shown in the graphs (n = 168 animals for correlation figures).

infected cattle were found to present increased AFB numbers in advanced-stage granulomas [19,21]. These data are in direct contrast with the findings obtained herein and could be explained by the employment of different models of infections, i.e. experimental vs natural infection. In addition, we have performed analysis of viable bacteria, which in comparison with AFB staining, more closely reflects the *M. bovis* loads present in the bTB lesions. The encapsulation response possibly may be induced by the bacillary burden in the granulomas. Nevertheless, animals with increased numbers of thickly encapsulated lesions were found to display lower bTB-lesions dissemination, suggesting induction of a mature connective tissue in the granulomas actively participates of anti-*M. bovis* immune responses during natural infection.

The majority of pulmonary granulomas investigated in our cattle cohort presented as encapsulated lesions with multiple intragranulomatous areas of caseous necrosis and the presence of dystrophic mineralization, which according to the criteria established for granuloma in lymphoid tissue during experimental infection, can be classified as chronic bTB-lesions (stage III/IV) [19,21]. Furthermore, histomorphological analysis of the lung granulomas revealed major differences in cell type counts **(Fig. 5)**. Consistent with these results, the process of granuloma maturation involves the migration of phagocytes and lymphocytes to the inflammation site in response to persistent mycobacterial stimuli [15,16,20,22,42]. An effective anti-mycobacteria host response primarily rely on cell-mediated immune response, controlled by cytokines such as IFN-γ produced by antigen-specific T cells [17,24,26,44,45]. Although the protective role of cell-mediated immune responses is unknown in cattle naturally infected with *M. bovis*, in the present study, we have observed significant correlations between neutrophil or Langhan's giant cell numbers and granuloma mycobacterial loads. Neutrophilic infiltrate was observed particularly in early stages of granuloma infection [19,21] and could be important for granuloma formation. Also, neutrophils have been suggested to play a regulatory anti-mycobacterial role [46,47]. We have a found a positive correlation between neutrophil numbers and CFU counts, suggesting that bacillary burden induce neutrophil recruitment and/or maintenance into the granulomas. In contrast, neutrophil could potentially play a detrimental role by favoring mycobacterial growth in granulomas during natural infection [48,49]. A negative correlation between multinucleated giant cell numbers and *M. bovis* CFU counts in granulomas suggests, as expected, that activated multinucleated macrophages contribute to the control of this important bovine pathogen. Data from experimental models have demonstrated Langhan's-type multinucleated giant cells can be found in all stages of development of lymph node granulomas [19,21]. Together, our findings indicate that *M. bovis*-induced granulomas in the lungs are dynamic lesions in which the cell populations change over the course of disease, stimulating a

diverse milieu during infection. The physiopathology of this complex structure during natural infection of *M. bovis* merits further investigation.

Cattle are natural hosts of *M. bovis*, which besides being an economically important pathogen for international trade, is an imminent risk to public health. The evidence presented in this study could reflect a situation of bTB found in Brazil, which may not be transferable to other countries. Nevertheless, the data a presented here offer basic information on the host response during the natural infection with *M. bovis*, which could be utilized as a potential source for biomarkers to test novel vaccine/adjuvant molecule candidates as well as efficient diagnostic methods. In addition, our findings may be important to reveal new components to understand the immunopathogenesis of the bTB and contribute to the establishment of rational strategies for bTB infection surveillance and control.

Materials and Methods

Animals and Ante-mortem Evaluation

The study obtained ethical clearance from the Universidade do Estado de Santa Catarina ethical review committee (P#1.13.10). Federal government inspection abattoirs comply with PNCETB 06/2004 and MAPA 03/2000, which follow International Ethical Guidelines of Animal Welfare. The study population was comprised of 247 crossbred Holstein/Jersey cows between the ages of ~1.6 to 11 years which were mandatorily conducted to abattoirs after a positive reaction for the single intradermal comparative cervical tuberculin test (SICTT; PPD) following Brazilian regulations [50]. These animals derived from 18 dairy farms with intensive husbandry systems, which experienced 23 bTB outbreaks between 2009 and 2011. Farms were located in Santa Catarina State, Brazil, and maintained under surveillance control against bTB following Brazilian's regulations. SICTT tests were performed in accordance with regulations set forth by the Brazilian Department of Agriculture (MAPA) [50]. Briefly, two sites located 12 cm to 15 cm apart on the cervical area of the mid-neck were shaved and skin thickness was measured using calipers. The first site was injected with 0.1 mL of bovine PPD (PPD-B - *M. bovis* strain AN5, 1 mg protein/mL), while the second site was injected with 0.1 mL of avian PPD (PPD-A - *Mycobacterium avium* strain D4, 0.5 mg protein/mL) [50]. After 72 hours, skin thickness at the injection sites was measured, and the difference between the reaction sizes for the two injection sites was determined. An animal was classified as PPD-positive if the skin thickness at the PPD-B injection site was at least 4 mm greater than the skin thickness at the PPD-A injection site [9].

During ante-mortem analysis, animals were classified into the following three clinical stages based on symptoms observed during clinical evaluation: *absence,* absence of clinical signs; *moder-*

Table 1. Distribution and stage of histological development of primary tuberculous granulomas in cattle naturally infected with *Mycobacterium bovis*.

Distribution of granulomas		Development stages of granulomas (%)			
		I	II	III	IV
Major organs/tissues					
Thorax	Lung	1.9 (3/159)	1.2 (2/159)	11.3 (13/159)	85.5 (136/159)
	Pleura	0	22.2 (4/18)	5.6 (1/18)	72.2 (13/18)
	Hearth		0	0	0
	Pericardia	0	0	0	100 (6/6)
Abdominal	Liver	0	12.5 (1/8)	0	87.5 (7/8)
	Spleen	0	0	16.7 (1/6)	83.3 (5/6)
	Intestine	0	0	28.6 (2/7)	71.4 (5/7)
	Mesentery	0	0	25 (2/8)	75 (6/8)
	Genito-urinary system	0	28.6 (2/7)	0	71.4 (5/7)
Carcass	Udder	0	0	0	100 (5/5)
	Other tissues	25 (1/4)	75 (3/4)	0	0
Lymph nodes					
Head	Parotid	0	16.7 (2/12)	0	83.3 (10/12)
	Retropharyngeal	4.2 (1/24)	0	16.7 (4/24)	79.2 (19/24)
	Mandibular	0	5.9 (1/17)	52.9 (9/17)	41.2 (7/17)
	Palatine tonsil	0	0	0	100 (3/3)
Thorax	Tracheobronchial	2.4 (1/42)	4.7 (2/42)	14.3 (6/42)	85.7 (36/42)
	Bronchial	1.6 (1/63)	3.2 (2/63)	4.7 (3/63)	90.5 (57/63)
	Mediastinal	4.3 (2/47)	2.1 (1/47)	4.3 (2/47)	89.4 (42/47)
Abdominal	Hepatic	0	0	22.2 (2/9)	77.8 (7/9)
	Mesenteric	0	9.1 (3/33)	12.1 (4/33)	69.7 (23/33)
Others	Iliac	0	0	0	100 (2/2)
	Sciatic	0	0	0	100 (3/3)
	Prescapular	0	14.3 (1/7)	0	85.7 (6/7)
	Precrural	0	0	0	100 (3/3)

ate, weight loss, hyporexia, coughing intermittently; and *severe,* extreme weight loss, weakness, hyporexia, hemoptysis, dyspnea, progressive cough and tuberculous mastitis.

Post-mortem Examination and Pathology Analysis

All major body organs and lymph nodes were examined for the presence of visible lesions suggestive of bTB disease. Organs and lymph nodes were cross-sectioned in 0.5 cm to 1 cm intervals and examined individually for the presence of lesions. Organ and tissue samples from animals with or without bTB visible lesions (VL) were collected for *M. bovis* culture and PCR analysis as well as for histopathological examination. Only animals displaying sample tissues positive for *M. bovis* by culture, PCR or direct examination (Ziehl-Neelsen – acid fast bacilli - staining) were included in the study. The anatomical dissemination of the visible gross patho-logical lesions in different organs and tissues were scored according to the following system: I = presence of bTB-lesions in the lymph nodes of the head, including the left and right medial and lateral retropharyngeal, left and right mandibular, and left and right parotid lymph nodes; II = presence of bTB-lesions in thoracic lymph nodes, including the cranial and caudal mediastinal, cranial tracheobronchial, left and right tracheobronchial lymph nodes, *or* in abdominal lymph nodes, including mesenteric, deep and

superficial inguinal, gastric, hepatic, splenic, renal, subiliac, medial and lateral iliac lymph nodes; III = simultaneous presence of bTB-lesions in thoracic *and* abdominal lymph nodes, including lymph nodes already mentioned above; IV = presence of bTB-lesions in organs of the thoracic *or* abdominal cavity, with or without the presence of lesions in the draining lymph nodes associated with the organ; and V = simultaneous presence of bTB-lesions in organs of thoracic *and* abdominal cavities, with or without the presence of lesions in the draining lymph nodes associated with the organ. Out of the cattle with score IV or V, most of them (85%) displayed also lesions in draining lymph nodes.

The severity of the visible gross pathological changes in the major body organs and lymph nodes were classified by applying the semi-quantitative scoring of gross lesions previously described by Vordermeier et al. [26]. Briefly, each lung lobe, including left cranial, left caudal, right cranial, right caudal/middle, and accessory lobes, was cross-sectioned at 0.5 to 1.0 cm intervals and scored from 0 to 5 depending on the number of lesions and extent of pathology observed, 0 being no visible lesions and 5 being coalescing gross lesions. The scores of the individual lobes were summed to calculate the lung score. The major **organs/ tissues,** including the pleura, pericardia, liver, spleen, intestine, mesentery, uterus, ovaries, kidney, bladder and muscular tissue, were scored as well. The **lymph nodes**, including the mandibular, parotid, medial retropharyngeal, palatine tonsil, bronchial, mediastinal and tracheobronchial, hepatic, mesenteric, iliac, sciatic, pre-scapular and pre-crural lymph nodes, were cross-sectioned at 0.5 cm intervals and were scored using a score of 0 to 3, 0 being no visible lesions and 3 being extensive or coalescing gross lesions. Pathology scores were combined to determine mean gross pathology severity score per animal.

Bacteriology and Molecular Typing of *M. bovis* from bTB Lesions

Tissue sections collected at post-mortem from lymph node and lung samples were individually homogenized using a rotating-blade macerator system (Tissue ruptor®). One milliliter of homogenate was decontaminated and concentrated by Petroff's Sodium Hydroxide method according to [9]. Culture and enumeration of bacteria ($CFU.mL^{-1}$ tissue homogenate) was performed by inoculating 100 µL of decontaminated tissue homogenate in Ogawa-Kudoh (OK) agar containing sodium pyruvate (12 mg/mL) and counting colonies after aerobic incubation at 37°C for 8 weeks. After growth in OK+pyruvate, colonies were molecularly typed by PCR. Briefly, purified mycobacterial DNA from colonies extracted as previously described [51] was used as template for PCR amplification of the following multi-copy insertion gene IS1081 (~135 bp), present in the *M. tuberculosis* complex organisms (Fig. 1B) [52] and RvD1Rv2031c (~500 bp) a polymorphic region of 2900 bp in the *M. bovis* genome which was not homologous in the genomes of *M. tuberculosis* and *M. avium* (Fig. 1C) [53]."

Histopathological Analysis

Tissues samples were fixed in 10% neutral buffered formalin and dehydrated in graded ethanol solutions. After dehydration, samples were paraffin-embedded, sectioned (4 µm), and stained by hematoxylin and eosin (H&E), Massons trichrome or AFB method. Microscopically, the granulomas from **lymph nodes** and major **organs/tissues** (pericardia, pleura, liver, spleen, intestine, mesentery, uterus, ovaries, kidney, bladder, adrenal and muscular tissue) were classified into the following four categories [21] according to the development of the lesion: stage I - initial or early lesions; stage II - solid granulomas; stage III - minimal necrosis; or stage IV - necrosis and mineralization. Additionally, three levels of granuloma encapsulation were identified following classification being proposed in this study: level I - thin encapsulation; level II - dense fibrous capsule; level III - thickly fibrous encapsulation. All **lung granulomas** were subjected to systemic histopathological examination. Specifically for the classification of lung granulomas, the following proposed criteria were used to classify in four different groups of lesions: **group I (score =1)** granulomas circumscribed by fibrous encapsulation with

caseous necrosis areas and presence of several scattered lymphocytes and dense clusters of neutrophils near the capsule. Epithelioid macrophages and low Langhans giant cell count, which surround the necrotic areas; **group II (score =2)** – granuloma circumscribe by fibrous encapsulation, with extensive areas of caseous necrosis. Granulomatous cellular response composed primarily of epithelioid macrophages, lymphocytes, moderate Langhans giant cell count and clusters of neutrophils, which surround the necrotic areas and extend until capsule; **group III (score =3)** – granulomas circumscribed by fibrous encapsulation, with extensive multicentric areas of caseous necrosis and centralized dystrophic mineralization. Granulomatous cellular response composed of epithelioid macrophages and moderate amount of scattered Langhan's giant cells, which surround the necrotic areas with dense clusters of lymphocytes and few or absent clustered neutrophils near the fibrous capsule; **group IV (score =4)** – granulomas encapsulated, with extensive multicentric areas of caseous necrosis and centralized dystrophic mineralization. Granulomatous cellular response composed of epithelioid macrophages admixed with large amount of Langhans giant cells, which surround the necrotic areas with dense clusters lymphocytes and few or absent neutrophils near the fibrous capsule. For the histopathological analysis, total number of granulomatous cellular response cells was counted in 10 microscope fields (1×100 magnification) per lung granuloma section. Mean and standard deviation were determined for each group. For coalescing or multicentric lesions in the histomorphological analysis, the primary lesion or more chronic/advanced lesion/stage was evaluated. The relative number of acid-fast bacilli (AFB) found in each ZN-stained section was estimated as well.

Statistical Analysis

Statistical analysis was carried out using GraphPad Prism 5 (GraphPad Software Inc., San Diego, CA, USA). Correlations between bacterial load, level of granuloma-encapsulation, histopathological lung-granulomatous response, gross pathology, and lesion distribution were assessed by nonparametrical analysis applying the Spearman rank correlation. Spearman's correlation coefficients (r_s) and p-values are provided.

Acknowledgments

We are grateful to CIDASC for allowing us to collect the samples used in this work.

Author Contributions

Conceived and designed the experiments: ÁM AB. Performed the experiments: ÁM RF CR PF. Analyzed the data: ÁM MM AB. Contributed reagents/materials/analysis tools: ÁM CP AB. Wrote the paper: AB ÁM.

References

1. World Health Organization (2008) Global tuberculosis control - surveillance, planning, financing: WHO report 2008. WHO/HTM/TB/2008 393: 1–304.
2. Thoen C, LoBue P, de Kantor I (2006) The importance of *Mycobacterium bovis* as a zoonosis. Vet Microbiol 112: 339–3345.
3. Cosivi O, Grange JM, Daborn CJ, Raviglione MC, Fujikura T, et al. (1998) Zoonotic tuberculosis due to *Mycobacterium bovis* in developing countries. Emerg Infect Dis 4: 59–70.
4. de Kantor IN, Ambroggi M, Poggi S, Morcillo N, Telles MADS et al. (2008) Human *Mycobacterium bovis* infection in ten Latin American countries. Tuberculosis 88: 358–365.
5. Berg S, Firdessa R, Habtamu M, Gadisa E, Mengistu A, et al. (2009) The Burden of Mycobacterial Disease in Ethiopian Cattle: Implications for Public Health. PLoS One 4: e5068. doi:10.1371/journal.pone.0005068.
6. Hlavsa MC, Moonan PK, Cowan LS, Navin TR, Kammerer JS, et al. (2008) Human tuberculosis due to *Mycobacterium bovis* in the United States, 1995–2005. Clin Infect Dis 47: 168–175.
7. Evans JT, Smith EG, Banerjee A, Smith RM, Dale J, et al. (2007) Cluster of human tuberculosis caused by *Mycobacterium bovis*: evidence for person-to-person transmission in the UK. Lancet 369: 1270–1276.
8. Renwick AR, White PCL, Bengis RG (2007) Bovine tuberculosis in southern African wildlife: a multi-species host-pathogen system. Epidemiol Infect 135: 529–540.
9. The World Organization for Animal Health (OIE) (2011) The manual of diagnostic tests and vaccines for terrestrial animals: Bovine tuberculosis. Paris: WAHID. 590 p.
10. Monaghan ML, Doherty ML, Collins JD, Kazda JF, Quinn PJ (1994) The tuberculin test. Vet Microbiol 40: 111–124.

11. Claridge J, Diggle P, McCann CM, Mulcahy G, Flynn R (2012) *Fasciola hepatica* is associated with the failure to detect bovine tuberculosis in dairy cattle. Nat Commun 3: 853 doi: 10.1038/ncomms1840.

12. de la Rua-Domenech R, Goodchild AT, Vordermeier HM, Hewinson RG, Christiansen KH, et al. (2006) Ante mortem diagnosis of tuberculosis in cattle: a review of the tuberculin tests, gamma-interferon assay and other ancillary diagnostic techniques. Res Vet Sci 81: 190–210.

13. Norby B, Bartlett PC, Fitzgerald SD, Granger LM, Brunning-Fann CS, et al. (2004) The sensitivity of gross necropsy, caudal fold and comparative cervical tests for the diagnosis of bovine tuberculosis. J Vet Diagn Invest 16: 126–131.

14. Volkman HE, Clay H, Beery D, Chang JCW, Sherman DR, et al. (2004) Tuberculous granuloma formation is enhanced by a *Mycobacterium* virulence determinant. PLoS Biol 2: e367. doi:10.1371/journal.pbio.0020367.

15. Cosma CL, Humbert O, Ramakrishnan L (2004) Superinfecting mycobacteria home to established tuberculous granulomas. Nat Immunol 5: 828–835.

16. Ulrichs T, Kaufmann SH (2006) New insights into the function of granulomas in human tuberculosis. J Pathol 208: 261–269.

17. Flynn JL, Chan J (2001) Immunology of tuberculosis. Annu Rev Immunol 19: 93–129.

18. Ramakrishnan L (2012) Revisiting the role of the granuloma in tuberculosis. Nat Rev Immunol 12: 352–366.

19. Palmer MV, Waters WR, Thacker TC (2007) Infected with *Mycobacterium bovis* lesion development and immunohistochemical changes in granulomas from cattle experimentally. Vet Pathol 44: 863 doi: 10.1354/vp.44-6-863.

20. Russell DG (2007) Who puts the tubercle in tuberculosis? Nat Rev Microbiol 5: 39–47.

21. Wangoo A, Johnson L, Gough J, Ackbar R, Inglut S, et al. (2005) Advanced granulomatous lesions in *Mycobacterium bovis*-infected cattle are associated with increased expression of type I procollagen, gammadelta (WC1+) T cells and CD 68+ cells. J Comp Pathol 133: 223–234.

22. Gil O, Díaz I, Vilaplana C, Tapia G, Díaz J, et al. (2010) Granuloma encapsulation is a key factor for containing tuberculosis infection in minipigs. PLoS One 5: e10030. doi:10.1371/journal.pone.0010030.

23. Thacker TC, Palmer MV, Waters WR (2007) Associations between cytokine gene expression and pathology in *Mycobacterium bovis* infected cattle. Vet Immunol Immunopath 10: 204–213.

24. Welsh MD, Cunningham RT, Corbett DM, Girvin RM, McNair J, et al. (2005) Influence of pathological progression on the balance between cellular and humoral immune responses in bovine tuberculosis. Immunology 114: 101–111.

25. Pollock JM, Neill SD (2002) *Mycobacterium bovis* infection and tuberculosis in cattle. Vet J 163: 115–127.

26. Vordermeier HM, Chambers MA, Cockle PJ, Whelan AO, Simmons J, et al. (2002) Correlation of ESAT-6-specific gamma interferon production with pathology in cattle following *Mycobacterium bovis* BCG vaccination against experimental bovine tuberculosis. Infect Immun 70: 3026–3032.

27. Finlay EK, Berry DP, Wickham B, Gormley EP, Bradley DG (2012). A genome wide association scan of bovine tuberculosis susceptibility in Holstein-Friesian dairy cattle. PLoS One 7: e30545. doi:10.1371/journal.pone.0030545.

28. Driscoll EE, Hoffman JI, Green LE, Medley GF, Amos W (2011) A preliminary study of genetic factors that influence susceptibility to bovine tuberculosis in the British cattle herd. PLoS One 6: e18806. doi:10.1371/journal.pone.0018806.

29. Phillips CJ, Foster CR, Morris PA, Teverson R (2002) Genetic and management factors that influence the susceptibility of cattle to *Mycobacterium bovis* infection. Anim Health Res Rev 3: 3–13.

30. Brotherstone S, White IMS, Coffey M, Downs SH, Mitchell AP, et al. (2009) Evidence of genetic resistance of cattle to infection with *Mycobacterium bovis*. J Dairy Sci 93: 1234–1242.

31. Liebana E, Johnson L, Gough J, Durr P, Jahans K, et al. (2008) Pathology of naturally occurring bovine tuberculosis in England and Wales. Vet J 176: 354–360.

32. Ameni G, Aseffa A, Engers H, Young D, Gordon SV, et al. (2007) High prevalence and increased severity of pathology of bovine tuberculosis in Holsteins compared to zebu breeds under field cattle husbandry in central Ethiopia. Clin Vaccine Immunol 14: 1356–1361.

33. Bermingham ML, More SJ, Good M, Cromie AR, Higgins IM, et al. (2009) Genetics of tuberculosis in Irish Holstein-Friesian dairy herds. J Dairy Sci 92: 3447–3456.

34. Widdison S, Watson M, Coffey TJ (2009) Correlation between lymph node pathology and chemokine expression during bovine tuberculosis. Tuberculosis 89: 17–422.

35. Neill SD, Bryson DB, Pollock JM (2001) Pathogenesis of tuberculosis in cattle. Tuberculosis 81: 79–86.

36. Ameni G, Vordermeier M, Firdessa R, Aseffa A, Hewinson G, et al. (2011) *Mycobacterium tuberculosis* infection in grazing cattle in central Ethiopia. Vet J 188: 359–361.

37. Corner LA (1994) Post-mortem diagnosis of *Mycobacterium bovis* infection in cattle. Vet Microbiol 40: 53–63.

38. Ameni G, Aseffa A, Sirak A, Engers H, Young DB, et al. (2007) Effect of skin testing and segregation on the prevalence of bovine tuberculosis, and molecular typing of *Mycobacterium bovis*, in Ethiopia. Vet Rec 161: 782–786.

39. Cassidy JP (2006) The pathogenesis and pathology of bovine tuberculosis with insights from studies of tuberculosis in humans and laboratory animal models. Vet Microbiol 112: 151–161.

40. Dean GS, Rhodes SG, Coad M, Whelan AO, Cockle PJ, et al. (2005) Minimum infective dose of *Mycobacterium bovis* in cattle. Infect Immun 73: 6467–6471.

41. Whipple DL, Bolin CA, Miller JM (1996) Distribution of lesions in cattle infected with *Mycobacterium bovis*. J Vet Diagn Investig 8: 351–354.

42. Egen JG, Rothfuchs AG, Feng CG, Horwitz MA, Sher A, et al. (2011) Intravital imaging reveals limited antigen presentation and T cell effector function in mycobacterial granulomas immunity 34: 807–819.

43. Wedlock DN, Aldwell FE, Collins DM, De Lisle GW, Wilson T et al. (1999) Immune responses induced in cattle by virulent and attenuated *Mycobacterium bovis* strains: correlation of delayed-type hypersensitivity with ability of strains to grow in macrophages. Infect Immun 67: 2172–2177.

44. Boom WH (1996) The role of T-cell subsets in *Mycobacterium tuberculosis* infection. Infect Agents Dis 5: 73–81.

45. Cooper AM, Dalton DK, Stewart TA, Griffin JP, Russell DG, et al. (1993) Disseminated tuberculosis in interferon gamma gene-disrupted mice. J Exp Med 178: 2243–2247.

46. Feng CG, Kaviratne M, Rothfuchs AG, Cheever A, Hieny S, et al. (2006) NK cell-derived IFN-gamma differentially regulates innate resistance and neutrophil response in T cell-deficient hosts infected with *Mycobacterium tuberculosis*. J Immunol 177: 7086–7093.

47. Seiler P, Aichele P, Bandermann S, Hauser AE, Lu B, Gerard NP, et al. (2003) Early granuloma formation after aerosol *Mycobacterium tuberculosis* infection is regulated by neutrophils via CXCR3-signaling chemokines. Eur J Immunol 33: 2676–2686.

48. Keller C, Hoffmann R, Lang R, Brandau S, Hermann C, et al. (2006) Genetically determined susceptibility to tuberculosis in mice causally involves accelerated and enhanced recruitment of granulocytes. Infect Immun 74: 4295–4309.

49. Eruslanov EB, Lyadova IV, Kondratieva TK, Majorov KB, Scheglov IV, et al. (2005) Neutrophil responses to *Mycobacterium tuberculosis* infection in genetically susceptible and resistant mice. Infect Immun 73: 1744–1753.

50. MAPA - Ministério da Agricultura, Pecuária e Abastecimento, Brasil (2006) Programa nacional de controle e erradicação da brucelose e da tuberculose animal (PNCEBT), MAPA/SDA/DSA, Brasília, 188 pp.

51. Wards BJ, Collins DM, de Lisle GW (1995) Detection of *Mycobacterium bovis* in tissues by polymerase chain reaction. Vet Microbiol 43: 227–240.

52. Taylor GM, Worth DR, Palmer S, Jahans K, Hewinson RG (2007) Rapid detection of *Mycobacterium bovis* DNA in cattle lymph nodes with visible lesions using PCR. BMC Vet Res 3: 12. doi:10.1186/1746-6148-3-12.

53. Rodríguez JG, Fissanoti JC, Del Portillo P, Patarroyo ME, Romano MI, et al. (1999) Amplification of a 500-basepair fragment from cultured isolates of *Mycobacterium bovis*. Eur J Clin Microbiol Infect Dis 37: 2330–2332.

3

Typing Late Prehistoric Cows and Bulls—Osteology and Genetics of Cattle at the Eketorp Ringfort on the Öland Island in Sweden

Ylva Telldahl[1]*, **Emma Svensson**[2], **Anders Götherström**[2], **Jan Storå**[1]

1 Osteoarchaeological Research Laboratory, Department of Archaeology and Classical Studies, Stockholm University, Stockholm, Sweden, 2 Department of Evolutionary Biology, Uppsala Universitet, Uppsala, Sweden

Abstract

Human management of livestock and the presence of different breeds have been discussed in archaeozoology and animal breeding. Traditionally osteometrics has been the main tool in addressing these questions. We combine osteometrics with molecular sex identifications of 104 of 340 morphometrically analysed bones in order to investigate the use of cattle at the Eketorp ringfort on the Öland island in Sweden. The fort is dated to 300–1220/50 A.D., revealing three different building phases. In order to investigate specific patterns and shifts through time in the use of cattle the genetic data is evaluated in relation to osteometric patterns and occurrence of pathologies on cattle metapodia. Males were genotyped for a Y-chromosomal SNP in *UTY19* that separates the two major haplogroups, Y1 and Y2, in taurine cattle. A subset of the samples were also genotyped for one SNP involved in coat coloration (*MC1R*), one SNP putatively involved in resistance to cattle plague (*TLR4*), and one SNP in intron 5 of the *IGF-1* gene that has been associated to size and reproduction. The results of the molecular analyses confirm that the skeletal assemblage from Eketorp is dominated by skeletal elements from females, which implies that dairying was important. Pathological lesions on the metapodia were classified into two groups; those associated with the use as draught animals and those lesions without a similar aetiology. The results show that while bulls both exhibit draught related lesions and other types of lesions, cows exhibit other types of lesions. Interestingly, a few elements from females exhibit draught related lesions. We conclude that this reflects the different use of adult female and male cattle. Although we note some variation in the use of cattle at Eketorp between Iron Age and Medieval time we have found little evidence for the use of different types of animals for specific purposes. The use of specific (genetic) breeds seems to be a phenomenon that developed later than the Eketorp settlement.

Editor: Vincent Laudet, Ecole Normale Supérieure de Lyon, France

Funding: Financial support to Emma Svensson from Birgit & Gad Rausing and Helge Axison Johnsson stiftelsen, P o Lundells, Lars Hiertas Minne. Financial support was received from Berit Wallenbergs Stiftelse and Birgit and Gad Rausings stiftelse to Ylva Telldahl. Anders Götherström was supported by the Royal Swedish Academy of Science. The funders had no role in study design, data collection and analysis, decision to publish, or preparation of the manuscript.

Competing Interests: The authors have declared that no competing interests exist.

* E-mail: ylva.telldahl@ofl.su.se

Introduction

Breeding of cattle has been suggested to have a long tradition in Europe [1]. For example in Italy (Etruria) some contemporary breeds are believed to predate the Roman age [2]. In Northern Europe there may be native breeds, which can be traced some 1000 years back in time [3]. Although farming was introduced to Scandinavia during the Neolithic it is from the Bronze Age and onwards that livestock was used more regularly in the cultivation of land [4] The interaction between farming and animal husbandry became more expressed during the Iron Age [4–7].

During the Viking Age and Medieval Age there were various trade markets in the Baltic region, organized through several ports. The ports also served as hubs for the spread of new agricultural technological innovations and often farms were located close to these ports. The Eketorp ringfort, in the southern parts of Öland, Sweden (Figure 1) offers a unique insight into Iron Age and medieval period husbandry. At an early stage the ringfort was a farming settlement, which over time developed to a garrison. Three settlement phases, I-III, have been identified. Phase I is

from Late Roman Iron Age ca. 300–400 A.D. and phase II from Germanic Iron Age ca.400–700 A.D. The ringfort was then abandoned and used again from about 1170–1220 A.D. [8,9]. The animal bones from the ringfort have previously been studied by Boessneck et al (1979). The vast majority of the osteological material is from the second and third phases of the settlement, and thus we have focused on these two periods.

Some of the 53 house foundations dating to phase II at Eketorp are remains of three-aisled houses [10] which were a new type that were built with a byre for stalling animals during winter [11–13]. The remains of 13 byres with stalls for approximately one hundred cattle have been excavated [14]. The faunal assemblage recovered at the Eketorp ringfort is one of the largest in Scandinavia from that time period; 0.5 tons from phase II and 1.3 tons from phase III [8,15]. The recovered bones represent food debris from domesticates such as cattle, sheep and pig, where cattle probably was the most important source of meat. Approximately 75% of the slaughtered adult animals were females [15,16], which illustrate the frequency bias in sex when females are kept to an adult age for milk production. In phase III the bones mainly represent debris of

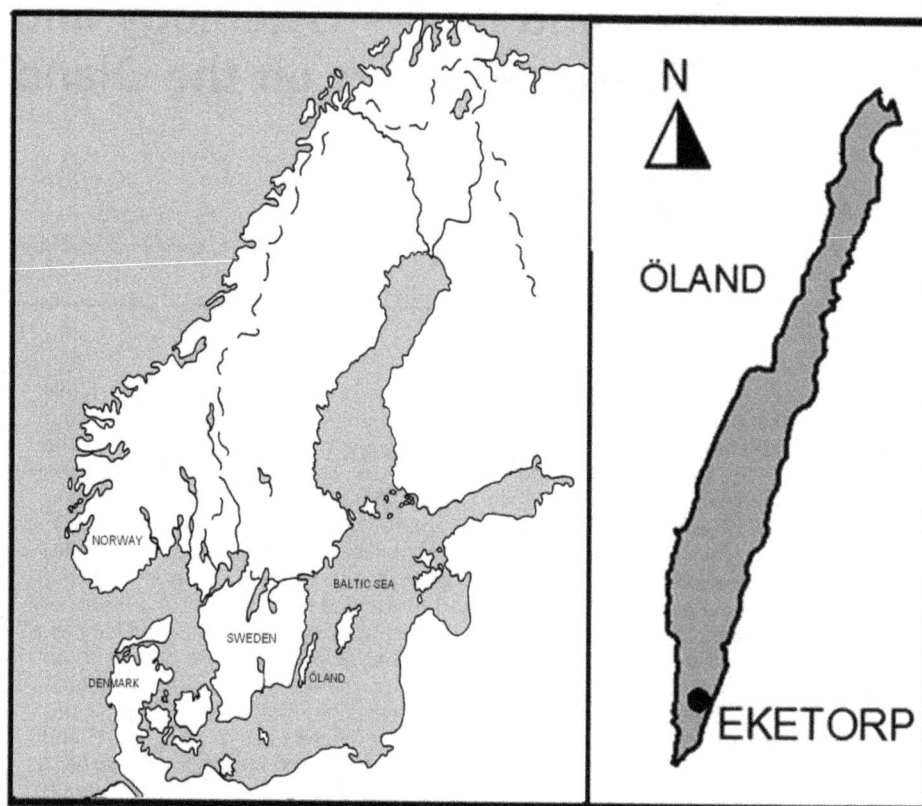

Figure 1. Map showing the location of Öland and Eketorp.

meat that had been brought to the site. Stables have been identified but they do not contain byres for cattle. The presence of long and slender metapodia shows that castration was practiced during both phases (II and III) [15,16]. Fifty-seven bones (23,1%) out of a total of 247 metatarsals and 41 bones (15,2%) of 269 metacarpals exhibit pathological lesions.

The mortality pattern for cattle shows a dominance of bones from sub adult animals in both phases. This is confirmed by Boessneck et al's data on tooth eruption and epiphysial closure on tibia and metapodials where 53.6% in phase II and 59.3% in phase III of the cattle were slaughtered before the age of 2 ½ years old. Boessneck et al also presents a size comparison of unfused first phalanx showing that the majority of sub adult cattle were slaughtered between 6–8 month and 1 ½ – 1 ¾ year of age. The calves were mainly slaughtered in the late autumn and early winter [15]. The average withers height for Eketorp bulls was 111 cm and for cows 109 cm in phase II while it in phase III was approximately two cm higher for both sexes. Compared to cattle from other Swedish and North European sites the Eketorp cattle from period III are among the largest [15,17].

Body size has been used to a wide extent to discuss prehistoric breeding and changes in body size have often been seen as a sign of improvement of livestock [18].Biomolecular analyses may provide complimentary data to the osteological data and holds the possibility to identify genetically different types of animals. Variation in genes coding for specific traits, such as, pigmentation, and muscle mass, may be used to detect breeding [19–21]. However, as breed identification of modern animals demands a panel of some 30 microsatellite markers [22] an even larger panel of SNPs suitable for degraded DNA would be needed [23]. This makes genetic breed identification based on ancient DNA (aDNA)

a challenging task given the poor preservation of the DNA and the techniques available at present. We choose to investigate size differences that may be related to genetic characteristics, and if such exist, it would be an indication of advanced animal husbandry. Also, changes in single genetic systems over time can be an indication of selection/breeding.

Here we use a combination of morphological data; sex, physical characteristics and pathological patterns (studied by Telldahl) with molecular data on sex and genetic variation to identify possible shifts in cattle breeding strategies at Eketorp. We consider Eketorp as a model site for northern European farming. If this is a key period in rapid sophisticated specialisation within farming, we expect to find a change in sex proportions and morphology. If, on the other hand, we do not find such change, it can be taken as support for continuity, or a slower rate of specialisation during this period.

Materials and Methods

Our study focuses on metapodia from cattle (*Bos taurus*) recovered at Eketorp. A total of 4470 metapodia have been identified at Eketorp whereof 1879 are from phase II and 2572 from phase III [15]. The bones are highly fragmented and from the assemblage we were able to retrieve 340 specimens of metapodia that offered possibilities for osteometric analyses and/ or analyses of specific skeletal lesions. The total sample comprises of 190 metatarsalia and 150 metacarpalia (McIII-IV and Mt III–IV – hereafter abbreviated Mc or Mt). Both complete and fragmentary metapodia from fully-grown and sub adult cattle were analysed. In cattle the distal epiphysis in metacarpals fuses at the age of 2–2 ½ and metatarsals fuses approximately ½ years later

[24–26]. In order to investigate the slaughter patterns of calves at Eketorp bones from sub adults were also selected for molecular sexing.

For size comparisons we use the breadth of the distal epiphysis (Bd) taken according to definitions from von den Driesch [27]. This measurement has proven useful for morphological sexing of male and female metapodia [28,29] and is commonly used in osteoarchaeological analyses. All measurements were documented using a digital calliper to the nearest 0.01 mm.

Seven different types of skeletal lesion on metapodia were identified in the Eketorp assemblage by Telldahl: lipping, new bone formation, eburnation, bone inflammation causing thickening of the diaphysis, depressions in articular facet, carpals/tarsals ankylosis and broadening of trochlea capitis medialis of metapodia. Lipping and broadening of trochlea capitis of metapodia is an overgrowth or bone modification beyond the joint margins. Exostosis is seen as new bone formation near the articular facets. Eburnation is seen as polished bone surface where the cartilage is damaged [30]. Thickening of the diaphysis could be the result of an inflammation where bacteria has access through the connective tissue[31]. The depressions are recorded in both proximal and distal articular facets. The etiology of carpal/tarsal ankylosis is uncertain but research have shown a correlation with age, conformation of the legs and increased load [32].

Two of these lesions, lipping and broadening of trochlea capitis medialis, are probably related to the use as draught animals [33,34,49] (Figure 2). In the present study the lesions are classified into two groups, lesions associated with draught use (workload related) and lesions with an unknown aetiology, i.e. not with certainty related to draught use. Here we report the lesions as present or absent.

A total of 133 metapodia dated to phase II and III were chosen for molecular analyses; 44 metacarpals and 89 metatarsals including 31 metatarsals from juvenile animals with an unfused distal epiphysis too young to be sexed morphometrically; 13 from phase II and 18 from phase III. The selection of the bones was conducted in order to gain a representative sample covering as completely as possible the full morphological size variation and also the presence of skeletal pathologies. A laboratory dedicated to work on aDNA, physically separated from work on modern DNA and PCR products, with positive air pressure and UV lightning was used for all aDNA extractions, a previously described method [21] was used and one extraction blank was included per every six extracts. PCR for sex identification was set up as in [28] using the forward sequencing system (F+R−biotinylated PCR primers and forward sequencing primer) S4 targeting a 63bp fragment. Positive PCR products were genotyped using pyrosequencing technology with a PSQ 96MA following guidelines from the manufacturer.

All samples identified as males were further genotyped for a Y chromosomal SNP in *UTY19*, this SNP has been shown to differentiate North and South European breeds in modern cattle, haplogroup Y1 and Y2 respectively [35]. A primer set targeting 74 base pairs was developed to increase the amplification success of the relatively degraded DNA (Figure S4). A subset of the samples genotyped for the sex identifying SNP were selected for further genotyping based on molecular preservation. Samples from both periods were genotyped in one SNP located in intron 5 of the *Insulin-like Growth Factor 1* (*IGF-1*) gene [38] (Figure S4). *IGF-1* is essential for in vivo follicular development in cattle [39,40] and it is also known to play an important role in various aspects of muscle growth and development [41,42]. The SNP is located in a QTL for twinning rate [38,43], and has been picked up in genome scans for selection in modern cattle [38,44,45]. Further one SNP involved in coat coloration in the *Melanocortin receptor 1* (*MC1R*) gene [36] and one SNP putatively involved in resistance to cattle plague, *Toll-like receptor 4* (*TLR4*) [37] were genotyped. These two

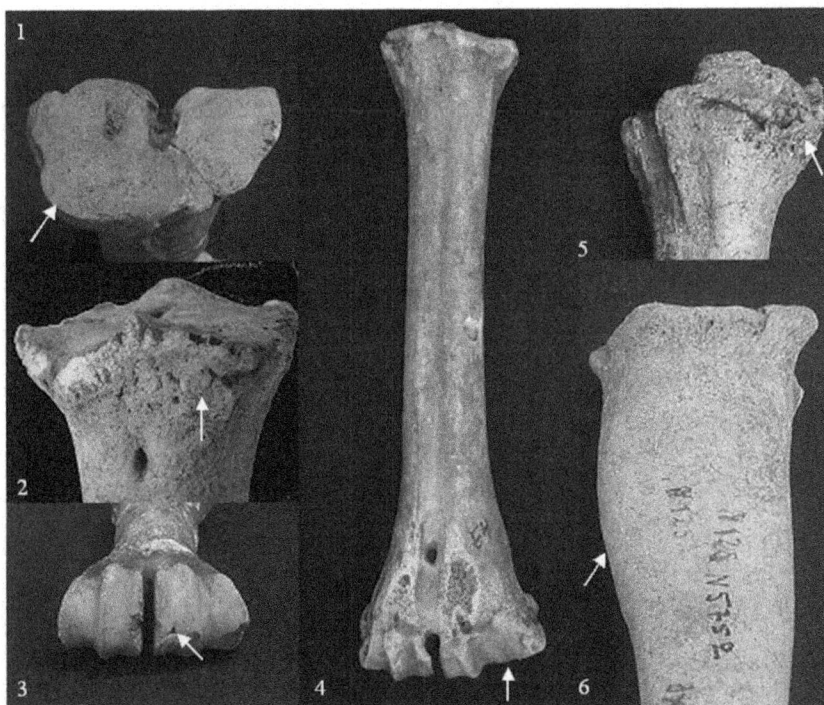

Figure 2. Six skeletal lesions in metapodials from Eketorp ringfort, Öland, Sweden. The lesions comprise of lipping (1), exostosis (2), depression on distal trochlea (3), broadening of the medial trochlea (4), tarsal ankylosis (5) and bone inflammation causing thickening of the diaphysis (6).

SNPs have been suggested to be under selection in northern European cattle (REF 21, Svensson et al, 2007 animal genetics) and the same PCR and sequencing conditions as in (21) was used.

All new primer systems were first blasted to ensure specificity to cattle, and tested on human DNA in the optimization process. The nature of pyrosequencing, where not only the SNP position, but also adjacent nucleotides is given also ensures that correct and specific results are obtained. Allelic dropout was assumed in cases where one or more replicates were homozygous while the other replicates were heterozygous or homozygous for another allele. An estimate of the probability of a false homozygote after (n) replicates was calculated according to [46]: P (false homozygote) = K x (K/2)$^{n-1}$, where K is the observed number of allelic dropouts divided by all heterozygous individuals. Allele frequencies were calculated by hand. Chi 2 test and Fisher's exact test as implemented in STATISTICA 9 were used to test for differentiation in allele frequencies between period II and III. Detailed descriptions information of each element is provided in the supporting information (Figures S1, S2, S3).

Results

DNA was successfully extracted from 104 of the 133 metapodia chosen for analysis, based on a minimum of 4 typings for females and 2 typings for males. However, 4 samples yielded insufficient data for a conclusive result. We were unable to extract DNA from 28 of the bones. The success rate was 78.9 % (Table 1). Allelic dropout was 0.33, providing significance with 4 observations for a female (p false homozygote = 0.001476). No bias was detected in which of the two alleles that was lost in male samples with allelic dropout. The osteological sex identification was confirmed by the molecular result in all cases.

The size distribution confirms that female animals dominate the Eketorp assemblage in both phase II and III. The distal breadth of the epiphysis of the metacarpal and metatarsal bone shows a good separation of the sexes with a small overlap around 53 mm for Mc and around 51 mm for Mt (Figure 3). Mean values and standard deviations of the distal breadth on successfully sexed metapodials confirm a minor overlap (Table 2). DNA analysis of young animals indicate that, more males were slaughtered at young age in period II compared to period III, however the differences is not significant, p = 0.09 (Chi2) (Table 1).

Table 1. Results of molecular sexing.

Adults	Phase	Female	Male	no result
Metacarpals	II	3	3	2
	III	11	14	10
	II/III			1
Total		**14**	**17**	**13**
Metatarsals	II	6	11	4
	III	16	15	4
	II/III	2	1	2
Total		**24**	**27**	**10**
Subadult metatarsals				
	II	2	7	3
	III	8	5	3
Total		**10**	**12**	**6**

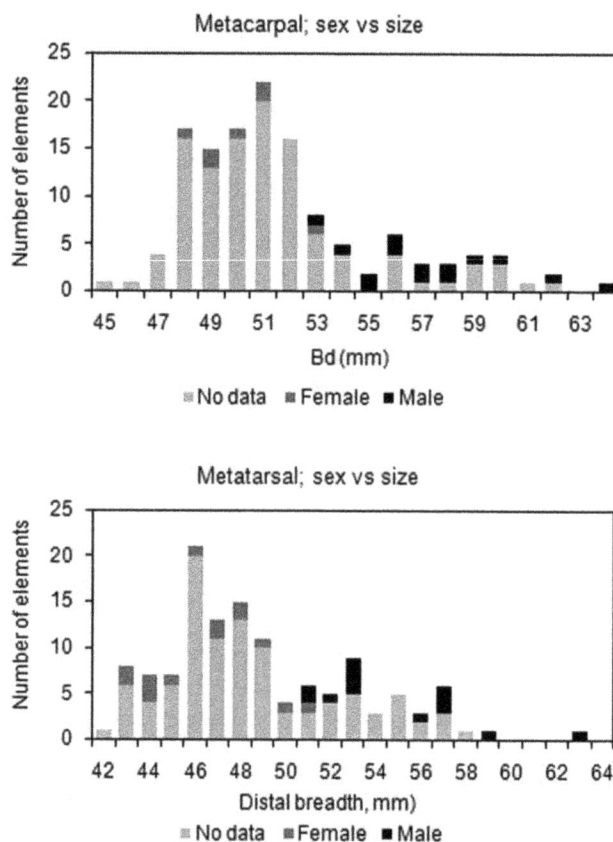

Figure 3. Histograms showing the size of cattle metatarsals and metatarsals according to the breadth of the distal epiphysis (Bd). Sex according to molecular analyses. Included are all available measurements.

The number of different fully grown elements identified was 135 metatarsals and 151 metacarpals. Twenty-three of the metatarsals elements exhibited pathological lesions of an unspecific aetiology while 13 elements (9.6%) exhibited draught related lesions. For metacarpals the corresponding frequencies were 20 unspecific and 8 (5.3%) draught related lesions. There is a slight difference in frequency of draught lesions between Mc and Mt in period II while the frequencies are more even in period III, the observations are too few for a more detailed interpretation, Table 3. The lesions associated to draught use were found mainly on metapodia from male animals while the other types of lesions are found on bones mainly coming from female animals (Figure 4). Noteworthy in

Table 2. Results of the mean value and standard deviation (s.d.) of the distal epiphysis (Bd) in molecular sexed metapodials from Eketorp ringfort, Öland in Sweden.

		Female			Male		
Adults	Phase	n	mean	s.d.	n	mean	s.d.
Metacarpals	II	2	52.61	1.52	3	57.53	1.27
	III	5	49.72	1.19	11	58.58	3.31
Metatarsals	II	2	45.28	2.79	4	57.06	2.50
	III	10	46.67	2.48	8	54.81	4.25

Table 3. Frequency of pathological lesions on cattle metapodia at Eketorp in phase II and III studied by molecular analyses.

Element	Phase	Female		Male		No result	
		Unspecificpat.	Workload related	Unspecific pat.	Workload related	Unspecificpat.	Workload related
Metacarpals	II	2		1	1	4	3
	III	10		4	4		
Metatarsals	II	3		3	5	1	
	III	8	1	7	3		2
	II/III	1		1			1

Phase III is that three metatarsals exhibiting workload related pathologies apparently come from female cattle on the basis of their distal breath measurement. Molecular sexing was inconclusive for two of the elements while the third one was not analysed (Figure S3).

Thirty-three male metapodia were successfully typed for the *UTY19* SNP, all but two have the Y2 defining allele (A). One sub adult from period II and one adult from period III belong to haplogroup Y1(C). The metapodia of the Y2 males exhibit a marked size variation (Figure 5). Only a limited number of animals were genotyped for the coat colour SNP *MC1R* (n = 34), but the result is interesting; no animals indicated the C/C genotype consistent with dominant black coat colour. Instead all animals

were either heterozygous (which also results in black pigmentation) or homozygous for the wild type allele, which suggests that the Eketorp cattle mainly were of red or light coat coloration. The *MC1R* results did not yield any significant difference between the two periods, possibly due to limited sample size, or because there was no difference in the coat coloration. When 85 animals were genotyped for the 2021C>T *TLR4* SNP putatively involved in resistance to cattle plague, no significant change in allele frequency over time p = 0.08 was found (Fishers exact two-tailed). The ancestral G allele (G is due to reverse sequencing of the SNP), linked to possible resistance to cattle plague that increases from 0.605 in period II to 0.769 in period III. Finally, 18 animals were typed for a C/T mutation in *IGF-1*, five from Eketorp II and 13 from Eketorp III. The difference between the two periods is on the verge of significant (p = 0.0532) indicating an increase of allele C, from 0.4 to 0.77, in phase III, but it should be noted that the sample set is relatively small. No obvious morphological trait could be assigned to the variation in *IGF-1*. However it should be noted that the frequency of the C allele in modern milk and meat breeds is 0.9 and 0.71 respectively, thus the allele frequency in Eketorp III is more similar to modern beef cattle. No size clusters correlated to *IGF-1* genotype are visible, since all genotyped animals fell within the same size range as the other animals (Figure 6).

Discussion

Our results confirm that the skeletal assemblage of cattle at Eketorp mainly consists of bones from female animals. The predominance of cows is by no means unusual as cows provided both milk and calves for breeding purposes. The need for bulls was not as great and only a handful was most likely enough in order to cover the need for breeding. The use of cattle was not restricted to dairying or meat procurement. At Eketorp the metapodia of males and females exhibit a different pattern of pathological lesions. Females exhibit a dominance of lesions with an unspecific etiology while males also exhibited lesions that may be associated to draught use.

Boessneck [15] observed that calves at Eketorp exhibited a seasonal pattern of slaughter (Figure 7). Phase II exhibits a roughly similar frequency of calves slaughtered in their first or second autumn while phase III shows a clear dominance of calves slaughtered in their first autumn (*ibid.*). The comparison is to some extent affected by the inclusion of both anterior and posterior elements, which may exhibit a slightly different growth pattern. This however is of no major consequence for the comparison. Furthermore, female and male cattle exhibit a different growth pattern. We show that the majority of the sub adult cattle were males, which is in accordance with the (opposite) sex distribution of the adults (Figure 8).

The difference in kill-off patterns between phases II and III is related to an increased reliance on meat, which is in line with the

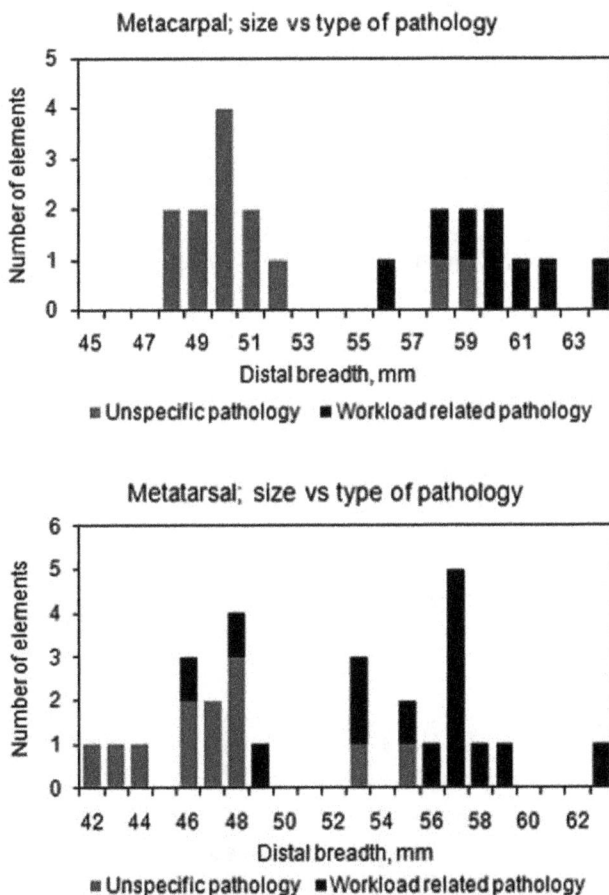

Figure 4. Histograms showing the size variation of metapodia with unspecific or workload related pathological lesions.

Metatarsal; size vs pathology and UTY19

Number of elements / Distal breadth, mm

■ Pathology ▨ Male Y2 pathology ▨ Male Y2 no pathology

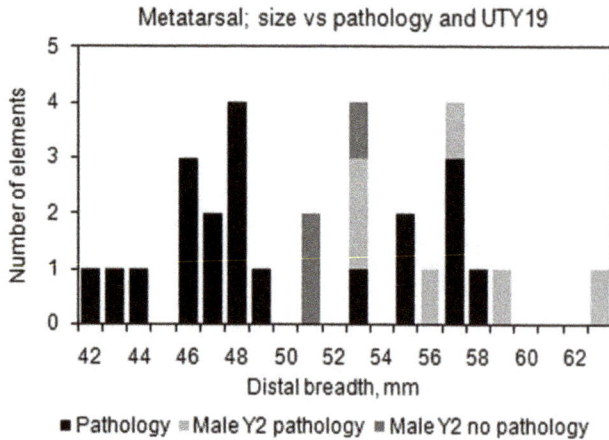

Figure 5. Histogram showing size variation and pathological lesions for males correlated with Y haplogroup.

Length of unfused first phalanx

Number of elements / GLoE, mm

◆ Phase II ■ Phase III

Figure 7. Line graph showing the size variation of unfused first phalanx at Eketorp, phases II and III. The GloE24-30 mm represent calves aged between 6–8 month and GloE 38–43 mm represents calves between 1 ½–1 ¾ years of age. Data are found in Boessneck (et al. 1979:tab 21).

change of the ringfort from a farming settlement to a fortified complex. However, the kill off pattern in phase III was not an ideal one towards husbandry practices focusing on milk production. Instead it indicates a specialization for meat production to the ringfort. The culling of many female calves is not commonly observed and, in fact, this may have led to a depletion of the cattle stock around Eketorp. Linked to this may have been the need to use females for draught purposes during phase III. Earlier studies [15,16] show that castration was most probably conducted on some male animals at Eketorp and thus a link between castration and draught use may be assumed. Systematic breeding of draught cattle is known in written sources in Sweden since the 16th Century when it became a profitable trade, especially in Southern Sweden when farming expanded [47]. We have no indications that the castrated males have been of a selected breed or specific type of animal. Bulls may have been chosen from a common pool of

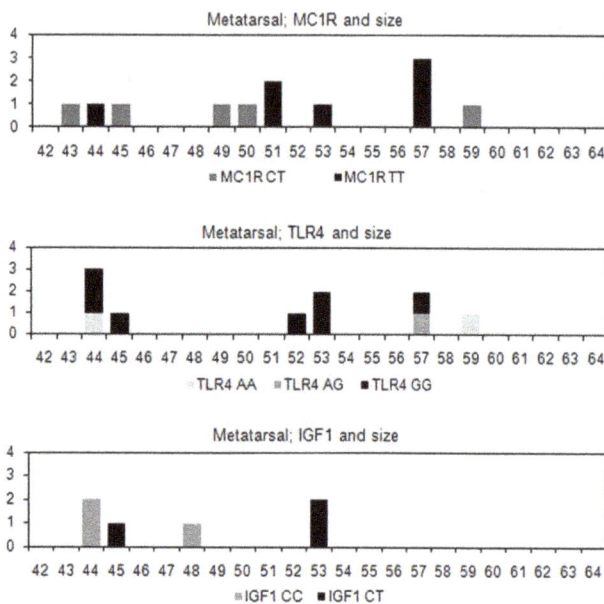

animals. All studied castrates belonged to haplogroup Y2, but note that we only observed two cases of Y1 among all males analysed.

The increase in body size observed by Boessneck et al. [15] might imply an introduction of a different type of livestock during phase III. However, we found no support for the use of different types of animals for specific purposes. The genetic data indicate that the cattle population at Eketorp was homogeneous both within each phase and between phase II and III, the latter also indicates that the population of cattle on Öland wasn't subjected to any major genetic changes for at least 400 years. There is no statistically significant difference in genetic data, but trends indicate possible differences. Taken together, the genetic result and the morphology suggest that there is a small but noticeable difference between the population from period II and that from period III. The resistance to cattle plague was possibly slightly higher in phase III. Only in less than one case out of ten would we expect to see the present difference *TLR4* by pure chance, the trend is even more obvious in *IGF-1*. If the trends are interpreted as true differences, then the animals were probably exposed to natural or artificial selection that is disease or breeding. However, given the time elapsed between the two periods and the relatively

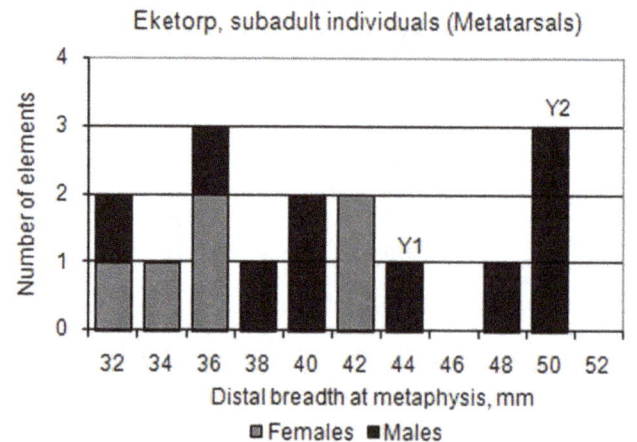

Metatarsal; MC1R and size

■ MC1R CT ■ MC1R TT

Metatarsal; TLR4 and size

▨ TLR4 AA ▨ TLR4 AG ■ TLR4 GG

Metatarsal; IGF1 and size

▨ IGF1 CC ■ IGF1 CT

Figure 6. Histograms showing the size variation of the genotyped animals (metatarsals) for the *MC1R*, *TLR4* and *IGF1* genes.

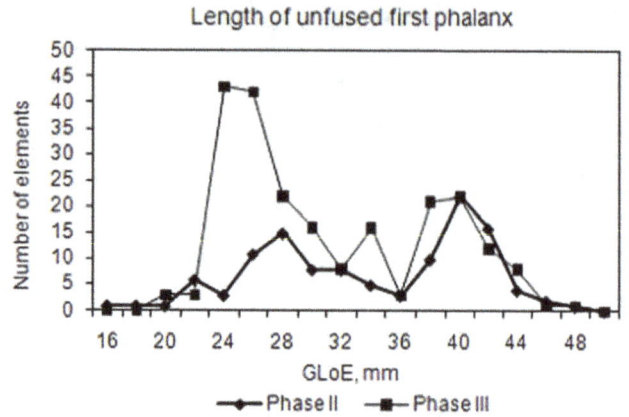

Eketorp, subadult individuals (Metatarsals)

Number of elements / Distal breadth at metaphysis, mm

▨ Females ■ Males

Figure 8. Histogram showing the size distribution of the sub adult metatarsals in phase III.

small sample set genetic drift could also explain the differences in allele frequencies.

Because of the relatively isolated location, the ringfort was probably dependent on local cattle. The military ringfort during phase III probably had to have some kind of organization to secure meat resources. But, it is unlikely that large numbers of cattle of different breeds were imported to Eketorp from other areas. However, it cannot be excluded that some animals or meat from animals that did not belong to the (local) breeding population were brought to the ringfort. Two of the male animals belong to a different Y-chromosomal haplogroup (Y1) than the majority of males, which similarly to other animals from early medieval northern Europe belong to haplogroup Y2 [48]. Although, this SNP is correlated with breeds in modern animals [35], we cannot claim that this is the case for the Eketorp cattle; since analysis of aDNA have shown temporal rather than geographical structure in historic populations [28]. It is therefore more appropriate to state that a minimum of two different male lineages were present at the site during both periods, one in majority and one very rare.

Summarizing our results, we uncovered trends that can be interpreted as a chronological shift, possibly towards a farming economy where cattle gained a new role. We also discovered patterns, compatible with early breeding and an increased level of specialisation in phase III, although these patterns were not obvious enough to be interpreted as undisputable evidence. We see a varied use of cattle at Eketorp and its surroundings, utilization strategies that require breeding efforts and conscious decisions on actions such as castration. In spite of this we have found little if any evidence of the use of genetically specific types of animals for specific purposes. The use of specific (genetic) breeds seems to be a later phenomenon. The usage of the bulk of the cattle seems to have been constant from period II to period III, indicating that the shift we describe was not a fast one.

Ethics statement

The animal bones used in this article are food debris from the excavated Eketorp ringfort on the Öland island in Sweden dated between 300–1200/50 A.D. The Museum of National Antiquities, Stockholm, Sweden, has permitted the analysis.

Supporting Information

Figure S1 Descriptive data on metatarsals including DNA results.

Figure S2 Descriptive data on metacarpals including DNA results.

Figure S3 Information on genotypic data, including number of successful genotypes for each SNP.

Figure S4 Primers and input data for the pyrosequencing software for PCR amplification and genotyping of IGF1, UTY19 and ZFX/Y.

Acknowledgments

We will thank the anonymous referees for their helpful comments.

Author Contributions

Conceived and designed the experiments: YT ES AG JS. Performed the experiments: YT . Analyzed the data: YT AG JS. Contributed reagents/materials/analysis tools: YT AG JS. Wrote the paper: YT ES AG JS. Performed the DNA analysis: ES.

References

1. Albarella U, Johnstone C, Vickers K (2008) The development of animal husbandry from the Late Iron Age to the end of the Roman period: a case study from South-East Britain. Journal of Archaeological Science 35; 1828–1848.
2. Pellecchia M, Negrini R, Colli L, Patrini M, Milanesi E, et al. (2007) The mystery of Etruscan origins: novel clues from Bos taurus mitochondrial DNA. Proceedings of the Royal Society B: Biological Sciences. 274: 1175.
3. Kantanen J, Olsaker I, LE Holm (2000) Genetic diversity and population structure of 20 North European cattle breeds. Journal of Heredity 91: 446.
4. Cserhalmi N (1998) Fårad mark: handbok för tolkning av historiska kartor och landskap: Sveriges hembygdsförb. 175 p.
5. Myrdal J (1985) Medeltidens åkerbruk: agrarteknik i Sverige ca 1000 till 1520 Nordiska museet. 294 p.
6. Sweeney D, Bailey M (1995) Agriculture in the middle ages: technology, practice, and representation. University of Pennsylvania Press.
7. Pedersen, EA, Widgren M (1998) Fähusdrift, järn och fasta åkrar. In: Welinder S, Pedersen EA, Widgren M, eds. Det svenska jordbrukets historia, Jordbrukets första femtusen år., Natur och Borås: Borås. pp 239–266.
8. Borg K (2000) Eketorp-III: Ett medeltidsarkeologiskt projekt: University of Lund, Institute of Archaeology. 188 p.
9. Borg K, Näsman U, Wegraeus E (1976) Eketorp: Fortification and Settlement on Öland, Sweden. The Setting. 127 p.
10. Näsman U (1976) Introduction to the Descriptions of Eketorp-I,-II &-III. In: Borg K, Näsman U, Wegreaus E, eds. Eketorp. Fortification and Settlement on Oland/Sweden The Monument. 215 p.
11. Zimmermann W (1988) Why was cattle-stalling introduced in prehistory? The significance of byre and stable and of outwintering, In: Fabech C, Ringtved J, eds. Settlement and landscape proceedings of a conference in Århus, Denmark, May 4-7, 1988 Jutland Archaeological Society.
12. Årlin C (1999) Under samma tak- Om "husstallets" uppkomst och betydelse under bronsåldern ur ett sydskandinaviskt perspektiv. In: Olausson, M, eds. Spiralens öga: tjugo artiklar kring aktuell bronsåldersforskning. pp 291–307.
13. Herschend F (2009) The Early Iron Age in South Scandinavia: Social Order in Settlement and Landscape. Uppsala: Institutionen för arkeologi och antik historia, Uppsala universitet. 449 p.
14. Näsman U (1981) Borgens Ö. Skal. 1: 19–27.
15. Boessneck J (1979) Eketorp: Befestigung und Siedlung auf Öland/Schweden; Die Fauna. Almqvist & Wiksell. 504 p.
16. Telldahl Y (2005) Can palaeopathology be used as evidence for draught animals, in: Diet and health in past animal populations. Oxford: Oxbow Books. pp 63–67.
17. Benecke N (1994) Archäozoologische Studien zur Entwicklung der Haustierhaltung: in Mitteleuropa und Südskandinavien von den Anfängen bis zum ausgehenden Mittelalter. Berlin.
18. Albarella U (1999) The animal economy of rural settlements: a zooarchaeological case study from Northamptonshire. Medieval Settlement Research Group Annual Report, 9: 16–17.
19. Schlumbaum A, Stopp B, Breuer G, Rehazek A, Blatter R, al et (2003) Combining archaeozoology and molecular genetics: the reason behind the changes in cattle size between 150BC and 700AD in Northern Switzerland. Antiquity 77: 298.
20. Schlumbaum A, Turgay M, Schibler J (2006) Near East mtDNA haplotype variants in Roman cattle from Augusta Raurica, Switzerland, and in the Swiss Evolene breed. Animal Genetics 37: 373–375.
21. Svensson E, Anderung C, Baubliene J, Persson P, Malmström H, et al. (2007) Tracing genetic change over time using nuclear SNPs in ancient and modern cattle. Animal Genetics 38: 378–383.
22. Wiener P, Burton D, Williams J (2004) Breed relationships and definition in British cattle: a genetic analysis. Heredity 93: 597–602.
23. McKay S, Schnabel RD, Murdoch BM, Matukumalli LK, Aerts J, et al. (2008) An assessment of population structure in eight breeds of cattle using a whole genome SNP panel. Bmc Genetics 9: 37.
24. Silver I (1969) The ageing of domestic animals. Science in archaeology 26: 283–302.
25. Habermehl KH (1961) Die Altersbestimmung bei Haustieren, Pelztieren und beim jagdbaren Wild Paul Parey.
26. Schmid E (1972) Atlas of animal bones: For prehistorians, archaeologists and Quaternary geologists. Knochenatlas. Für Prähistoriker, Archäologen und Quartärgeologen Elsevier Science Ltd. 159 p.
27. Von Den Driesch A (1976) A guide to the measurement of animal bones from archaeological sites. Cambridge MA. 101 p.
28. Svensson E, Götherström A, Vretemark M (2008) A DNA test for sex identification in cattle confirms osteometric results. Journal of Archaeological Science 35: 942–946.
29. Mennerich G (1968) Römerzeitliche Tierknochen aus drei Fundorten des Niederrheingebiets Universität Munchen. 176 p.

30. Roberts C, Manchester K (1997) The Archaeology of Disease. 243 p.
31. Hoerr NL, Osol A (1956) Blakiston's new Gould medical dictionary. McGraw-Hill. 1528 p.
32. Axelsson M (2000) Bone spavin. Clinical and epidemiological aspects of degenerative joint disease in the distal tarsus in Icelandic horses .Acta Universitatis Agriculturae Sueciae. Veterinaria (Sweden).
33. Bartosiewicz L, Van Neer W, Lentacker A (1997) Draught cattle: their osteological identification and history. Annales-Musee Royal de l'Afrique Centrale Sciences Zoologiques (Belgium). 147 p.
34. Cupere BDe, Lentacker A, Neer WVan, Waelkens M, et al. (2000) Osteological evidence for the draught exploitation of cattle: first applications of a new methodology. International Journal of Osteoarchaeology 10: 254–267.
35. Götherström A, Anderung C, Hellborg L, Elburg R, Smith C, al et (2005) Cattle domestication in the Near East was followed by hybridization with aurochs bulls in Europe. Proceedings of the Royal Society B: Biological Sciences 272: 2345.
36. Klungland H, Vage DI, Gomez-Raya L, Adalsteinsson S, Lien S (1995) The role of melanocyte-stimulating hormone (MSH) receptor in bovine coat color determination. Mammalian Genome 6: 636–639.
37. White S, Kata S, Womack J (2003) Comparative fine maps of bovine toll-like receptor 4 and toll-like receptor 2 regions. Mammalian Genome 14: 149–155.
38. Lien S, Karlsen A, Klemetsdal G, Våge DI, Olsaker, et al (2000) A primary screen of the bovine genome for quantitative trait loci affecting twinning rate. Mammalian Genome 11: 877–882.
39. Beg M, Bergfelt DR, Kot K, Ginther OJ (2002) Follicle selection in cattle: dynamics of follicular fluid factors during development of follicle dominance. Biology of reproduction 66: 120.
40. Ginther O, Bergfelt DR, Beg MA, Meira C, Kot K (2004) In vivo effects of an intrafollicular injection of insulin-like growth factor 1 on the mechanism of follicle deviation in heifers and mares. Biology of reproduction 70: 99.
41. Bunter K, Hermesch S, Luxgford BG, Graser HU, Crump RE (2005) Insulin-like growth factor-I measured in juvenile pigs is genetically correlated with economically important performance traits. Australian Journal of Experimental Agriculture 45: 783–792.
42. Davis M, Simmen R (2006) Genetic parameter estimates for serum insulin-like growth factor I concentrations, and body weight and weight gains in Angus beef cattle divergently selected for serum insulin-like growth factor I concentration. Journal of animal science 84: 2299.
43. Meuwissen T, Karlsen, A, Lien S, Olsaker, I, Goddard ME (2002) Fine mapping of a quantitative trait locus for twinning rate using combined linkage and linkage disequilibrium mapping. Genetics 161: 373.
44. Flori L, Fritz, S, Jaffrézic F, Boussaha M, Gut I, al et (2009) The genome response to artificial selection: a case study in dairy cattle. PLoS One 4: 6595.
45. Qanbari S, Pimentel ECG, Tetens J, Thaller G, Lichtner P, et al. (2009) A genome-wide scan for signatures of recent selection in Holstein cattle. Animal Genetics;doi:10.1111/j.1365-2052.2009.02016.x.
46. Gagneux P, C Boesch, Woodruff D (1997) Microsatellite scoring errors associated with noninvasive genotyping based on nuclear DNA amplified from shed hair. Molecular Ecology 6: 861–868.
47. Myrdal J (1999) Jordbruket under feodalismen 1000-1700. Natur och kultur/LTs förlag. 407 p.
48. Svensson E, Götherström A (2008) Temporal fluctuations of Y-chromosomal variation in Bos taurus. Biology Letter 4: 752–754.
49. Johannsen Nørkjær N (2006) Draught cattle and the South Scandinavian economies of the 4th millennium BC. Environmental archaeology 11: 35–48.

4

Choriodecidual Group B Streptococcal Inoculation Induces Fetal Lung Injury without Intra-Amniotic Infection and Preterm Labor in *Macaca nemestrina*

Kristina M. Adams Waldorf[1]*, Michael G. Gravett[1,2], Ryan M. McAdams[3], Louis J. Paolella[2], G. Michael Gough[4], David J. Carl[5], Aasthaa Bansal[6], H. Denny Liggitt[7], Raj P. Kapur[8], Frederick B. Reitz[9], Craig E. Rubens[2,10]

1 Department of Obstetrics & Gynecology, University of Washington, Seattle, Washington, United States of America, 2 Global Alliance to Prevent Prematurity & Stillbirth, Seattle, Washington, United States of America, 3 Department of Pediatrics, University of Washington, Seattle, Washington, United States of America, 4 Washington National Primate Research Center, Seattle, Washington, United States of America, 5 Ross University School of Medicine, Dominica, West Indies, 6 Department of Biostatistics, University of Washington, Seattle, Washington, United States of America, 7 Department of Comparative Medicine, University of Washington, Seattle, Washington, United States of America, 8 Department of Laboratories, Seattle Children's, Seattle, Washington, United States of America, 9 Center on Human Development and Disability, University of Washington, Seattle, Washington, United States of America, 10 Division of Infectious Disease, Seattle Children's, Seattle, Washington, United States of America

Abstract

Background: Early events leading to intrauterine infection and fetal lung injury remain poorly defined, but may hold the key to preventing neonatal and adult chronic lung disease. Our objective was to establish a nonhuman primate model of an early stage of chorioamnionitis in order to determine the time course and mechanisms of fetal lung injury *in utero*.

Methodology/Principal Findings: Ten chronically catheterized pregnant monkeys (*Macaca nemestrina*) at 118–125 days gestation (term = 172 days) received one of two treatments: 1) choriodecidual and intra-amniotic saline (n = 5), or 2) choriodecidual inoculation of Group B *Streptococcus* (GBS) 1×10^6 colony forming units (n = 5). Cesarean section was performed regardless of labor 4 days after GBS or 7 days after saline infusion to collect fetal and placental tissues. Only two GBS animals developed early labor with no cervical change in the remaining animals. Despite uterine quiescence in most cases, blinded review found histopathological evidence of fetal lung injury in four GBS animals characterized by intra-alveolar neutrophils and interstitial thickening, which was absent in controls. Significant elevations of cytokines in amniotic fluid (TNF-α, IL-8, IL-1β, IL-6) and fetal plasma (IL-8) were detected in GBS animals and correlated with lung injury ($p < 0.05$). Lung injury was not directly caused by GBS, because GBS was undetectable in amniotic fluid (~10 samples tested/animal), maternal and fetal blood by culture and polymerase chain reaction. In only two cases was GBS cultured from the inoculation site in low numbers. Chorioamnionitis occurred in two GBS animals with lung injury, but two others with lung injury had normal placental histology.

Conclusions/Significance: A transient choriodecidual infection can induce cytokine production, which is associated with fetal lung injury without overt infection of amniotic fluid, chorioamnionitis or preterm labor. Fetal lung injury may, thus, occur silently without symptoms and before the onset of the fetal systemic inflammatory response syndrome.

Editor: Markus M. Heimesaat, Charité, Campus Benjamin Franklin, Germany

Funding: This work was supported by the March of Dimes (21-FY06-77) and the National Institutes of Health (AI067910). The funders had no role in study design, data collection and analysis, decision to publish, or preparation of the manuscript.

Competing Interests: The authors have declared that no competing interests exist.

* E-mail: adamsk@u.washington.edu

Introduction

Preterm birth and the resulting neonatal morbidity and mortality represent a significant public health and economic burden to our society [1]. Intrauterine infection is present in most cases of the earliest preterm births and incites an inflammatory response believed to result in preterm labor and fetal lung injury [2]. Biological mechanisms initiating and propagating inflammation, preterm birth and fetal lung injury remain ill-defined and represent a major barrier to finding an effective treatment. The currently accepted paradigm is that bacteria ascend from the lower genital tract and sequentially colonize the choriodecidual space (external to the membranes and amniotic fluid) followed by trafficking into the amniotic fluid. Bacteria then induce cytokines, including interleukin-1β (IL-1β) and interleukin-8 (IL-8), which are thought to be a critical trigger of preterm labor and fetal lung injury predisposing the neonate to chronic lung disease [3,4,5].

Studying early events in microbial invasion of the amniotic cavity may help determine how a therapeutic might be best administered to successfully prevent preterm birth. An intramuscular or intravenous medication might be ideal to target choriodecidual bacteria and downregulate immune effectors. Recently, intra-amniotic infection has been suggested as an earlier step in the process, followed by secondary bacterial colonization of the fetal membranes (chorioamnion) resulting in chorioamnionitis [6]. If this scenario is more typical, then direct administration of a drug into the amniotic fluid via amniocentesis may be required. Both microbial and host factors, as well as inoculum size, are likely to play a role in whether bacterial colonization of the choriodecidual space results in intra-amniotic infection. In a pilot study in rhesus macaques, we have shown that Group B *Streptococcus* (GBS) inoculated into the choriodecidual space can traffic into the amniotic fluid, but required large and sometimes several inoculations [7]. The extent to which a small inoculum or transient infection might impact the mother or fetus' health is unknown, but may reflect the most common event leading to preterm birth in the setting of intrauterine inflammation [elevated amniotic interleukin-6 (IL-6)] and a negative amniotic fluid culture [8,9,10,11].

Controversy also exists as to whether inflammation in the fetal membranes (chorioamnionitis) is associated with the most common form of neonatal chronic lung disease, bronchopulmonary dysplasia (BPD) [12,13]. Although infection and inflammation can incite lung injury, the inflammatory response may also be protective by accelerating lung maturation and surfactant production. A recent meta-analysis of more than 15,000 subjects concluded that the pooled adjusted odds ratio for an association between BPD and chorioamnionitis was 1.58 (95% CI 1.1–2.2) [14]. Considerable study heterogeneity and publication bias, however, prevented the authors from concluding that chorioamnionitis was a definite risk factor for BPD. Understanding the relationship between inflammation and fetal lung injury has greater significance, because the prevalence of BPD is increasing, particularly in very immature infants who may have little or no

evidence of respiratory distress syndrome. This variant has been called "new BPD" and is thought to be triggered by inflammation and intrauterine cytokines, which arrest alveolarization and inhibit growth of pulmonary vasculature [15,16].

To investigate early factors involved in the initiation of intrauterine inflammation and fetal lung injury, we used a chronically catheterized pregnant nonhuman primate model (pigtail macaque; *Macaca nemestrina*). The nonhuman primate shares many important features with human pregnancy including uterine anatomy, singleton gestation, hemochorial placentation, and microbial communities within the vagina. We infused GBS, an organism known to cause preterm birth and neonatal invasive disease [17,18], into the choriodecidual space via a catheter placed between the uterine muscle and membranes (external to amniotic fluid) overlying the lower uterine segment. We performed Cesarean section in the first week after choriodecidual inoculation to study early events associated with intrauterine infection.

Results

Uterine Activity

The mean gestational age of inoculation was 136 days (range: 131–139 days) and delivery was 141 days from conception (range: 134–145 days) corresponding to approximately 80% of a typical *M. nemestrina* pregnancy in our colony delivering at 172 days. Prior to GBS or saline inoculation, the uterus was quiescent in all animals. Peak uterine activity after inoculation was not significantly different between GBS and saline groups, but two GBS animals developed labor based on the finding of cervical change associated with more intense contractions (Table 1). In one case, a building contraction pattern (4,000–5,000 mmHg•sec/hr) and cervical change prompted Cesarean section three days after GBS infusion. In the second animal, slow cervical change occurred in the setting of episodic contractions. No cervical change or

Table 1. Uterine Activity, Cytokines and Prostaglandins.

Measure	Post-inoculation Peak		p-value
	Saline (n = 5)	GBS (n = 5)	
Uterine activity (mmHg•sec/hr)	1,533.4 (880.6)	2,453.5 (2,362.5)[†]	0.70
	Amniotic Fluid (ng/ml)		
IL-1β	0.004 (0.006)	0.1 (0.2)	0.04*
TNF-α	0.02 (0.03)	0.6 (0.7)	0.01*
IL-6	9.9 (4.8)	72.6 (34.3)	0.003*
IL-8	1.3 (0.6)	13.0 (9.9)	0.001*
PGE₂	0.6 (0.8)	0.7 (0.7)	0.71
PGF₂α	0.6 (0.4)	1.2 (1.3)	0.48
Total MMP activity (pmol/min)	25.9 (5.3)	29.1 (11.6)	0.59
	Fetal Plasma (pg/ml)		
IL-1β	0.0 (0.0)[‡]	0.0 (0.0)	-
TNF-α	0.7 (1.2)[‡]	0.1 (0.2)	-
IL-6	1.8 (0.8)[‡]	4.9 (4.5)	0.06
IL-8	309.5 (186.3)[‡]	1,569.2 (1,081.2)	0.03*

Table presents the mean (SD). Values for amniotic fluid analyses are ng/ml or pmol/min (MMP activity) and for fetal analyses are pg/ml. P-values are based on ANOVA models fit on log-transformed data except total MMP activity, which did not require log transformation.
*p<0.05.
[†]N = 4 for uterine activity in GBS group due to technical issues and insufficient data collection in one case.
[‡]N = 3 for fetal plasma of saline controls.

evidence of labor occurred in the remaining three GBS animals or any saline controls.

Cultures and GBS PCR

Cultures of the amniotic fluid and fetal membranes, lungs, blood and cerebrospinal fluid were performed to correlate findings with bacterial trafficking (Table 2). Culture of the chorioamnion at the inoculation site revealed low-level GBS [100–1,000 colony forming units/milliliter (CFU)] in two cases; one animal had no evidence of labor and the second had slow cervical change with episodic contractions. The inoculation site was culture negative in the other GBS animal in labor. Cultures of the amniotic fluid (~10 samples tested/animal) and fetal tissues were negative in all animals, with the exception of suspected contaminants in a few cases (e.g. *Streptococcus viridans*). To determine whether low levels of GBS might be present in the amniotic fluid that was not detected by culture, quantitative real-time PCR was performed on serially sampled amniotic fluid at three points in the course of the experiment including the day prior to inoculation, day of Cesarean section and once during the course of the experiment. All amniotic fluid samples were negative with the lower limit of assay detection being 10 copies per PCR reaction.

Fetal Lung Injury

A representative fetal lung section from a GBS and saline control animal is shown in Figure 1. Fetal lung histology was scored on a scale of 0 (normal) to 4 (severe injury) by a board certified veterinary pathologist (H.D.L.) blinded to group assignment as previously reported [19]. There was evidence of fetal lung injury in four of the five GBS animals (lung scores = 2, 3, 3, and 4), as well as one control (lung score = 2). Fetal lung injury varied in severity and distribution. Injury was defined as an aggregate of histologic changes including accumulation of inflammatory cells, evidence of necrosis, inflammatory related tissue thickening, collapse or other injury such as fibrin exudation or hemorrhage. The distribution of injury varied with severity but involved vascular and perivascular compartments as well as airway and alveolar compartments. In one control, fetal lung injury was an infarction of a lung tip and appeared histologically

very different from controls and GBS lungs. In this case, hemorrhage was the predominant finding and thought to have occurred peri-mortem.

Inflammatory cells observed in the fetal lungs from GBS group included high numbers of neutrophils and macrophages, which is consistent with the pattern described in preterm infants at different stages of developing BPD [20]. In addition, there was increased staining density and thickened septa that was absent in saline controls. The most severe cases of fetal lung injury (fetal lung scores = 3, 3, and 4) correlated with the highest levels of amniotic fluid and fetal IL-8, but not other cytokines or prostaglandins tested (Table 1).

Cytokines, Prostaglandins, and MMP

Temporal relationships between uterine activity, amniotic fluid cytokines and prostaglandins are depicted in one animal after GBS inoculation with moderate fetal lung injury and minimal uterine activity and a representative saline control (Figure 2). Saline infusion in either the choriodecidual space or the amniotic fluid of controls was not associated with an elevation in amniotic fluid cytokines. Following GBS choriodecidual infusion, amniotic fluid IL-1β, IL-8, IL-6 and TNF-α increased significantly compared to controls (Table 1; all p<0.05). GBS inoculation was not associated with a significant change in amniotic fluid prostaglandins or total matrix metalloproteinase activity during this four day experiment.

In two controls, fetal samples for cytokine analysis were not obtained due to either an inability to place the fetal catheter or clotting of the catheter. Fetal plasma IL-8 was significantly higher in GBS animals versus controls and correlated best with fetal lung injury of the fetal cytokines measured (p = 0.03). The GBS animal with the greatest degree of fetal lung injury (lung score = 4) also developed preterm labor and had a fetal IL-6 level of 11.3 pg/ml, which is diagnostic of the fetal systemic inflammatory response syndrome (FIRS) in humans [21]. In the other three GBS animals with fetal lung injury, the fetal IL-6 level (2.6, 3.1, 7.5 pg/ml) was below the threshold for FIRS. Fetal plasma IL-1β was undetectable in all but one animal and fetal plasma TNF-α was undetectable in all but two animals.

Table 2. Amniotic Fluid and Fetal Cultures.

Group	AF	Membrane		Fetal Meninges	Fetal Lung	Fetal CSF	Fetal blood
		Inoculation site	Fundus				
Saline 1	None	None	None	None	None	None	None
Saline 2	None*	None	None	None	None	None	None
Saline 3	None	None	None	None	None	None	None
Saline 4	None*	None	None	None	None	None	None
Saline 5	None	None	None	None	None	None	None
GBS 1	None*	None	None	None	None	None	None
GBS 2	None	None	None	None	None	None	None
GBS 3	None	None	None	None	None	None	None
GBS 4	None	1,000 GBS, <100 *S. aureus*	None	None	None	None	None
GBS 5	None	100 GBS	None	None*	None*	None	None

Above values represent CFU/ml.
*A suspected contaminant (coagulase negative *Staphylococcus*, *S. viridians*) was noted in one AF culture of two saline controls and one GBS animal with all subsequent cultures being negative. Multiple suspected contaminants were noted in fetal tissue cultures from GBS #5 collected at the time of necropsy by an ill pathologist, who was coughing and wearing a mask (e.g. *Streptococcus gordonii*, *Neisseria* species).
AF, amniotic fluid; CSF, cerebrospinal fluid.

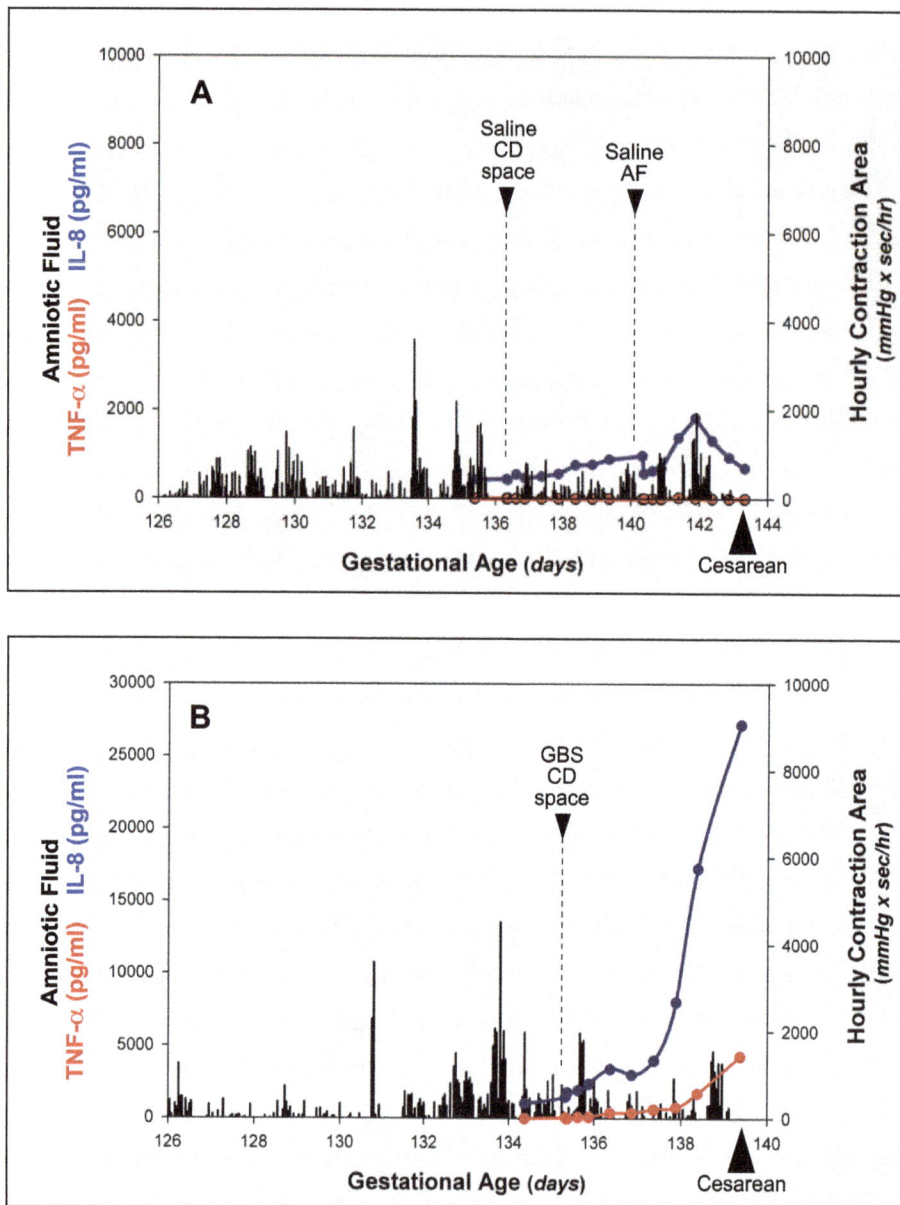

Figure 1. Histopathology of the fetal lungs. Hematoxylin and eosin stained histologic sections of fetal lung are shown for a saline control (A; lung score = 0) and GBS animal with severe fetal lung injury (B; lung score = 4).

Placental Histopathology

Histopathology of the chorioamnion was reviewed by a pathologist (R.P.K.) blinded to group assignment. Representative tissues are shown in Figure 3 and results correlated with fetal lung score and labor in Table 3. Chorioamnionitis was diagnosed in two GBS animals with evidence of fetal lung injury (lung scores = 4 and 2); only one of these animals was in labor. Funisitis (inflammation of the umbilical cord) also occurred in one case, which correlated with the lung score of four. As previously noted, GBS was not detected in the amniotic fluid by either culture or PCR. Normal placental histology was noted in all controls and the remaining three GBS animals, two of which had signs of moderate fetal lung injury (lung score = 3 in both cases). In one GBS animal with fetal lung injury and a final diagnosis of normal histology, there were very rare scattered degenerating neutrophils within the

membranes; this finding was subtle and not sufficient for making the diagnosis of chorioamnionitis.

Discussion

Our study objective was to determine early biological events in choriodecidual infection and temporal relationships between bacterial trafficking, chorioamnionitis and fetal lung injury. We, therefore, performed Cesarean section a few days after initial inoculation and in the absence of labor in all but two cases. Despite relative uterine quiescence and minimal numbers of GBS organisms cultured from membranes at the inoculation site, significant fetal lung injury was detected in four of five animals just four days after choriodecidual inoculation. The lung injury could not be attributed to live bacteria, because amniotic fluid cultures

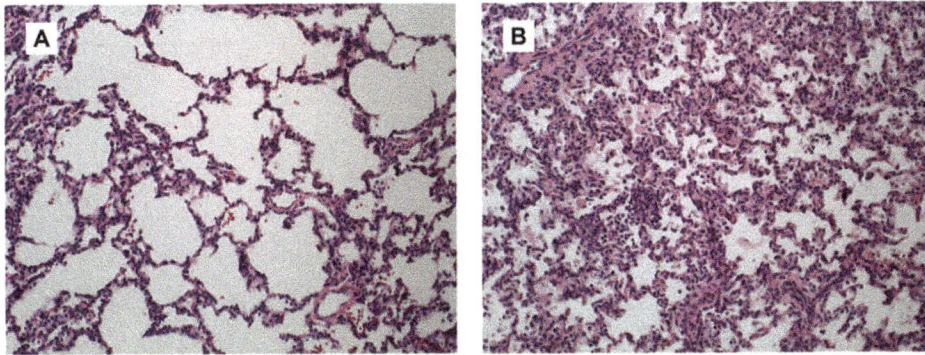

Figure 2. Uterine activity and amniotic fluid cytokines. Temporal relationships among inoculation of GBS or saline, uterine activity, and amniotic fluid (AF) cytokines (TNF-α, IL-8) are shown in a representative animal after saline inoculation (A) and in an animal after GBS inoculation (B), which developed moderate lung injury in the setting of minimal uterine activity. The x-axis represents gestational age in days ranging from the vascular implantation surgery until cesarean section. The y-axis is hourly contraction area (HCA; gray bars), or the level of amniotic fluid TNF-α (red line) or IL-8 (blue line). CD, choriodecidual; AF, amniotic fluid.

and PCR were negative in all animals. This suggests that fetal lung injury may occur silently, predisposing the neonate to bronchopulmonary dysplasia, without presenting any warning signs to the obstetrician until the relatively late development of preterm labor.

Elevation of amniotic fluid cytokines in GBS animals of our study is consistent with the hypothesis of others that aspiration of inflammatory mediators from the amniotic fluid is a key factor contributing to the fetal lung injury leading to BPD, the leading cause of chronic lung disease in infancy in the United States [5,16,22,23,24]. Our study extends this work by revealing that fetal lung injury may occur without clinical signs or symptoms of preterm labor and no microbiologic or pathologic evidence of infection. This suggests that a placental or membrane immune response may clear a choriodecidual infection to allow the pregnancy to continue, but results in production of inflammatory mediators that induce fetal lung injury in a paracrine response (Figure 4). This may occur through diffusion of inflammatory mediators into the amniotic fluid and direct contact with fetal lungs or via diffusion into fetal blood at the maternal-fetal interface [25,26]. The mechanisms involved in the pathway linking antenatal inflammation and chorioamnionitis to fetal lung injury remain unclear.

How fetal lung injury is initially mediated has not been explored previously, because amniotic fluid and cord blood samples are generally collected at the time of preterm labor and delivery, which our study suggests may be quite late in the process. The

relatively low levels of fetal plasma cytokines in most GBS animals with fetal lung injury suggest that in the early stages, fetal lung injury may be more likely to occur through direct contact of the fetal lung with inflammatory mediators in the amniotic fluid. In one animal receiving two GBS inocula, an elevated fetal plasma IL-6 (11.3 pg/ml) meeting criteria for FIRS occurred; this level of fetal IL-6 has been reported to better predict BPD than inflammatory mediators in the amniotic fluid [27,28]. However, marked fetal lung injury was noted in three other GBS animals despite fetal IL-6 levels that were fairly low in two cases (2–3 pg/ml). In contrast, amniotic fluid peak IL-6 levels were relatively high in all animals with lung injury (range: 77.9–102.6 ng/ml). Whether an elevated amniotic fluid IL-6 or another inflammatory mediator initiates fetal lung injury is unknown, but this pattern of inflammation may be a biomarker for the early stages of fetal lung injury; interestingly, it also models the clinical condition in up to 25% of preterm labor cases with an elevated amniotic fluid IL-6 and a negative culture and/or PCR result [8,9,10,11]. This suggests that *in utero* fetal lung injury of some degree may be much more common than previously recognized.

The role of IL-8 as a biomarker or initiator of BPD is also unclear. IL-8 is a plausible candidate as a key trigger of injury, because it is a chemoattractant for neutrophils, which were the predominant leukocyte in affected fetal lungs. In our study, amniotic fluid and fetal plasma IL-8 was significantly elevated in the GBS group

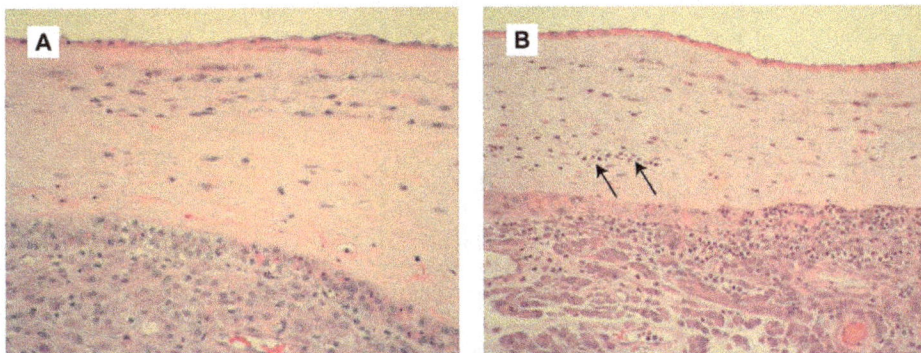

Figure 3. Histopathology of chorioamnion. Hematoxylin and eosin stained histologic sections of chorioamnion (fetal membranes) are shown for a saline control (A) and GBS animal with chorioamnionitis (B). Neutrophils in the chorion are indicated with arrows in panel B, as well as being abundant in the decidua.

Table 3. Fetal Lung Score, Cytokines and Chorioamnionitis in Each Animal.

Group	Fetal Lung Score	Peak AF		Peak Fetal Plasma		Inoculation Site Culture	Chorio-amnionitis	Labor
		IL-6 (ng/ml)	IL-8 (ng/ml)	IL-6 (pg/ml)	IL-8 (pg/ml)			
Saline 1	0	8.3	1.0	*	*	No growth	NO	NO
Saline 2	2	16.0	1.6	2.0	523.4	No growth	NO	NO
Saline 3	0	3.0	0.5	*	*	No growth	NO	NO
Saline 4	0	10.3	1.6	0.9	182.3	No growth	NO	NO
Saline 5	0	11.7	1.9	2.4	223.0	No growth	NO	NO
GBS 1	0	13.8	3.6	0	3,142.8	No growth	NO	NO
GBS 2	2	102.6	6.3	7.5	558.1	No growth	YES	YES
GBS 3	3	80.8	8.5	2.6	1,606.5	No growth	NO	NO
GBS 4	3	88.1	27.2	3.1	1,975.2	1,000 GBS	NO	NO
GBS 5	4	77.9	19.3	11.3	563.5	100 GBS	YES	YES

*In these two animals, fetal samples were not obtained.

compared to controls. Two of the four GBS animals had an amniotic fluid IL-8 greater than 10.7 ng/ml, which is a threshold previously associated with BPD (range: 6.3–27.2 ng/ml) [24]. In a prior study in rhesus macaques, we have shown that daily infusions of a single cytokine including IL-8 and others (IL-6, IL-1β, TNF-α) were associated with neutrophil infiltrates in the fetal lungs; IL-8 and IL-6 infusions were also associated with interstitial lymphocytic aggregates, but this may have been a function of a longer exposure duration [29]. In the preterm fetal sheep model, infusion of recombinant sheep IL-8 induced a fivefold increase in monocytes and neutrophils, but did not induce lung maturation associated with arrest of lung development and BPD [30]. Blockade of lipopoly-saccharide-induced IL-8 signaling (CXCR2 blocker) was also not effective in decreasing leukocytes in the bronchoalveolar lavage or cytokines in the fetal lung. These studies in sheep suggest that IL-8 may be more accurately described as a biomarker.

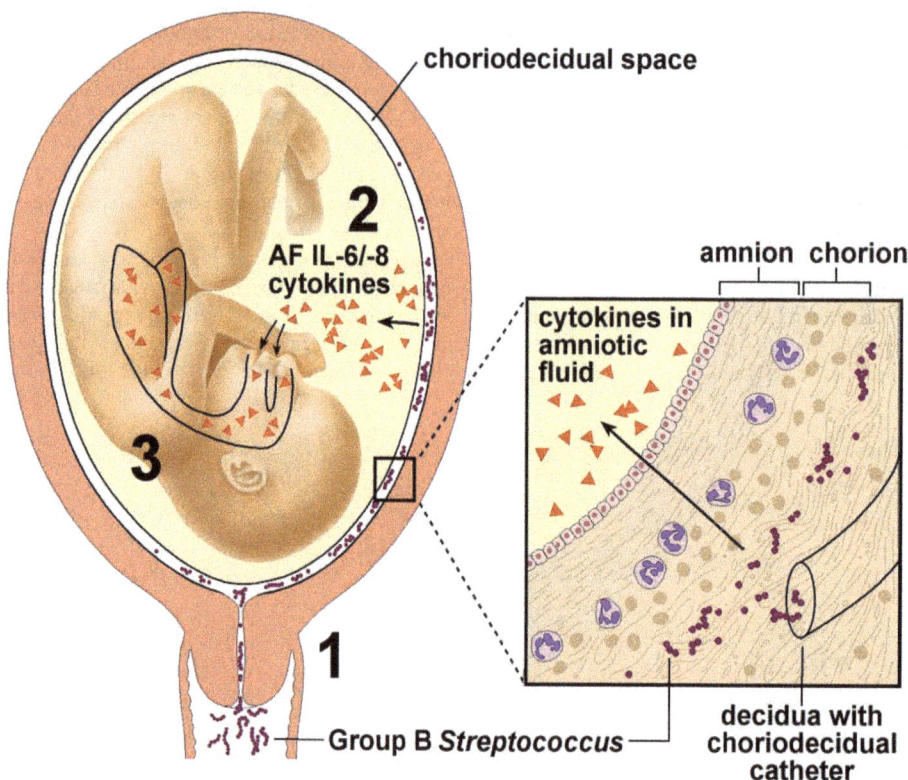

Figure 4. Our conceptual model. 1. Bacteria from the lower genital tract ascends into the choriodecidual space. 2. Inflammatory mediators (e.g. IL-8) produced by decidua and/or membranes diffuse into amniotic fluid and the fetal lung. 3. Fetal lung injury is induced by inflammatory mediators. IL, Interleukin; AF, amniotic fluid.

Matrix metalloproteinases have been linked to bronchopulmonary dysplasia and degradation of the fetal membrane extracellular matrix [31,32]. Increased activity of matrix metalloproteinase-9 (MMP-9) likely plays a role in fetal lung injury, because elevated cord blood MMP-9 has been correlated with bronchopulmonary dysplasia severity and oxygen supplementation [33]. We found no changes in total matrix metalloproteinase activity in the amniotic fluid, which is consistent with both *ex vivo* and *in vivo* data suggesting that increased matrix metalloproteinase activity is localized within the membranes and fetus [34,35]. In a pilot study of GBS choriodecidual infection in rhesus macaques, active MMP-9 only became elevated in the amniotic fluid of a single animal after a high dose GBS inoculum that resulted in preterm labor [36]. In early choriodecidual infection, local production and conversion to active enzyme within the fetal lungs may be a more likely mechanism of injury than direct exposure of the fetal lungs to matrix metalloproteinases in amniotic fluid.

The absence of chorioamnionitis in two cases with fetal lung injury sheds light on an important controversy surrounding whether chorioamnionitis is a risk factor for BPD [14,23,37,38,39]. Although early observational studies suggested an association, a subsequent cohort found no association [14]. Bronchopulmonary dysplasia began to be viewed as requiring "multiple hits", which included an antenatal inflammation component, as well as postnatal factors like oxidative stress, ventilator injury, and proteases [38]. Likewise, studies have reported chorioamnionitis to be associated with both increased production and depletion of surfactant [40]. These conflicting reports suggest that the degree and duration of inflammation may be important in determining the outcome on surfactant production and possibly the outcome of fetal lung injury. Our results suggest that a normal histologic appearance of the fetal membranes does not preclude the possibility of a transient choriodecidual infection that may have triggered fetal lung injury. As we ended these experiments after four days, it is unclear whether the fetal lung injury observed would progress or resolve with further time *in utero* [41,42]. Only survival studies with measurements of lung function after birth would address the question of whether this lung injury develops into a condition similar to human bronchopulmonary dysplasia with accelerated lung maturation, disordered structural development and impaired function.

Animal models have previously been used to model lung injury often by inducing end-stage disease. In the preterm fetal sheep model, the time course and major inflammatory effectors of endotoxin-induced fetal lung injury have been defined [41,43,44]. In contrast, this study focused on early events in lung injury, which may have significant relevance in investigation directed towards prevention. A major strength of this work is the use of an animal model with many similarities to both human pregnancy and fetal lung development. The nonhuman primate has a singleton fetus with a long gestational period (160–170 days), hemochorial placentation, and maternal-fetal inflammatory responses induced by infection and parturition, which mimic human pregnancy. Fetal lung injury in our model also occurs in the saccular stage of fetal lung development, which replicates the timing of human fetal lung injury leading to neonatal chronic lung disease. Other animal models (sheep, mice) are in a more advanced stage of lung development (alveolar) at the time of experimental injury, which may limit translation of results to human disease. Pulmonary morphologic and immune features in our model also emulate that in humans, but differ from many other species [45]. Both humans and nonhuman primates lack pulmonary intravascular macrophages present in the lungs of many species, making their lungs less susceptible to injury than other species (e.g. sheep, cattle, pigs).

One important study limitation is that microbial invasion of the amniotic cavity is likely a chronic process and the time course of infection depends on the organism and inoculum. Our results are more likely to reflect events associated with an immune response to a small or limited choriodecidual infection. A second limitation is that we terminated our experiments at 4 days; thus, we may have truncated a process leading to further fetal lung injury or maturation as the repair process begins. Third, the small sample size for fetal cytokine data in the saline group precluded confirming a possible association between fetal IL-8 and lung injury as suggested by our data and prior reports [5,23,46].

Mechanisms initiating and propagating fetal lung injury *in utero* are difficult to study after birth due to the many confounding clinical variables in the intensive care of preterm infants, such as the use of mechanical ventilation. Further studies at different time points may elucidate the natural course of fetal lung inflammation induced by choriodecidual bacteria and provide insight into how this response potentially contributes to neonatal lung injury. Additional soluble effectors associated with this process remain to be defined and could include previously implicated biomarkers of fetal lung injury including many chemokines (e.g. MCP-1, MIP-1β) [47], elastase [48], leukotriene B$_4$ [48], fibronectin [49], MMP-8 [12], MMP-9 [50,51], and complement C5a anaphylatoxin [52]. Overall, our model provides a unique opportunity to study the fetal origins of neonatal chronic lung disease induced by amniotic fluid inflammatory mediators, which can be triggered by many types of bacteria.

Materials and Methods

Ethics Statement

This study was carried out in strict accordance with the recommendations in the Guide for the Care and Use of Laboratory Animals of the National Research Council and the Weatherall report, "The use of non-human primates in research". The protocol was approved by the Institutional Animal Care Use Committee of the University of Washington (Permit Number: 4165-01). All surgery was performed under general anesthesia and all efforts were made to minimize suffering.

Animals and Study Groups

Ten chronically catheterized pregnant monkeys (*Macaca nemestrina*) at 118–125 days gestation (term = 172 days) received one of two experimental treatments: 1) choriodecidual and intra-amniotic saline infusions (n = 5), or 2) GBS choriodecidual inoculation (n = 5). Saline infusions were performed separately in the choriodecidual and amniotic fluid to confirm that saline would not stimulate cytokine production in either compartment. In two saline controls, fetal samples were not collected due to either an inability to place the fetal catheter during initial surgery or clotting of the fetal catheter. This resulted in three fetal cytokine analyses in the saline group. In one GBS case, technical problems led to only intermittent data collection and so the remaining uterine activity data was excluded for this animal.

In our model, pregnant pigtail macaques were time-mated and fetal age determined using early ultrasound. The tethered chronic catheter preparation was used for all *in vivo* experiments and is a major breakthrough in studying maternal-fetal immunologic responses [53,54]. The animal was first conditioned to a nylon jacket/tether system for several weeks before surgery, which allowed free movement within the cage, but protected the catheters. On day 118–125 of pregnancy (term = 172 days) catheters were implanted into the maternal femoral artery and vein, fetal internal jugular vein, amniotic cavity, and choriodecidual interface in the lower uterine segment (between uterine muscle and fetal membranes, external to amniotic fluid). Fetal

ECG electrodes and a maternal temperature probe were also implanted. After surgery, the catheters/electrodes were tracked through the tether system and cefazolin and terbutaline sulfate were administered to reduce postoperative infection risk and uterine activity. Both cefazolin and terbutaline were stopped at least 72 hours before experimental start (~5 half-lives for terbutaline, 40 half-lives for cefazolin, >97% of both drugs eliminated). Cefazolin 1 gram was administered intravenously each day in saline controls to minimize chances of a catheter-related infection. Experiments began approximately two weeks after catheterization surgery to allow recovery (~30–31 weeks human gestation). At our center, term gestation in the non-instrumented pigtail macaque population averages 172 days.

Uterine Activity, Labor and Delivery

Intraamniotic pressure, fetal heart rate and maternal temperature were continuously recorded and digitized with a Powerlab System (AD Instruments, Colorado Springs, CO) connected to an Intel computer. Amniotic fluid pressure signals were processed after delivery using custom software to eliminate noise due to respiration or position changes. The area under each contraction (mmHg•sec/hr) was summed for each hour allowing calculation of the hourly contraction area, which is a measure of uterine activity. Labor was defined as progressive uterine activity associated with cervical effacement and dilatation. In the GBS group, Cesarean section was performed when uterine activity exceeded a 12,000 hourly contraction area for more than two hours and/or cervical change indicated labor. Cervical exams were performed on all animals the day prior to inoculation and then daily in the GBS group or every other day in the saline group until Cesarean section. Cesarean section was performed in all animals in order to optimize the collection of intact gestational tissues. In order to study early events following a choriodecidual infection, a Cesarean section was planned 4 days after the GBS inoculation. In saline controls the Cesarean section was performed 7 days after initial inoculation; saline was inoculated twice (day 0 and day 4) in alternating order into the choriodecidual space and amniotic fluid. This protocol was chosen to determine if saline inoculation induced production of inflammatory mediators when inoculated into either the amniotic fluid or choriodecidual space; no significant elevation was detected. In one GBS animal with no cervical change during the experiment, technical difficulties resulted in insufficient collection of data for analysis of uterine activity.

Pathology and Lung Injury

After cesarean section, fetuses were euthanized by barbiturate overdose followed by exsanguination and fetal necropsy. Complete gross and histopathologic examination was performed on infants and placentas. The placenta was examined by a board-certified pediatric pathologist (R.P.K.) and fetal lungs examined by a board-certified veterinary pathologist (H.D.L.) with the each pathologist blinded to group assignment. Lung histologic sections were evaluated and scored, as previously described, using a semi-quantitative scale [19]. Components were scored on a scale of 0–4 (0 = normal) for inflammatory cells, necrosis, and inflammation including tissue thickening, collapse or other injury (e.g. fibrin exudation). Lung compartments scored were (1) vascular/perivascular; (2) bronchial/peribronchial; (3) alveolar wall; and (4) trichrome stain intensity positivity. Mononuclear inflammatory cells and neutrophils (Leder stain) within alveolar spaces were counted (5 random 40× fields). An overall severity score was generated.

GBS and Bacterial Cultures

The microbiologist preparing the GBS and performing the bacterial cultures participates in a laboratory quality assurance program through the College of American Pathologists (CAP) and is licensed through the American Society of Clinical Pathologists (ASCP) and the American Society of Microbiologists (ASM). We inoculated a clinical isolate of GBS (Type III, COH-1) using 1×10^6 of freshly grown mid-log phase bacteria inoculated into the choriodecidual space of the lower uterine segment. The COH-1 isolate was recovered from a neonate with meningitis and is highly virulent; it is the same strain used in prior experiments of intra-amniotic infection and pilot studies of choriodecidual GBS infection [7,53]. Single colonies of minimally-passaged GBS from blood agar plates were transferred to sterile Todd Hewitt Broth and grown overnight. The GBS inoculum was prepared to a concentration of 10^6 CFU/mL using the McFarland standard and a spectrophotometer. Bacterial concentration and purity was confirmed by colony counts on sheep blood agar with an average inoculum of 4.6×10^6 CFU (range: 3.5–6.3×10^6). In one GBS animal, the inoculum was inadvertently administered simultaneously with cefazolin. This GBS strain (COH-1) is rapidly killed by cefazolin, therefore the cefazolin was stopped. Three days later a second inoculum of GBS was given to the same animal.

Amniotic fluid was collected daily into anaerobic culture vials and equal volumes were sterilely inoculated in chopped-meat anaerobic broth as well as streaked for isolation on Brucella H/K and Chocolate agar plates. An additional volume was added to a glass microscope slide and allowed to air dry for Gram staining. Cultures grown anaerobically were placed within anaerobic culture jars and the anoxic environment was confirmed by aerobic indicators. Anaerobic plates were read after 5–7 days and chocolate plates grown under aerobic conditions were read after 72 hours. Any growth was subcultured and characterized according to established microbiological techniques.

Additional cultures were collected at the end of the experiment during Cesarean section and fetal necropsy. The maternal membrane fundus and inoculation site in the choriodecidual space were swabbed and placed in anaerobic culture tubes. Cerebral spinal fluid was aspirated in a sterile fashion and collected in anaerobic culture vials. Fetal lungs and meninges were sterilely swabbed and placed within anaerobic culture tubes. Fetal CSF and blood cultures were cultured as conducted with amniotic fluid. The above swab cultures were streaked for isolation on Brucella H/K and chocolate agar plates, and then placed in chopped meat broth for culture and grown according the procedure described above.

Quantitation of Amniotic Fluid Cytokines, Prostaglandins, and Matrix Metalloproteinases

Amniotic fluid and maternal and fetal blood were sampled frequently before (−24 and −1 hour) and after GBS inoculation (+1, +6, +12, +24 hours, and then daily until delivery). Amniotic fluid and blood samples were centrifuged for 5 minutes at 1200 RPM and the supernatant frozen and stored at −80°C. Prior to freezing, ethylene diamine tetraacetic acid (EDTA) (8.7 mM) and indomethacin (0.3 mM) was added to samples saved for cytokine and prostaglandin quantitation, respectively. Cytokine (IL-1β, IL-6, IL-8, and TNF-α) levels were determined by Luminex multiplex technology using commercially available non-human primate cytokine kits (Millipore, Billerica, MA). Quantities of PGE_2, and $PGF_{2\alpha}$ were determined using commercially available human ELISA EIA kits (Cayman Chemical, Ann Arbor, MI). Values were converted to pg/ml by comparison to a standard curve.

Analysis of matrix metalloproteinase activity was performed on amniotic fluid sampled and stored as described above using P126 (BioMol, Plymouth Meeting, PA), a MMP fluorogenic substrate [Mca-Pro-Leu-Gly-Leu-Dpa-Ala-Arg-NH₂·AcOH, Mca = (7-methoxycoumarin-4-yl)acetyl; Dpa = N-3-(2,4-dinitrophenyl)-L-α,β-diaminopropionyl]. Briefly, samples were diluted in activity buffer (500 mM HEPES, 100 mM CaCl$_2$, 0.05% w/v Brij-35, pH 7), pre-warmed to 37°C, and added to the fluorogenic substrate (10 µM). Quantification of the activity (pmol/min) was achieved using a standard curve generated with the cleaved fluorogenic product, P127 (BioMol, Plymouth Meeting, PA). Plate fluorescence (Ex.: 328 nm, Em.: 393 nm) was measured serially for four hours at 37°C and a standard curve generated of the cleaved fluorogenic product (P127; pmol/min). The units of total MMP activity are reported as pmol/min of cleaved product. Positive controls were run for each plate with either human recombinant MMP-9 or lysed fibroblasts.

Quantitative Real-Time PCR

All primers were designed using Primer 3 software (Whitehead Institute for Biomedical Research, NJ). A standard curve was prepared by amplifying $CPSH_{III}$ sequence specific to the GBS strain, COH1. First, genomic DNA was purified from 500 µL of overnight GBS culture in TSB using the Gentra Puregene Yeast/Bact. Kit (Qiagen, Valencia, CA). Primers, 5′-CTT TGG AAG AGT GAG TTA G-3′ and 5′-TGA CCA ATT AGT GTA GCA TA-3′, were used to generate a 389-bp product from the $CPSH_{III}$ sequence [55]. The PCR amplification was performed in 25 µL reactions using MyTaq (Bioline, Taunton, MA, USA). The PCR conditions were as follows: initial DNA denaturation at 95°C for 60 sec followed by 35 cycles of 95°C for 30 s, 52°C for 30 sec, and 72°C for 40 sec. Primer specificity and quality was confirmed by gel electrophoresis of 5 µL PCR product on 1.5% agarose gel, stained with 0.02 µg/mL ethidium bromide. The PCR product was purified using MinElute Reaction Cleanup Kit (Qiagen, Valencia, CA) and the concentration was determined by Nanodrop. Amplicon concentration (amp/µL) was determined using the molecular weight of amplified product calculated with sequence manipulation suite and the DNA concentration [56].

For quantitative real-time PCR, 500 µL of amniotic fluid was centrifuged at 15,000×g for 5 minutes. Supernatant was removed and the pellet resuspended in 40 µL of cell lysis buffer (20% sucrose, 10 mM MgCl, 10 mM Tris pH 7.0, 0.05% Triton X-100, 0.5 units/µL mutanolysin). Cells were lysed at 37°C for 2-3 hours.

Quantitative real-time PCR was conducted in 25 µL reactions consisting of 5 µL of above cell lysate, respective standard, or PCR-grade water (Ambion, Austin, TX); 0.25 µM primers: 5′-CAG TTG TAA GGA ATG TGG TAA AGG-3′ and 5′-AAA GTT GGC TTC AGC ATA GG-3′; and 1× SensiMix SYBR and Fluoroscein qRT-PCR Kit Mix (Bioline, Taunton, MA). A 500 seq/µL standard and 1,000 CFU/µL were used as positive controls for unknowns. The reaction conditions were as follows: DNA was denatured at 95°C for 10 minutes followed by 40 cycles at 95°C for 15 seconds, 55°C for 15 seconds, and 72°C for 15 seconds. Specificity of primers was confirmed with melting curve of product and gel electrophoresis with 10 µL of reaction product on a 2% agarose gel.

Statistical Analysis

Study outcomes were quantities of uterine activity (mean 24-hour HCA), cytokines in amniotic fluid and fetal plasma (IL-1β, TNF-α, IL-6, IL-8), and amniotic fluid prostaglandins (PGE$_2$, PGF$_{2\alpha}$) and matrix metalloproteinases (total MMP activity). Data was transformed by natural logarithm prior to analysis with the exception of matrix metalloproteinase data. We used one-way analysis of variance (ANOVA) to assess differences between the control and GBS groups with respect to each outcome. IL-1β and TNF-α in fetal plasma could not be assessed due to a large number of 0 values. All statistical analyses were conducted using Intercooled STATA 8.2 for Windows 2000 (StatCorp, College Station, TX). Significance was considered at p<0.05.

Acknowledgments

The authors gratefully acknowledge the technical assistance of Jan Hamanishi and Jennifer Summers in preparing the figures and Dr. Marie-Térèse Little for manuscript editing.

Author Contributions

Conceived and designed the experiments: KAW MG CR. Performed the experiments: LP GG DC KAW. Analyzed the data: RM AB HL RK KAW. Contributed reagents/materials/analysis tools: FR. Wrote the paper: KAW.

References

1. (2006) Preterm Birth: Causes, Consequences, and Prevention; Behrman RE, Stith Butler A, eds. Washington, D.C.: The National Academies Press.
2. Goldenberg RL, Hauth JC, Andrews WW (2000) Intrauterine infection and preterm delivery. N Engl J Med 342: 1500–1507.
3. Romero R, Brody DT, Oyarzun E, Mazor M, Wu YK, et al. (1989) Infection and labor. III. Interleukin-1: a signal for the onset of parturition. Am J Obstet Gynecol 160: 1117–1123.
4. Romero R, Ceska M, Avila C, Mazor M, Behnke E, et al. (1991) Neutrophil attractant/activating peptide-1/interleukin-8 in term and preterm parturition. Am J Obstet Gynecol 165: 813–820.
5. Yoon BH, Romero R, Jun JK, Park KH, Park JD, et al. (1997) Amniotic fluid cytokines (interleukin-6, tumor necrosis factor-alpha, interleukin-1 beta, and interleukin-8) and the risk for the development of bronchopulmonary dysplasia. Am J Obstet Gynecol 177: 825–830.
6. Kim MJ, Romero R, Gervasi MT, Kim JS, Yoo W, et al. (2009) Widespread microbial invasion of the chorioamniotic membranes is a consequence and not a cause of intra-amniotic infection. Lab Invest 89: 924–936.
7. Grigsby PL, Novy MJ, Waldorf KM, Sadowsky DW, Gravett MG (2010) Choriodecidual inflammation: a harbinger of the preterm labor syndrome. Reprod Sci 17: 85–94.
8. Yoon BH, Romero R, Moon JB, Shim SS, Kim M, et al. (2001) Clinical significance of intra-amniotic inflammation in patients with preterm labor and intact membranes. Am J Obstet Gynecol 185: 1130–1136.
9. Shim SS, Romero R, Hong JS, Park CW, Jun JK, et al. (2004) Clinical significance of intra-amniotic inflammation in patients with preterm premature rupture of membranes. Am J Obstet Gynecol 191: 1339–1345.
10. Oh KJ, Yoon BH, Romero R, Park CW, Lee SM, et al. (2009) The frequency and clinical significance of intra-amniotic inflammation in twin pregnancies with preterm labor and intact membranes. Am J Obstet Gynecol 201: S166.
11. Maymon E, Romero R, Chaiworapongsa T, Berman S, Conoscenti G, et al. (2001) Amniotic fluid matrix metalloproteinase-8 in preterm labor with intact membranes. Am J Obstet Gynecol 185: 1149–1155.
12. Lee J, Oh KJ, Yang HJ, Park JS, Romero R, et al. (2009) The importance of intra-amniotic inflammation in the subsequent development of atypical chronic lung disease. J Matern Fetal Neonatal Med 22: 917–923.
13. Kramer BW, Kallapur S, Newnham J, Jobe AH (2009) Prenatal inflammation and lung development. Semin Fetal Neonatal Med 14: 2–7.
14. Hartling L, Liang Y, Lacaze-Masmonteil T (2011) Chorioamnionitis as a risk factor for bronchopulmonary dysplasia: a systematic review and meta-analysis. Arch Dis Child Fetal Neonatal Ed.
15. Speer CP (2003) Inflammation and bronchopulmonary dysplasia. Semin Neonatol 8: 29–38.
16. Jobe AH (2011) The new bronchopulmonary dysplasia. Curr Opin Pediatr 23: 167–172.
17. Anderson BL, Simhan HN, Simons KM, Wiesenfeld HC (2007) Untreated asymptomatic group B streptococcal bacteriuria early in pregnancy and chorioamnionitis at delivery. Am J Obstet Gynecol 196: 524 e521–525.
18. Hillier SL, Krohn MA, Kiviat NB, Watts DH, Eschenbach DA (1991) Microbiologic causes and neonatal outcomes associated with chorioamnion infection. Am J Obstet Gynecol 165: 955–961.
19. Morris AE, Liggitt HD, Hawn TR, Skerrett SJ (2009) Role of Toll-like receptor 5 in the innate immune response to acute P. aeruginosa pneumonia. Am J Physiol Lung Cell Mol Physiol 297: L1112–1119.
20. Speer CP (2006) Inflammation and bronchopulmonary dysplasia: a continuing story. Semin Fetal Neonatal Med 11: 354–362.
21. Romero R, Gomez R, Ghezzi F, Yoon BH, Mazor M, et al. (1998) A fetal systemic inflammatory response is followed by the spontaneous onset of preterm parturition. Am J Obstet Gynecol 179: 186–193.

22. Rojas MA, Gonzalez A, Bancalari E, Claure N, Poole C, et al. (1995) Changing trends in the epidemiology and pathogenesis of neonatal chronic lung disease. J Pediatr 126: 605–610.

23. Watterberg KL, Demers LM, Scott SM, Murphy S (1996) Chorioamnionitis and early lung inflammation in infants in whom bronchopulmonary dysplasia develops. Pediatrics 97: 210–215.

24. Ghezzi F, Gomez R, Romero R, Yoon BH, Edwin SS, et al. (1998) Elevated interleukin-8 concentrations in amniotic fluid of mothers whose neonates subsequently develop bronchopulmonary dysplasia. Eur J Obstet Gynecol Reprod Biol 78: 5–10.

25. Kent AS, Sullivan MH, Elder MG (1994) Transfer of cytokines through human fetal membranes. J Reprod Fertil 100: 81–84.

26. Zaga V, Estrada-Gutierrez G, Beltran-Montoya J, Maida-Claros R, Lopez-Vancell R, et al. (2004) Secretions of interleukin-1beta and tumor necrosis factor alpha by whole fetal membranes depend on initial interactions of amnion or choriodecidua with lipopolysaccharides or group B streptococci. Biol Reprod 71: 1296–1302.

27. Gomez R, Romero R, Ghezzi F, Yoon BH, Mazor M, et al. (1998) The fetal inflammatory response syndrome. Am J Obstet Gynecol 179: 194–202.

28. Yoon BH, Romero R, Kim KS, Park JS, Ki SH, et al. (1999) A systemic fetal inflammatory response and the development of bronchopulmonary dysplasia. Am J Obstet Gynecol 181: 773–779.

29. Sadowsky DW, Adams KM, Gravett MG, Witkin SS, Novy MJ (2006) Preterm labor is induced by intraamniotic infusions of interleukin-1beta and tumor necrosis factor-alpha but not by interleukin-6 or interleukin-8 in a nonhuman primate model. Am J Obstet Gynecol 195: 1578–1589.

30. Kallapur SG, Moss TJ, Auten RL, Jr., Nitsos I, Pillow JJ, et al. (2009) IL-8 signaling does not mediate intra-amniotic LPS-induced inflammation and maturation in preterm fetal lamb lung. Am J Physiol Lung Cell Mol Physiol 297: L512–519.

31. Davey A, McAuley DF, O'Kane CM (2011) Matrix metalloproteinases in acute lung injury: mediators of injury and drivers of repair. Eur Respir J 38: 959–970.

32. Vadillo-Ortega F, Estrada-Gutierrez G (2005) Role of matrix metalloproteinases in preterm labour. Bjog 112 Suppl 1: 19–22.

33. Fukunaga S, Ichiyama T, Maeba S, Okuda M, Nakata M, et al. (2009) MMP-9 and TIMP-1 in the cord blood of premature infants developing BPD. Pediatr Pulmonol 44: 267–272.

34. Gomez-Lopez N, Vadillo-Perez L, Hernandez-Carbajal A, Godines-Enriquez M, Olson DM, et al. (2011) Specific inflammatory microenvironments in the zones of the fetal membranes at term delivery. Am J Obstet Gynecol 205: 235 e215–224.

35. Zaga-Clavellina V, Garcia-Lopez G, Flores-Pliego A, Merchant-Larios H, Vadillo-Ortega F (2011) In vitro secretion and activity profiles of matrix metalloproteinases, MMP-9 and MMP-2, in human term extra-placental membranes after exposure to Escherichia coli. Reprod Biol Endocrinol 9: 13.

36. Vadillo-Ortega F, Sadowsky DW, Haluska GJ, Hernandez-Guerrero C, Guevara-Silva R, et al. (2002) Identification of matrix metalloproteinase-9 in amniotic fluid and amniochorion in spontaneous labor and after experimental intrauterine infection or interleukin-1 beta infusion in pregnant rhesus monkeys. Am J Obstet Gynecol 186: 128–138.

37. Van Marter LJ, Dammann O, Allred EN, Leviton A, Pagano M, et al. (2002) Chorioamnionitis, mechanical ventilation, and postnatal sepsis as modulators of chronic lung disease in preterm infants. J Pediatr 140: 171–176.

38. Speer CP (2009) Chorioamnionitis, postnatal factors and proinflammatory response in the pathogenetic sequence of bronchopulmonary dysplasia. Neonatology 95: 353–361.

39. Thomas W, Speer CP (2011) Chorioamnionitis: important risk factor or innocent bystander for neonatal outcome? Neonatology 99: 177–187.

40. Been JV, Rours IG, Kornelisse RF, Jonkers F, de Krijger RR, et al. (2010) Chorioamnionitis alters the response to surfactant in preterm infants. J Pediatr 156: 10–15 e11.

41. Kallapur SG, Willet KE, Jobe AH, Ikegami M, Bachurski CJ (2001) Intra-amniotic endotoxin: chorioamnionitis precedes lung maturation in preterm lambs. Am J Physiol Lung Cell Mol Physiol 280: L527–536.

42. Jobe AH, Newnham JP, Willet KE, Moss TJ, Gore Ervin M, et al. (2000) Endotoxin-induced lung maturation is not mediated by cortisol. Am J Respir Crit Care Med 162: 1656–1661.

43. Kramer BW, Moss TJ, Willet KE, Newnham JP, Sly PD, et al. (2001) Dose and time response after intraamniotic endotoxin in preterm lambs. Am J Respir Crit Care Med 164: 982–988.

44. Kramer BW, Kramer S, Ikegami M, Jobe AH (2002) Injury, inflammation, and remodeling in fetal sheep lung after intra-amniotic endotoxin. Am J Physiol Lung Cell Mol Physiol 283: L452–459.

45. Matute-Bello G, Frevert CW, Martin TR (2008) Animal models of acute lung injury. Am J Physiol Lung Cell Mol Physiol 295: L379–399.

46. Munshi UK, Niu JO, Siddiq MM, Parton LA (1997) Elevation of interleukin-8 and interleukin-6 precedes the influx of neutrophils in tracheal aspirates from preterm infants who develop bronchopulmonary dysplasia. Pediatr Pulmonol 24: 331–336.

47. Baier RJ, Majid A, Parupia H, Loggins J, Kruger TE (2004) CC chemokine concentrations increase in respiratory distress syndrome and correlate with development of bronchopulmonary dysplasia. Pediatr Pulmonol 37: 137–148.

48. Bagchi A, Viscardi RM, Taciak V, Ensor JE, McCrea KA, et al. (1994) Increased activity of interleukin-6 but not tumor necrosis factor-alpha in lung lavage of premature infants is associated with the development of bronchopulmonary dysplasia. Pediatr Res 36: 244–252.

49. Watts CL, Fanaroff AA, Bruce MC (1992) Elevation of fibronectin levels in lung secretions of infants with respiratory distress syndrome and development of bronchopulmonary dysplasia. J Pediatr 120: 614–620.

50. Curley AE, Sweet DG, Thornton CM, O'Hara MD, Chesshyre E, et al. (2003) Chorioamnionitis and increased neonatal lung lavage fluid matrix metalloproteinase-9 levels: implications for antenatal origins of chronic lung disease. Am J Obstet Gynecol 188: 871–875.

51. Schock BC, Sweet DG, Ennis M, Warner JA, Young IS, et al. (2001) Oxidative stress and increased type-IV collagenase levels in bronchoalveolar lavage fluid from newborn babies. Pediatr Res 50: 29–33.

52. Groneck P, Oppermann M, Speer CP (1993) Levels of complement anaphylatoxin C5a in pulmonary effluent fluid of infants at risk for chronic lung disease and effects of dexamethasone treatment. Pediatr Res 34: 586–590.

53. Gravett MG, Witkin SS, Haluska GJ, Edwards JL, Cook MJ, et al. (1994) An experimental model for intraamniotic infection and preterm labor in rhesus monkeys. Am J Obstet Gynecol 171: 1660–1667.

54. Adams Waldorf KM, Persing D, Novy MJ, Sadowsky DW, Gravett MG (2008) Pretreatment with toll-like receptor 4 antagonist inhibits lipopolysaccharide-induced preterm uterine contractility, cytokines, and prostaglandins in rhesus monkeys. Reprod Sci 15: 121–127.

55. Borchardt SM, Foxman B, Chaffin DO, Rubens CE, Tallman PA, et al. (2004) Comparison of DNA dot blot hybridization and lancefield capillary precipitin methods for group B streptococcal capsular typing. J Clin Microbiol 42: 146–150.

56. Stothard P (2000) The sequence manipulation suite: JavaScript programs for analyzing and formatting protein and DNA sequences. Biotechniques 28: 1102, 1104.

5

Mites Parasitic on Australasian and African Spiders Found in the Pet Trade; a Redescription of *Ljunghia pulleinei* Womersley

Peter Masan[1,2]*, **Christopher Simpson**[1], **M. Alejandra Perotti**[3], **Henk R. Braig**[1]

1 School of Biological Sciences, Bangor University, Bangor, Wales, United Kingdom, **2** Institute of Zoology, Slovak Academy of Sciences, Bratislava, Slovakia, **3** School of Biological Sciences, University of Reading, Reading, United Kingdom

Abstract

Parasitic mites associated with spiders are spreading world-wide through the trade in tarantulas and other pet species. *Ljunghia pulleinei* Womersley, a mesostigmatic laelapid mite originally found in association with the mygalomorph spider *Selenocosmia stirlingi* Hogg (Theraphosidae) in Australia, is redescribed and illustrated on the basis of specimens from the African theraphosid spider *Pterinochilus chordatus* (Gerstäcker) kept in captivity in the British Isles (Wales). The mite is known from older original descriptions of Womersley in 1956; the subsequent redescription of Domrow in 1975 seems to be questionable in conspecificity of treated specimens with the type material. Some inconsistencies in both descriptions are recognised here as intraspecific variability of the studied specimens. The genus *Arachnyssus* Ma, with species *A. guangxiensis* (type) and *A. huwenae*, is not considered to be a valid genus, and is included in synonymy with *Ljunghia* Oudemans. A new key to world species of the genus *Ljunghia* is provided.

Editor: Dirk Steinke, Biodiversity Insitute of Ontario – University of Guelph, Canada

Funding: These authors have no support or funding to report.

Competing Interests: The authors have declared that no competing interests exist.

* E-mail: peter.masan@savba.sk

Introduction

Close inspection of spiders often reveals mites associated with various body parts. Although these associations are most frequently reported from tropical spider families, mites are not uncommon on temperate spider species. Deutonymphs of Astigmata mites and Heterostigmata mites can be found phoretic on spiders; larvae of the Prostigmata families Erythraedae, Trombiculidae and Trombidiidae (chigger mites) can be parasitic on spiders, while Mesostigmata mites in the family Laelapidae often occur both as immature stages and adults on spiders [1–3]. Mites on spiders go back in time at least 50 Ma. Baltic amber shows phoretic and parasitic Acari together with jumping and cell spiders [4], [5]. In addition, free-living mites (Asigmata and Mesostigmata) can become a problem for captive tarantulas when high numbers start to occlude the moist surfaces of the book lungs [6]. The large number of saprophilous and predatory Mesostigmata might overshadow the host-specific associations particularly between spider and mites of the mesostigmatic family Laelapidae. However, specific associations are well documented. For example, all life stages of *Androlaelaps pilosus* Baker (Laelapidae) can be found on the hexathelid spider *Macrothele calpeiana* (Walckenaer), the only European tarantula [7]. Here we report laelapid mites living on captive *Pterinochilus chordatus* Gerstäcker, the Kilimanjaro mustard baboon spider.

The laelapid genus *Ljunghia* includes species that have established close associations with various mygalomorph spiders in Indonesia [8,9], Malaysia [10], Australia [11–13], New Caledonia [14], Africa [15], and China [16]. It is assumed that they have developed obligatory parasitic relationships with their hosts [1]. To date, there is only one comprehensive review of *Ljunghia*, which includes a description of a new species from a Central American mygalomorph spider kept in captivity in Spain, a key for their identification and an enumeration of their host species [17].

Although there is no published record of an *Ljunghia* species from the British Isles, reports of mites parasitizing captive spiders is a common occurrence, often owing to contamination [17]. The presence of a seemingly Australian mite species on an African spider on the territory of the UK is interesting and might be either a consequence of the brisk business of tarantulas as pets including the wide-spread exchange of spiders among the breeders or an indication for a wider geographical distribution of *Ljunghia*.

The main aim of this study was a morphological redescription of *Ljunghia pulleinei*. Detailed observations of the most important morphological features of this mite allowed to discern more details than those reported in the original descriptions [11]. Generally, the original description of Womersley does not include illustrations of diagnostic morphologies as well as important metric data of some idiosomal structures and setae. There is one redescription of this species, that of Domrow [12], based on specimens that differ in some characters, e.g. distinctly shorter idiosomal setae when compared with the type specimens. Inconsistencies in the descriptions of Womersley and Domrow are another good reason for the following redescription.

Results and Discussion

Genus *Ljunghia* Oudemans

Ljunghia Oudemans, 1932: 204 [8]. Type species *Ljunghia selenocosmiae* Oudemans, 1932; by monotypy [8].

Ljunghia (Metaljunghia) Fain, 1989: 158 [9]. Type species *Ljunghia rainbowi* Domrow, 1975; by original designation [12].

Arachnyssus Ma, 2002: 8 [16]. Type species *Ljunghia guangxiensis* Ma, 2002; by original designation [16]. New synonymy.

Diagnosis (Adults). Chelicerae chelate-dentate in female, with fixed digit usually reduced in size; cheliceral digits of male subequal in length, with curved spermatodactyl slightly exceeding the tip of the movable digit. Dorsal shield entire, not covering the whole dorsal surface, and with hypotrichous setation (at most, 32 pairs of setae present). Sternal shield with three pairs of setae, metasternal shields and setae often absent. A pair of genital setae present or absent, usually placed on epigynal shield. Anal shield relatively small, elongate, bearing three circum-anal setae. Leg setation holotrichous to markedly hypotrichous.

Notes on the genus. The genus *Ljunghia* was proposed by Oudemans [8], based on adults and deutonymphs collected from the theraphosid spider of the genus *Selenocosmia* Ausserer in Sumatra. Oudeman's genus *Ljunghia* has gained broad acceptance [9], [12], [15], [17], [20], mostly as a member of the subfamily Iphiopsinae within the family Laelapidae, and is currently divided into two subgenera, *Ljunghia* and *Metaljunghia*. We agree with Moraza *et al.* that this subgeneric structure is not useful, and it is not used here [17].

A new separate genus *Arachnyssus* was erected [16] to accommodate two mesostigmatic mite species associated with the mygalomorph theraphosid spider *Selenocosmia huwena* Wang, Peng & Xie (= *Haplopelma schmidti* von Wirth, based on the newest taxonomic revision [21]) in China. The most important features that define the genus *Arachnyssus*, classified within the family Macronyssidae, are: (1) entire dorsal shield; (2) idiosomal setae very long, with tips reaching far beyond the insertions of following setae; (3) anus with anterior position to adanal setae; (4) coxae I–IV not armed with spines; (5) sternal shield saddle-shaped, with posterior margin deeply concave; (6) epigynial shield short, tongue-shaped; (7) anal shield drop-shaped; (8) epigynial and anal shields well separated [16].

It is obvious that the author who erected *Arachnyssus* neglected the existence of the genus *Ljunghia* because there is no reference to this genus in his paper [16] and all of the above characters enumerated for *Arachnyssus* can be found in *Ljunghia* [17]. Therefore *Arachnyssus* is here regarded as synonymous with *Ljunghia*, and the two species, namely *A. guangxiensis* and *A. huwenae* are therefore, newly transferred to the genus *Ljunghia*.

Ljunghia pulleinei Womersley

Ljunghia pulleini Womersley, 1956: 591–593 [11].

Ljunghia pulleini – Domrow, 1975: 35–37 (in part: only specimens of the type series) [12].

Ljunghia pulleinei (emend. nov.) s. str. – Fain, 1991: 78–79 [13].

Ljunghia (Metaljunghia) pulleini – Fain, 1989: 159 [9]; Moraza *et al.*, 2009: 125 (in part) [17].

Material examined. 4 females, 2 males – on *Pterinochilus chordatus* (det. R. C. Gallon) kept in captivity in the Laboratory of Molecular Parasitology, School of Biological Sciences, Bangor University, Gwynedd, NW Wales. The mites were collected by one of the authors, MAP, following the technique described aboved; October 2006.

Description (Adults). Female. Dorsal idiosoma (Figure 1A). Idiosoma oblong, egg-shaped, 810–860 µm long and 610–635 µm wide (650 µm long and 443 µm wide in freshly moulted and poorly sclerotized specimen). Dorsal shield entire, oblong, suboval, 560–595 µm long and 320–355 µm wide nearly at level of setae z5, usually not completely covering dorsal surface, with regularly rounded posterior margin and smooth surface. The shield free of anterior sections of peritremes, anterior ends of peritremes reaching close to paravertical setae z1. Podonotal region of the shield with 15 pairs of setae (j1–j6, z1, z2, z4–z6, s1–s4), opisthonotum with reduced complement of three setal pairs (J4, Z4 and Z5). Most dorsal shield setae simple, smooth, needle-like, sinuous and considerably elongated, the longest setae up to 270 µm in length and with thread-like distal part reaching far beyond the insertions of following setae; only setae j1, z1 and J4 short. Metric data for some selected dorsal setae as follows: j1 33–44 µm, j4 220–230 µm, j5 136–153 µm, j6 230–260 µm, J4 25–31 µm, z5 170–190 µm, Z4 142–152 µm, Z5 152–162 µm, the longest setae situated on soft membranous dorsal integument 220–255 µm. Dorsolateral membranous integument with 13 pairs of setae.

Ventral idiosoma (Figure 1B). Presternal platelets absent. Sternal shield almost quadrangular, longitudinally narrowed, 30–40 µm long in midline, 120–132 µm wide at level of setae st2 and 149–158 µm at level of setae st3, smooth on surface, deeply concave posteriorly; anterolateral corners well developed, slender and obtusely acuminate; the shield bearing two pairs of lyrifissures and three pairs of setae, length of sternal shield setae slightly increasing posteriorly: st1 100–115 µm, st2 105–122 µm, st3 150–170 µm. Metasternal platelets and setae st4 absent, a pair of metasternal lyrifissures placed on soft membrane close to posterolateral corners of sternal shield. Endopodal sclerites absent. Epigynal shield tongue-shaped, elongated, slightly constricted between coxae IV, hyaline anteriorly, rounded posteriorly, 238–252 µm long, 75–83 µm wide at level of genital setae, with a pair of genital setae st5 (166–184 µm) inserted in posterior part and a pattern of weak longitudinal lines on medial surface; associate genital pores not detected. Peritrematal shields almost fully reduced, only short and narrow poststigmatic section present; peritremes well developed, long and with stigma between coxae III and IV. Exopodal sclerites absent, parapodal sclerites developed, crescent. A pair of small and suboval metapodal platelets present. Anal shield pear-shaped, rounded anteriorly and posteriorly, 74–82 µm wide, smooth, bearing rounded anus and three circum-anal setae; postanal seta (64–77 µm) shorter than adanals (80–90 µm); anus with posterior position on the shield. Ventral and ventrolateral membranous integument with 10 pairs of setae. All ventral setae similar to those on dorsal idiosoma.

Gnathosomal structures (Figures 2B, 2C, 2E). Anterior ventral part of hypostome as in Figure 2B, with three pairs of simple hypostomal setae h1–h3; posterior setae h3 longest; posterior surface bearing a pair of simple postcoxal setae. Deutosternal groove relatively narrow and difficult to examine posteriorly, with only three detectable transverse rows of denticles on its anterior section. Corniculi obscure and covered by hypertrophied, lobe-like projection. Chelicerae chelate-dentate (Figure 2C); fixed digit reduced in size, markedly shorter and thiner than movable digit, and armed with distal hook; movable digit relatively robust, with distal hook and two massive subsidtal teeth. Epistome rounded and serrate on anterior margin (Figure 2D).

Legs. All legs with a well developed pretarsus and ambulacral apparatus (including pulvillus and two claws), shorter than idiosoma. Leg segments without specific projections or macro-setae, with the chaetotactic pattern as previously described. Coxae IV associated with relatively thin and long tubular structures of insemination apparatus (Figure 2F).

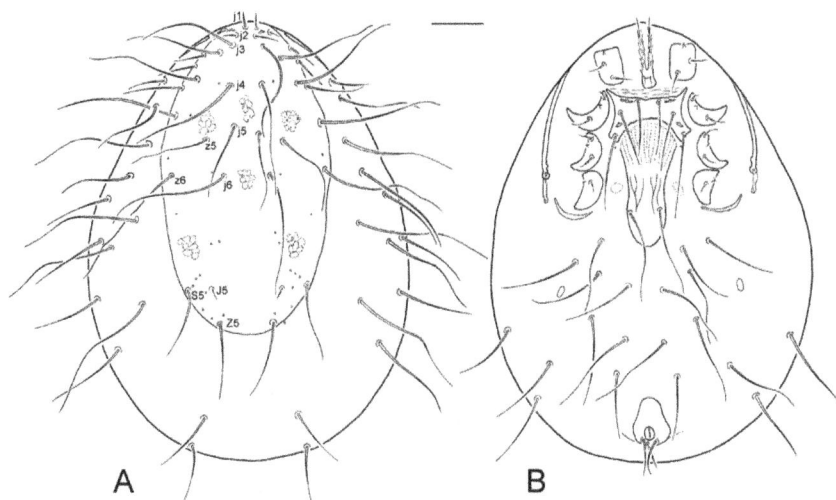

Figure 1. *Ljunghia pulleinei*, **female.** A, dorsal idiosoma (with setal notation of some dorsal setae); B, ventral idiosoma. Scale: 100 µm.

Male (Figures 2A, 2D). Idiosoma 540–590 µm long and 360–395 µm wide, dorsal shield 490–515 µm long and 285–325 µm wide. Dorsum with a compact holodorsal shield. Metric data for some selected dorsal setae as follows: j1 23–29 µm, j3 177 µm, j4 200 µm, j5 110–115 µm, J4 12–19 µm, z5 134–158 µm, z6 184–207 µm, Z4 120–126 µm, Z5 126–132 µm. Venter with separate sternogenital (Figure 2A), and anal shields. Sternogenital shield oblong, subtruncate anteriorly, rounded posteriorly, 250–270 µm long in midline, 130–138 µm wide at level of setae st3 and 94–99 µm at level of setae st5, smooth on surface; the shield bearing three pairs of lyrifissures and four pairs of setae (st1–st3, st5), length of sternogenital shield setae slightly increasing posteriorly: st1 75–81 µm, st2 99–105 µm, st3 122–141 µm, st5 150 µm.

Cheliceral digits subequal in length, without striking dentation; spermatodactyl hook-like, robust in basal part, curved distally (Figure 2D). Other characters almost identical as in female, including those on opisthogastric region.

Taxonomic notes. The original description of *Ljunghia pulleinei* was inadequately illustrated, the description itself was insufficient [11]; therefore, amendments followed in the redescription of Domrow [12], especially in the dorsal shield setation. For example, Womersley stated only 14 pairs of setae on the dorsal shield instead of 17–18 pairs documented by Domrow who examined three series of specimens: (1) the type material collected from theraphosid spider *Selenocosmia stirlingi* Hogg in South Australia; (2) specimens from a nemesiid spider of the genus

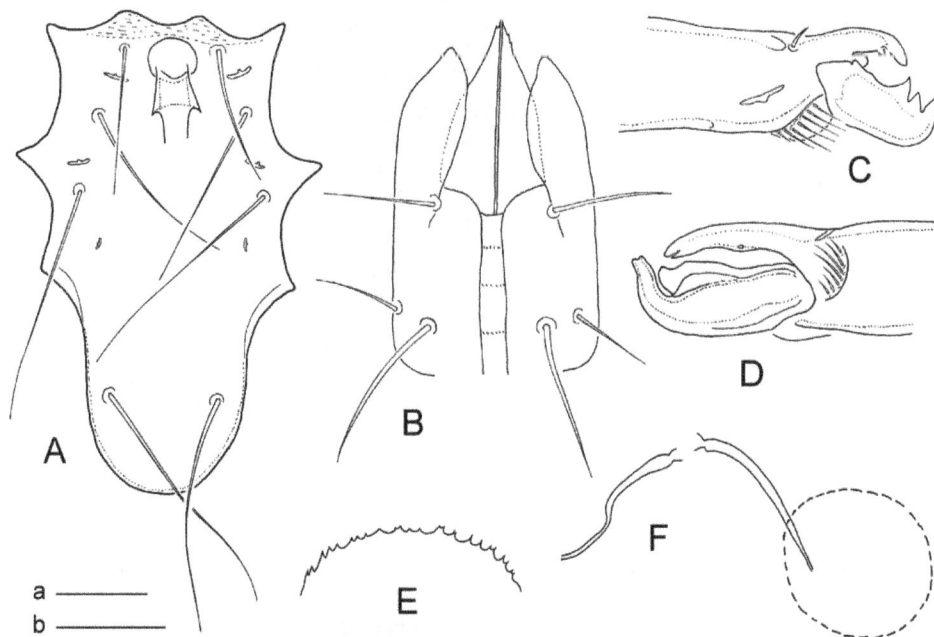

Figure 2. *Ljunghia pulleinei*. A, sternogenital shield of male; B, ventral hypostome of female (anterior part); C, cheliceral digits of female; D, cheliceral digits of male; E, epistome of female; F, tubular structures of insemination apparatus associated with coxae IV in female. Scales: a = 50 µm (Figs 2A, 2F), b = 25 µm (Figs 2B–E).

Aname L. Koch found in South Australia; (3) specimens from an unidentified diplurid spider in Queensland. All three series were keyed out together by Domrow and, despite the presence of some morphological differences, indicative of a mixture of three species, they were declared to be conspecific [12]. We now know that the specimens from the spiders of the genus *Aname*, which differ from the typical series mainly by the lack of the subterminal pair of setae on the dorsal shield, belong to the species *Ljunghia aname*, which was originally described as a new subspecies of *L. pulleinei* [13], [14]. A third unknown species is being described by Bruce Halliday (personal communication).

Unfortunately, the description and figures of adults given by Domrow [12] and of deutonymphs of *Ljunghia pulleinei* by Fain [14]) did not apply to the mites of the type series but to those of an unknown diplurid spider. The type specimens and specimens introduced by Domrow (and Fain) can be easily distinguished from each other by the length of setae situated on medial surface of the dorsal shield. They belong to two species, and show a certain degree of interspecific variability not only in the length of idiosomal setae but also in position of some dorsal shield setae (especially in J4 and Z4). So, two main patterns of chaetotaxy can be distinguished: (1) type species with longer idiosomal setae, e.g. setae j5 and z5 with tips reaching far beyond the insertions of j6, setae j6 beyond the insertions of J4, and setae z5 beyond the lateral margin of dorsal shield; (2) species illustrated by Domrow and Fain with shorter idiosomal setae, e.g. setae j5 and z5 with tips not reaching the insertions of j6, setae j6 hardly reaching to the insertions of J4, and setae z5 clearly not reaching the lateral margin of dorsal shield.

Ljunghia pulleinei bearing the longer setae cannot be reliably identified in the newest key of the genus [17]; where some statements are solely applicable to the form exhibiting short setae as described by Domrow [12]. In addition there is a mistake in their key in relation to both setal forms: "setae j4 do not reach the tips of j6". With exception of this inaccuracy and a pair of additional setae present on the opisthogastric ventral surface in our individuals, our description generally agrees with most of the published morphological characters given by Womersley and Domrow [11], [12]. In addition, we have included in our redescription new metric data for some idiosomal setae, and the shields.

Ljunghia pulleinei s. str. has here been collected from the Kilimanjaro mustard baboon spider from East Africa and previously from the common whistling spider from Australia. This is the first time that one and the same *Ljunghia* species has been associated with two different host species suggesting that *Ljunghia* species are not strictly species-specific. *Ljunghia* is well known from mygalomorph spiders but has also been reported from a more primitive liphistiid Malaysian trap door spider belonging to the Mesothelae [10]. Recently, new *Ljunghia* species have been retrieved from more liphistiid spiders from Vietnam and Thailand [22]. The female spiders showed clear bite marks of the mites on their prosomata emphasising the parasitic nature of *Ljunghia*.

Key to the species now known in *Ljunghia* Oudemans

1. Opisthonotal region of dorsal shield with strongly suppressed setation, only 2–5 pairs of setae present 2

   – Setation of opisthonotal region moderately suppressed, 7–14 pairs of setae present 7

2. Opisthonotal region with two pairs of setae, podonotal region with 14 pairs of setae . . . . *Ljunghia aname* Fain, 1991

   – Opisthonotal region with at least three pairs of setae . . . 3

3. Genital setae (st5) absent; podonotal region with 20 pairs of setae, male sternogenital shield with three pairs of setae (st1–st3) . . . . *Ljunghia novaecaledoniae* Fain, 1991

   – Genital setae present; podonotal region with at most 18 pairs of setae, male sternogenital or sternogenito-ventral shield with at least four pairs of setae 4

4. Podonotal region of dorsal shield with strongly suppressed setation, only 11 pairs of setae present, opisthonotal region with 4–5 pairs of setae 5

   – Setation of podonotal region moderately suppressed, 17–18 pairs of setae present, opisthonotal region with 3 pairs of setae 6

5. Opisthonotal region with 5 pairs of setae, setae J4 absent . . . . *Ljunghia bristowi* (Finnegan, 1933)

   – Opisthonotal region with 4 pairs of setae, setae J4 present . . . . *Ljunghia rainbowi* Domrow, 1975

6. Podonotal region with 14 pairs of setae, setae j5 absent; setae j6 and z5 relatively short and subequal in length . . . . *Ljunghia africana* Fain, 1991

   – Podonotal region with 15 pairs of setae, setae j5 present; setae j6 relatively long, obviously longer than setae z5 . . . . *Ljunghia pulleinei* Womersley, 1956

7. Metasternal setae absent; opisthonotal region with 8 pairs of setae 8

   – Metasternal setae present; opisthonotal region with at least 11 pairs of setae 9

8. Podonotal region with 17 pairs of setae; setae J4 present, minute; sternal shield subrectangular; male with sternogenital shield . . . . *Ljunghia hoggi* Domrow, 1975

   – Podonotal region with 20 pairs of setae; setae J4 absent; sternal shield saddle-like, deeply concave posteriorly; male with holoventral shield . . . . *Ljunghia guangxiensis* (Ma, 2002) comb. nov.

9. Opisthonotal region with 14 pairs of setae; male with sternogenital shield bearing five pairs of setae (st1–st5) . . . . *Ljunghia minor* Fain, 1989

   – Opisthonotal region with 11 pairs of setae; male with sternogenital-ventral or holoventral shield bearing five pairs of setae together with a number of additional ventral setae 10

10. Setae J4 not modified, subequal with most of other dorsal setae; male with sternogenital-ventral shield, ventral part of the shield with 5–7 setae . . . . *Ljunghia selenocosmiae* Oudemans, 1932

   – Setae J4 reduced in length, conspicuously shorter than other dorsal setae; male with holoventral shield bearing at least 13 setae in ventral part 11

11. Podonotal region with 21 pairs of setae; setae J4 shorter, with tips not reaching the posterior margin of dorsal shield;

holoventral shield of male with 20–21 setae in ventral part
. . . .*Ljunghia luciae* Moraza, Iraola & Alemany, 2009

- Podonotal region with 20 pairs of setae; setae J4 longer, with
tips reaching beyond the posterior margin of dorsal shield;
holoventral shield of male with about 13 setae in ventral part
. . . . *Ljunghia huwenae* (Ma, 2002) comb. nov.

Materials and Methods

All examined specimens of *Ljunghia pulleinei* were obtained from
the mygalomorph spider *Pterinochilus chordatus* kept in captivity in
Gwynedd, North Wales. *P. chordatus* is an East African theraphosid
species distributed in Ethiopia, Kenya, Somalia, Sudan, Tanzania
and Uganda [18].

The collection of mites was carried out on the living spider. Due
to the aggressivity of the spider it was necessary to develop a
technique to collect the mites attached to the dorsal parts of the
cephalothorax and the abdomen. The spider was reared in a
plastic container covered by a plastic lid. Small holes of 2 mm
where made in the lid to allow breading but also to allow insertion
of a wire to touch the mites. The tip of the wire was soaked in
100% glycerol (glycerin) and then directed inside the cage towards
every single mite. Due to the sticky nature of glycerol, the mites
were instantly glued to the tiny tip of the wire and extracted from
the cage by slowly moving the tip out to avoid distressing the
spider. Once outside the cage, the tip of the wire with a glued mite
was submerged in 96% ethanol where the mites detached and
became fixed and preserved for further analysis.

The mites were mounted on permanent microscope slides using
Swan medium. Illustrations were made by using a high
magnification microscope equipped with a drawing tube. Measurements were made from slide-mounted specimens with stage-
calibrated ocular micrometers. Lengths of shields and leg segments
were measured along their midlines, and widths were measured at
the widest point. Dorsal setae were measured from the bases of
their insertions to their tips. Measurements are mostly presented as
ranges (minimum to maximum). The terminology of dorsal and
ventral chaetotaxy follows Lindquist & Evans [19]. For the specific
chaetotactic notation of some dorsal shield setae, see Figure 1A.
The redescribed specimens are deposited at the Institute of
Zoology, Slovak Academy of Sciences, Bratislava, and the
Australian National Insect Collection, Canberra, Australia (2♀♀,
1♂).

Acknowledgments

We are very grateful to Bruce Halliday, of the CSIRO Ecosystem Sciences
and Australian National Insect Collection, Canberra, for his review of
some of our mite specimens and the very valuable discussions on *Ljunghia
pulleinei* morphology.

Author Contributions

Conceived and designed the experiments: HRB MAP. Performed the
experiments: MAP. Analyzed the data: PM. Contributed reagents/
materials/analysis tools: HRB. Wrote the paper: PM MAP HRB.
Collected and illustrated specimens examined: CS.

References

1. Welbourn W, Young OP (1988) Mites parasitic on spiders, with a description of a new species of *Eutrombidium* (Acari, Eutrombidiidae). J Arachnol 16: 373–385.
2. Baker A (1992) Acari (mites and ticks) associated with other arachnids. In: Cooper JE, Pearce-Kelly P, Williams DL, editors. Arachnida: Proceedings of a Symposium on Spiders and Their Allies. London: Chiron Press. pp. 126–131.
3. Ebermann E, Goloboff PA (2002) Association between neotropical burrowing spiders (Araneae: Nemesiidae) and mites (Acari: Heterostigmata, Scutacaridae). Acarologia 42: 173–184.
4. Wunderlich J (2004) Fossil jumping spiders (Araneae: Salticidae) in Baltic and Dominican amber, with remarks on Salticidae subfamilies. Beitr Araneol 3B: 1761–1819.
5. Dunlop JA, Wirth S, Penney D, McNeil A, Bradley RS, et al. (2012) A minute fossil phoretic mite recovered by phase-contrast X-ray computed tomography. Biol Lett 8: 457–460.
6. Pizzi R (2009) Parasites of tarantulas (Theraphosidae). J Exot Pet Med 18: 283–288.
7. Baker A (1991) A new species of the mite genus *Androlaelaps* Berlese (Parasitiformes: Laelapidae) found in association with the spider *Macrothele calpeiana* (Walckenaer) (Mygalomorphae: Hexathelidae). Bull Br Arachnol Soc 8: 219–223.
8. Oudemans AC (1932) Opus 550. Tijdschr Entomol 75: 202–210.
9. Fain A (1989) Notes on the genus *Ljunghia* Oudemans, 1932 (Acari, Mesostigmata) associated with mygalomorph spiders from the Oriental and Australian Regions. Bull Inst R Sci Nat Belg Entomol 59: 157–160.
10. Finnegan S (1933) A new species of mite parasitic on the spider *Liphistius malayanus*, from Malaya. Proc Zool Soc London 1993: 413–417.
11. Womersley H (1956) On some Acarina Mesostigmata from Australia, New Zeland and New Guinea. J Linn Soc Zool 42: 505–599.

12. Domrow R (1975) *Ljunghia* Oudemans (Acari: Dermanyssidae), a genus parasitic on mygalomorph spiders. Rec S Aust Mus 17: 31–39.
13. Fain A (1991) Notes on mites parasitic or phoretic on Australia centipedes, spiders and scorpions. Rec West Aust Mus 15: 69–82.
14. Fain A (1991) A new species of *Ljunghia* Oudemans, 1932 (Acari, Laelapidae) from a New-Caledonian spider. Bull Inst R Sci Nat Belg Entomol 61: 199–205.
15. Fain A (1991) Notes on some new parasitic mites (Acari, Mesostigmata) from Afrotropical region. Bull Inst R Sci Nat Belg Entomol 61: 183–191.
16. Ma LM (2002) A new genus and two new species of gamasid mites parasitic on spiders (Acari: Macronyssidae). Acta Arachn Sinica 11: 8–13.
17. Moraza ML, Iraola V, Alemany C (2009) A new species of *Ljunghia* Oudemans, 1932 (Arachnida, Acari, Laelapidae) from a mygalomorph spider. Zoosystema 31: 117–126.
18. Gallon RC (2002) Revision of the African genera of *Pterinochilus* and *Eucratoscelus* (Araneae, Theraphosidae, Harpactirinae) with description of two new genera. Bull Br Arachnol Soc 12: 201–232.
19. Lindquist EE, Evans GO (1965) Taxonomic concepts in the Ascidae, with a modified setal nomenclature for the idiosoma of the Gamasina (Acarina: Mesostigmata). Mem Ent Soc Can 47: 1–64.
20. Casanueva MA (1993) Phylogenetic studies of the free-living and arthropod associated Laelapidae (Acari: Mesostigmata). Gayana Zool 57: 21–46.
21. Zhu MS, Zhang R (2008) Revision of the theraphosid spiders from China (Araneae: Mygalomorphae). J Arachnol 36: 425–447.
22. Schwendinger PJ, Ono H (2011) On two *Heptathela* species from southern Vietnam, with a discussion of copulatory organs and systematics of the Liphistiidae (Araneae: Mesothelae). Rev Suisse Zool 118: 599–637.

6

Using Animal Performance Data to Evidence the Under-Reporting of Case Herds during an Epizootic: Application to an Outbreak of Bluetongue in Cattle

Simon Nusinovici[1,2]*, Pascal Monestiez[3], Henri Seegers[1,2], François Beaudeau[1,2], Christine Fourichon[1,2]

1 INRA, UMR1300 Biology, Epidemiology and Risk Analysis in animal health, Nantes, France, 2 LUNAM Université, Oniris, Ecole nationale vétérinaire, agroalimentaire et de l'alimentation Nantes-Atlantique, Nantes, France, 3 INRA, UR 546, Biostatistics and Spatial Processes, Avignon, France

Abstract

Following the emergence of the Bluetongue virus serotype 8 (BTV-8) in France in 2006, a surveillance system (both passive and active) was implemented to detect and follow precociously the progression of the epizootic wave. This system did not allow a precise estimation of the extent of the epizootic. Infection by BTV-8 is associated with a decrease of fertility. The objective of this study was to evaluate whether a decrease in fertility can be used to evidence the under-reporting of cases during an epizootic and to quantify to what extent non-reported cases contribute to the total burden of the epizootic. The cow fertility in herds in the outbreak area (reported or not) was monitored around the date of clinical signs. A geostatistical interpolation method was used to estimate a date of clinical signs for non-reported herds. This interpolation was based on the spatiotemporal dynamic of confirmed case herds reported in 2007. Decreases in fertility were evidenced for both types of herds around the date of clinical signs. In non-reported herds, the decrease fertility was large (60% of the effect in reported herds), suggesting that some of these herds have been infected by the virus during 2007. Production losses in non-reported infected herds could thus contribute to an important part of the total burden of the epizootic. Overall, results indicate that performance data can be used to evidence the under-reporting during an epizootic. This approach could be generalized to pathogens that affect cattle's performance, including zoonotic agents such as *Coxiella burnetii* or Rift Valley fever virus.

Editor: Houssam Attoui, The Pirbright Institute, United Kingdom

Funding: Financial support for this research was provided by INRA, Cemagref and Basse-Normandie, Bretagne, Pays de le Loire and Poitou-Charentes Regional Councils under SANCRE project, in the framework of "For and About Regional Development" programs. The authors gratefully acknowledge the Centre de Traitement de l'Information Génétique (INRA, Jouy-en-Josas, France) for providing the performance data and the Ministry of Agriculture (Direction Générale de l'Alimentation) for the BTV case herds data. The funders had no role in study design, data collection and analysis, decision to publish, or preparation of the manuscript.

Competing Interests: The authors have declared that no competing interests exist.

* E-mail: simon.nusinovici@oniris-nantes.fr

Introduction

Following the emergence of the Bluetongue virus serotype 8 (BTV-8) in France in 2006, a surveillance system was implemented to detect and follow precociously the progression of the epizootic wave. This system was composed of both passive (detection of clinical signs of the disease by farmers) and active surveillance (blood sampling and diagnostic tests in targeted populations). This system did not allow a precise estimation of the extent of the epizootic. A cross-sectional serologic study conducted in 2007 showed that only a low proportion of seropositive herds reported clinical cases, indicating a high under-reporting rate of clinical cases [1]. Several reasons could explain the fact that some herds infected by BTV-8 were not reported during the epizootic. Firstly, because most infected cattle herds showed no evidence of clinical signs, their infection was not systematically noticed by farmers and veterinary practitioners [1,2,3]. Secondly, the fact that BTV-8 recently emerged in this part of Europe complicated the identification of the disease because of the low level of awareness (only 6 case herds were reported in 2006 in mainland France). Therefore, even in case of clinical expression of the disease,

farmers could not have detected them. Moreover, they could have detected clinical signs but not notified them. As suggested, there is some reluctance to report suspect clinical situations in general by farmers and veterinary practitioners to the veterinary authorities in fear of anticipated social and economic consequences [3]. Finally, most clinical signs of the disease are not specific, and therefore could have been detected but not attributed by farmers to BTV-8 infection. Concerning the active surveillance system, the objective was to detect the virus in areas previously free of virus, using very small samples. The surveillance was stopped in a given area once the virus was detected. This system was thus not designed to quantify the incidence of the infection. These facts highlight the limits of surveillance systems performance in the event of an emerging disease.

Infection by BTV-8 is associated with a decrease of fertility [4,5]. For cows in herds reported after clinical signs suspicion during the BTV-8 epizootic in 2007 in France, fertility was adversely affected around the date of detection of clinical signs in the herd [5]. A decreased fertility can be expected for cows in herds not reported during the epizootic, if a proportion of these herds are in fact infected. It can be assumed that the magnitude of

(a)

(b)

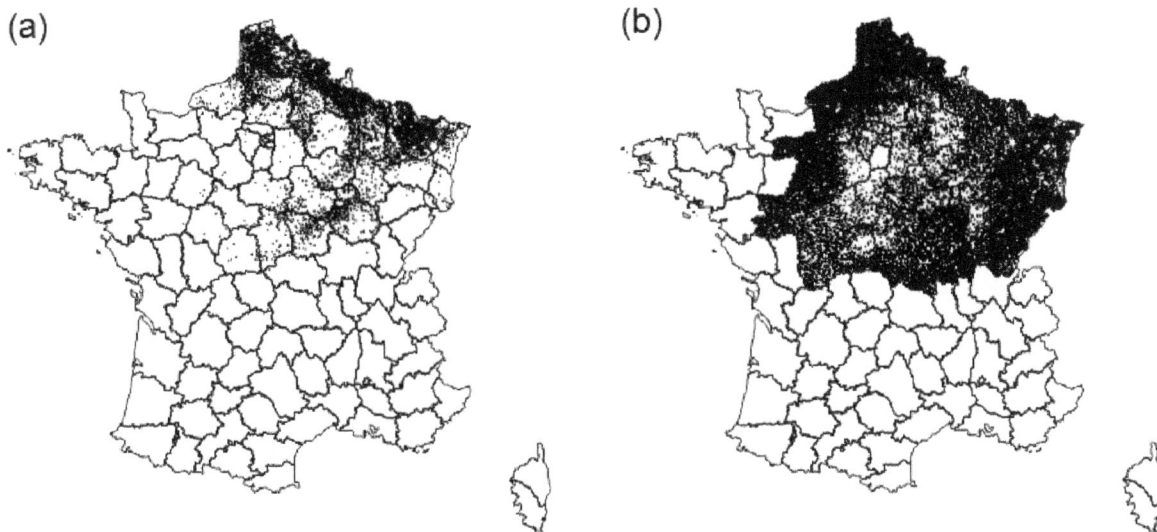

Figure 1. Geographical location of cattle herds in the outbreak area: (a) 8,313 case herds reported after clinical signs of Bluetongue virus serotype 8 (BTV-8) in 2007, (b) 74,169 non-reported herds (e.g., herds with an interpolated date of BTV-8 exposure); 2007; France.

the decrease in undetected herds depends on the proportion of herds that were infected. The magnitude is likely to be lower compared to the variations quantified in reported herds.

In most dairy cattle, artificial inseminations (AI) are used for reproduction. This information on individual cow reproduction is centralized in a national data base. The monitoring of these events can be used to evaluate reproduction performance at the cow level. For example, the occurrence of repeated AI can be used as proxy of cow fertility disorders [6,4,7,8].

Decrease in fertility could be used as non-specific indicator to evaluate the existence of under-reporting of BTV-8 cases in exposed areas. Moreover, quantifying such losses in non-reported herds would enable to obtain a more comprehensive evaluation of the burden of an epizootic in a newly infected area than when accounting only for case herds. The objective of this study was to evaluate whether a decrease in fertility can be used to evidence the under-reporting of cases during an epizootic and to quantify to what extent non-reported cases contribute to the total burden of the epizootic.

Materials and Methods

General Study Design and Available Data

Decrease in fertility was quantified for cows in reported case herds and cows in non-reported herds located in the 2007 outbreak area (herds with uncertain infectious status). These quantifications were performed using cows in herds unexposed to BTV-8 in 2007 as reference population.

Information about exposure of herds to BTV-8 during 2007 was obtained from the official veterinary surveillance system. Herds were reported in 2 distinct situations: (i) in the event of clinical signs detected by the farmer or the veterinary practitioner, subsequently confirmed by a diagnostic test and (ii) in the event of a positive serological test performed either before animal transfer or sale, or in sentinel herds. Among herds reported during 2007, only herds with a confirmed detection reported after clinical suspicion (situation (i)) were included as the date of a positive serological test did not necessarily identify the possible date of BTV-8 exposure of the herd. Information about BTV-8 exposure was available at the herd level only. Thus, a herd was considered exposed if at least 1 animal with clinical signs had tested positive for BTV-8. The proportion of infected animals in reported herds was unknown. Herds reported after clinical suspicion and

Table 1. Return-to-service rates and distribution of cantons, herds and cows according to herds Bluetongue virus serotype 8 (BTV-8) exposure statuses, 2007, France.

	Number of cantons	Number of herds	Number of cows	90-day-return-to-service rates (%)
Reported case herds with clinical signs	408	2,646	43,786*	56.9
Non-reported herds located in the 2007 outbreak area	648	5,237	78,293*	56.0
Unexposed herds in 2007	312	9,485	211,578**	54.2
Herds in 2005 that were located in the 2007 outbreak area	715	8,215	126,362*	54.3

*Cows with first artificial insemination (AI) between 10 weeks before and 4 weeks after the observed date of clinical detection (case herds), the interpolated date of clinical detection (non-reported herds) and the transposed date in a year free of BTV-8 (herds in 2005 located in the 2007 outbreak area).
**Cows with first AI performed during the same period in the year than herds located in the outbreak area.

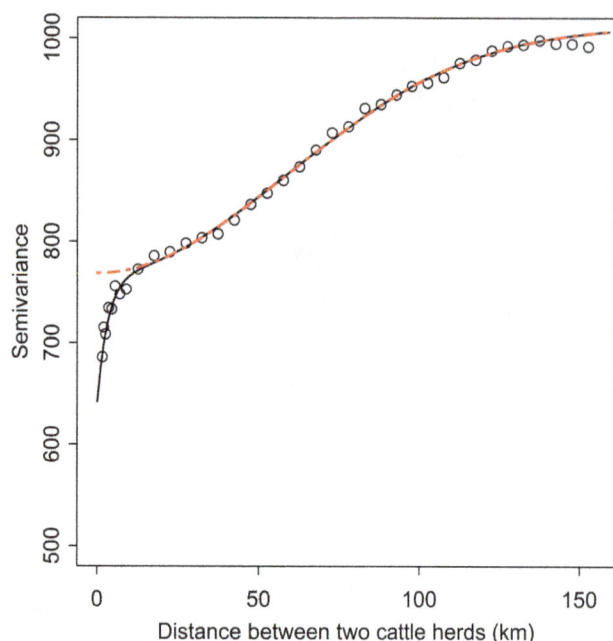

Figure 2. Experimental variogram of the observed dates of detection of Bluetongue virus serotype 8 clinical signs of reported case herds (dots) and the fitted nested model of semivariogram (solid black line) which is the sum of a nugget effect, an exponential and a Gaussian variogram model. The gaussian component which is kept for kriging is shown in red dashed line.

subsequently selected for this study will be referred to as 'case herds'. Case herds located in 23 departments were selected (n = 8,494), corresponding to 96% of all cattle herds reported due to clinical suspicion during the 2007 epizootic. Cattle herds that were not reported during 2007 and located in these departments were considered to have an uncertain infectious status, and were thus referred as 'herds with uncertain BTV-8 status' (n = 46,569).

The performance data were obtained in dairy herds enrolled in the official Milk Recording Scheme and where artificial insemination was used. For each cow, obtained data were dates of AIs, rank of service (number of AI within lactation), date of culling (if it had occurred during the study period) and data used to adjust for factors known to influence fertility: cow and bull breeds, lactation number, calving date, milk production data at each milk record (record date, milk yield, protein content, fat content). After selection of dairy herds that use AI for reproduction, populations of case herds and herds with uncertain BTV-8 status were composed of 4,392 and 13,804 herds respectively.

A date of exposure to BTV-8 was either estimated from recorded data for cows in case herds, or interpolated for cows in herds with uncertain BTV-8 status. This interpolation was based on the spatio-temporal dynamics of detection of confirmed case herds that reported clinical signs in 2007. Decrease in fertility in both case herds and herds with uncertain BTV-8 status were quantified around the date of exposure (observed or predicted). The geographical coordinates of herds were available at the municipality level.

Estimated Date of Exposure for Reported Case Herds

For each case herd, available data included the date at which clinical signs of disease were first suspected and the date at which disease was confirmed via diagnostic tests. The estimated date of

exposure for reported herds was defined as the recorded date of suspicion which corresponded to the first detection of clinical signs in the herd. The same date of exposure was assigned to all cows in a herd. For 6.1% of the case herds, the date of clinical suspicion was missing but the date of confirmation by a diagnostic test was known. In order to assign a date of suspicion, an imputation method based on the distribution of the time interval between dates of suspicion and confirmation was applied (values selected at random around a median interval of 4 days). Moreover, 181 case herds that had a non-plausible time interval between dates of suspicion and confirmation (interval >30 days or date of suspicion posterior to the date of confirmation) were excluded.

Interpolation of a Date of Detection of Clinical Signs for Herds Not Reported and Located in Exposed Areas

A date of exposure to BTV-8 for each cattle herd with uncertain BTV-8 status during 2007 was interpolated.

Kriging, a geostatistical interpolation method, was used to estimate a date of detection of clinical signs for herds with uncertain BTV-8 status. Dates were expressed as the number of days since the first case herd reported in 2007. Kriging uses data sample (cattle case herds) to predict values at unsampled locations (herds with uncertain BTV-8 status). All the cattle herds (dairy and beef) were included because they could have all played a role in the epizootic wave diffusion. Both beef and dairy herds are exposed to *Culicoïdes*. Densities of beef and dairy herds widely vary among French areas. This method is based on assumptions regarding the form of the trend of the sample data, its variance and spatial correlation. The first step consisted in modelling the spatial correlation of the data. Two models were compared. A cross-validation process with observed data was used to determine each model's goodness of fit and to compare their predictions. Spatial variation in detection dates were modelled using a gaussian semivariogram – for smooth long-range propagation waves - and an exponential semivariogram - for short-range random propagation between neighbouring herds - models. To account for the non stationarity of the BTV-8 spreading process, the gradient of the viral diffusion was also included in the model by the use of Universal Kriging in place of Ordinary Kriging. For the final interpolation of detection dates, only the gaussian-model spatial component was kept for filtering the random local component.

Selection of Unexposed Herds and Cows

A reference population was used to quantify both decrease in fertility of cows in case herds and cows in herds with uncertain BTV-8 status. It was composed of cows located in 2 French regions unexposed to BTV-8 during 2007: Brittany and a south-western area. In France, herd management varies between areas. Therefore, unexposed cows from 2 different parts of France were selected in order to better represent the unexposed population. This comparison limited the impact of any possible confounding factors due to variations of herd management over time.

The month of AI is known to influence fertility [7,8]. Consequently, unexposed cows were selected according to the date of AI such that cows from exposed herds and unexposed cows underwent AI during the same period in the year.

Fertility Parameter and Data Selection

Fertility was assessed by the occurrence of a repeat AI after the first AI. In case of a return-to-oestrus after the first AI in a lactation, most farmers are likely to decide to reinseminate the cow. In such a context, the occurrence of a repeat AI (return-to-service) after a first AI can be used as a proxy for infertility. The

Using Animal Performance Data to Evidence the Under-Reporting of Case Herds during an Epizootic...

47

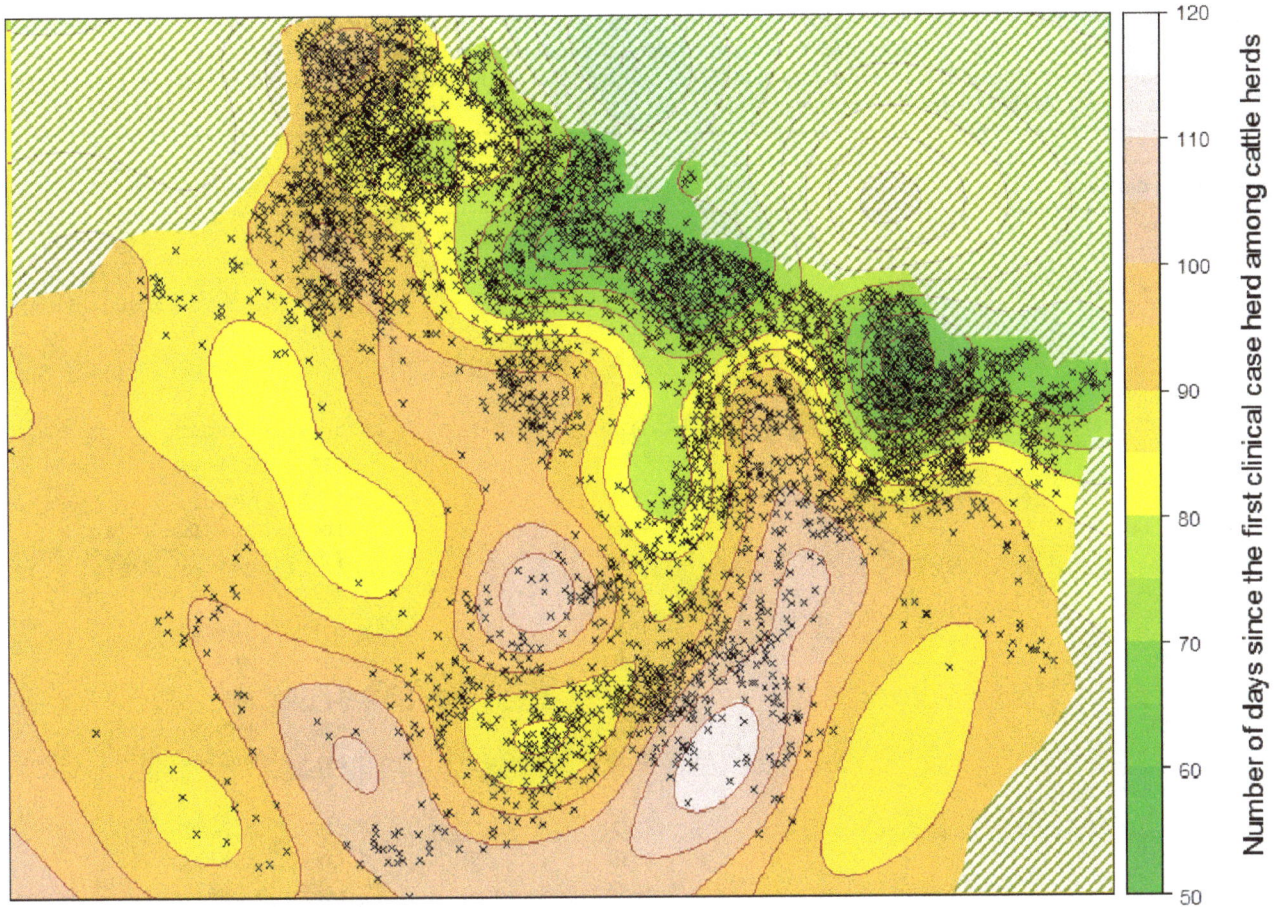

Figure 3. Kriging map of the dates of detection of Bluetongue virus serotype 8 clinical signs, expressed as a number of days since the first clinical case herd during the 2007 epizootic in France (31st July 2007), and location of reported case herds (black crosses). The hatched areas correspond to regions with no data.

criteria used to quantify effect of BTV-8 exposure on fertility was the 90-d-return-to-service, defined as a return-to-service occurring between 18 and 90 d after AI (binary variable). It was assumed that BTV-8 exposure could have 3 possible effects on fertility:

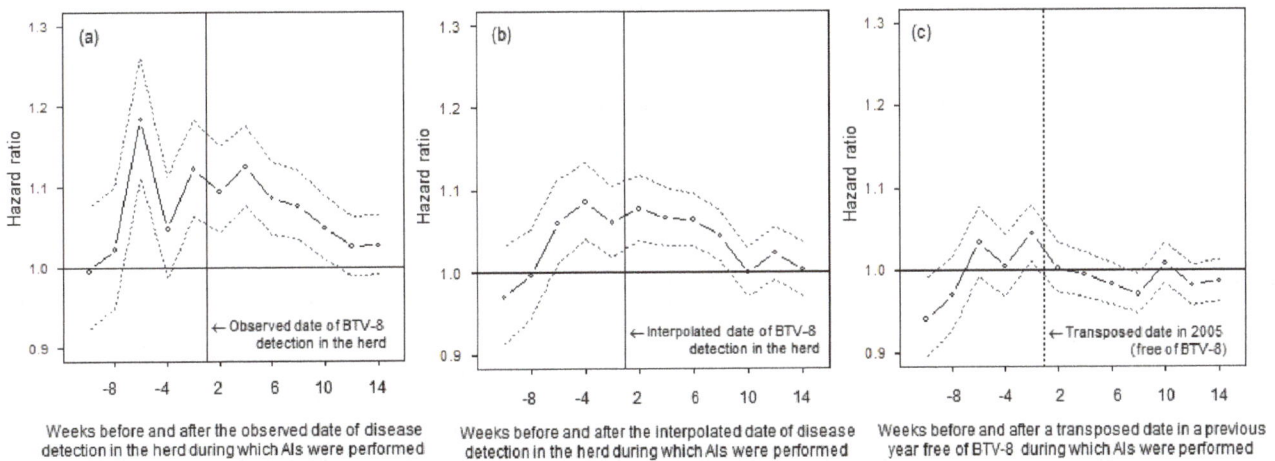

Figure 4. Hazard Ratio (HR) of 90-d-return-to-service before and after (a) the date of Bluetongue virus serotype 8 (BTV-8) clinical detection for case herds reported during the 2007 epizootic, (b) the interpolated date of BTV-8 clinical detection for non-reported herds located in the 2007 outbreak area, (c) the transposed date in a previous year free of BTV (2005) for herds in 2005 located in the 2007 outbreak area, France.

Table 2. Effect of adjustment variables on risk of 90-day-return-to-service for cows which underwent artificial insemination (AI) between 10 weeks before and 14 weeks after the observed date of Bluetongue virus serotype 8 (BTV-8) detection (2,646 case herds), the interpolated date of BTV-8 clinical detection (5,237 non-reported herds) and the transposed date in a year free of BTV-8 (8,215 herds in 2005 located in the 2007 outbreak area).

Variable and classes	Number of AI	HR	95% CI*
Lactation number			
1	179,508	1	Ref
2	120,951	1.10	[1.09–1.12]
3	77,463	1.12	[1.11–1.13]
4 or more	82,137	1.21	[1.19–1.22]
Peak milk yield (category)#			
1	58,772	0.94	[0.93–0.95]
2	115,175	0.97	[0.96–0.98]
3	140,240	1	Ref
4	96,807	1.04	[1.03–1.05]
5	49,065	1.10	[1.08–1.11]
Protein:Fat ratio			
>0; ≤0.58	47,239	1.04	[1.02–1.05]
>0.58; ≤0.66	93,475	1.03	[1.02–1.04]
>0.66; ≤0.75	159,567	1	Ref
>0.75; ≤0.83	105,573	0.98	[0.97–0.99]
>0. 83; ≤1.5	54,205	0.97	[0.96–0.99]
Calving-to-AI interval (days)			
>35; ≤50	35,134	1.25	[1.23–1.27]
>50; ≤62	85,366	1.13	[1.12–1.15]
>62; ≤80	133,327	1.07	[1.05–1.08]
>80; ≤102	109,056	1	Ref
>102; ≤125	55,126	0.95	[0.94–0.97]
>125; ≤150	26,909	0.92	[0.90–0.94]
>150; ≤180	14,366	0.88	[0.86–0.91]
Month of service§			
May	16,198	0.92	[0.90–0.95]
June	16,167	0.89	[0.87–0.92]
July	21,238	0.95	[0.93–0.97]
August	34,268	0.96	[0.94–0.98]
September	46,444	1	Ref
October	71,011	1.01	[0.99–1.02]
November	99,904	0.97	[0.95–0.99]
December	86,194	0.98	[0.96–1.01]
January	45,041	0.98	[0.96–0.99]
February	23,594	1.01	[0.99–1.03]

*95% Confidence interval.
#Classes were constituted according to the distribution of the milk yield production and the lactation number.
§Month of service in 2007 for cows in herds located in the 2007 outbreak area; month of service in 2005 for cows inseminated in 2005 in herds located in the 2007 outbreak area.
The unexposed population was composed of 211,578 cows in 9,485 herds, 2005–2007, France.

conception failure, embryonic death and fetal death in early gestation, all resulting in the same outcome. Cows with non-plausible or extreme data (checked for consistency of calving to first AI interval, AI to calving interval, interval between AI, interval between 2 test-days, peak milk yield and minimum Protein:Fat ratio) and herds with unusual management (unusual demographic structure, delayed first service or very small herds,

low rate of IA indicative of the use of a bull) were excluded. After these exclusions, the study population was composed of 122,079 cows with a first AI performed in 2007 (43,786 cows in case herds and 78,293 in herds with uncertain BTV-8 status) in 7,883 herds located in the epizootic area (2,646 case herds and 5,237 herds with uncertain BTV-8 status). The reference population was composed of 211,578 cows in 9,485 herds located in regions unexposed to BTV-8.

Selection and Classification of AIs to Evaluate the Under-reporting

To evaluate the under-reporting of BTV-8 exposure, 90-d-return-to-service of cows in case herds and cows in herds with uncertain BTV-8 status were compared to those of cows in the reference population. All first AIs performed from 10 weeks before to 14 weeks after the date of BTV-8 exposure (observed or predicted) in herds were selected. The AIs were classified into categories according to the time interval between the date of the AI of cows and the date of exposure (observed or predicted). Intervals of 15 d were considered (see results for categories).

Statistical Models

The relationship between exposure and occurrence of a possible return-to-service was assessed with multivariate Cox models. To account for factors likely to influence the probability of return-to-service, the association between BTV-8 exposure and occurrence of return-to-service was adjusted for several independent variables already described as risk factors for fertility traits in the literature [6,7,8,9,10] as described by Eq. (1):

$$\lambda_{ij}(t|X, HERD) = \lambda_0(t) \times \exp(\beta_i X_i + HERD_j)$$
$$HERD \sim N\left(0, \sum\right) \tag{1}$$

where λ_{ij} is the hazard function at time t for the probability of 90-d-return-to-service following the first AI for the ith cow in the jth herd, X is the vector of the 6 following fixed effect variables: the exposure status (36 classes corresponding to 12 periods of 2 weeks for 3 populations); the lactation number (4 classes); the maximum milk production in kg at the 3 first milk records in the lactation used as a proxy for peak milk yield (5 classes); the minimum of Protein:Fat ratio out of the first 3 milk records (5 classes); the calving-to-AI interval (7 classes) and the month of AI (8 or 10 classes), β is a vector which contains the coefficients for the 6 fixed effect variables and HERD is the random effect term corresponding to the herd number which follow a normal distribution $(0,\sum)$. The random effect term made it possible to adjust for clustering within the data using frailty model. The effects in percentage points of return rate were calculated from estimated hazard ratio (HR). All statistical analyzes were performed by using R software [11], Cox models were performed using the survival package (Therneau T, 2008. A package for survival analysis in S) and kriging map using gstat package (Pebesma, EJ, 2004. Multivariable geostatistics in S).

Selection of a Cow Population to Check the Specificity of the Fertility Decreases

To check whether decreases in fertility in both case herds and herds with uncertain BTV-8 status can be attributable to BTV-8 exposure, possible decrease was also quantified for cows in herds that were not exposed to BTV-8. Indeed, decrease could be related to the climate or diet. This population was considered to demonstrate the specificity of the fertility decreases regarding the BTV-8 exposure, reported or not. This population was composed of cows inseminated in 2005 in herds that were located in the 2007 outbreak area (reported or not). The date around which fertility decreases were quantified corresponded to the same day within the year (called 'transposed date') than the date of exposure (observed or predicted). This population (after the same exclusions than the

exposed and unexposed populations) was composed of 211,578 cows with a first AI in 9,485 herds.

Results

Location of Herds and Unadjusted Return-to-service Rates

Cattle case herds reported after clinical signs in 2007 were located in the north-eastern part of France (Figure 1(a)). The overall 90-day-return-to-service rates were 56.9% for cows in case herds and 56.0% for cows in herds with uncertain BTV-8 status. The overall 90-day-return-to-service rate was 54.2% in the reference population and 54.3% for cows inseminated in 2005 in herds that were located in the 2007 outbreak area (Table 1).

Interpolated Date of Clinical Signs Detection for Herds with Uncertain BTV-8 Status

Figure 2 shows the experimental semivariogram of the observed dates of clinical signs detection in case herds. Some case herds located in the same municipality were detected at different periods of the epizootic. These point pairs had thus a large semivariance, giving a pure random term (nugget effect) of 640 day^2 and a fitted exponential semivariogram model with a semi-variance of 127 day^2 and a range of 9.9 km. The fitted gaussian semivariogram model had a semi-variance of 243 day^2 for a scale parameter (sd) of 82 km that is equivalent to an effective range of about 160 km. The fitted nested semivariogram model, plotted in black in Figure 2, shows the suitability of the fitted model for all distances larger than 10 km. The Gaussian component of the variogram model, in red dashed line, was used to map mid-to-long-range variation by Universal Kriging, filtering short range variation (5 to 10 km) and semivariance due to location uncertainty inside the municipality level. Figure 3 shows the location of the 8,313 cattle herds used as the data sample and the predicted values of the kriging model for the dates of clinical detection of the disease in the outbreak area. Predicted dates of clinical suspicion were expressed as a number of days since the first clinical case detected the 31st July 2007 among cattle herds.

Under-reporting Evidenced Using Performance Data

As expected, exposure to BTV-8 at the time were clinical signs were observed was associated with an increase of 90-d-return-to-service rate for cows in case herds (Figure 4-a). The period of fertility decrease corresponded to AIs performed between 6 weeks before to 10 weeks after the date of clinical detection (HR between 1.05 and 1.18). More interestingly, for cows in herds with uncertain BTV-8 status, an increase of the 90-day-return-to-service rate was also found (Figure 4-b). The period of decreased fertility corresponded to AIs performed between 6 weeks before and 8 weeks after the interpolated date (HR between 1.04 and 1.08). Finally, for cows inseminated in 2005 in herds that were located in the 2007 outbreak area, only a very slight increase of 90-day-return-to-service rate was observed for AIs performed 2 weeks before the date in a previous year free of BTV-8 (HR = 1.04) (Figure 4-c). These fertility decreases corresponded to an increase of 5.2 and 3.0 percentage points of 90-day-return-to-service for cows in case herds and cows in herds with uncertain BTV-8 status, respectively.

The following adjustment variables were significantly associated with a risk of 90-day-return-to-service: lactation number, milk yield, Protein:Fat ratio and calving-to-AI interval. The risk was higher for multiparous cows and for cows with a higher milk yield. In contrast, the risk was lower for cows with a higher Protein:Fat ratio and for cows with a higher calving-to-AI interval (Table 2).

Discussion

The results indicate that fertility data can be used to evidence the under-reporting of cases during an epizootic. Indeed, an decrease in fertility was found for cows in non-reported herds located in the 2007 outbreak area in France, corresponding to 60% of the effect for cows in case herds. Only a very slight decrease in fertility was found when comparing two populations of cows in unexposed herds, indicating that the episodes of fertility decreases quantified in this study were likely attributable to BTV-8 exposure. Moreover, the fertility decreases were precocious relative to the date of clinical suspicion.

The magnitude and duration of the episode of fertility decrease for cows in non-reported herds suggested that some of these herds have been infected by the virus during 2007. If assuming a similar average effect of infection between case herds and non-reported herds, around 60% of non-reported herds located in the 2007 outbreak area would have been infected (if the effect is lower in these herds, the percentage would be greater). This result indicates that production losses in non-reported infected herds could contribute to an important part of the total burden of the epizootic.

Results found in this study are consistent with other publications. A follow-up survey of 50 dairy herds in Belgium conducted between December 2007 and February 2008 indicated that only 20 herds were officially notified as BTV outbreaks whereas all had been infected with BTV-8. The authors indicated that similar discrepancies occurred in all provinces [2]. A study conducted in the Netherlands in 2007 quantified an increase in mortality of dairy cows in non-reported herds located in areas exposed to BTV-8 [12]. This effect corresponded to an increase of 1.11 (95% CI: 1.08–1.13) of the mortality rate ratio for cows >1 year while for cows in confirmed herds, the mortality rate ratio was equal to 1.41 (95% CI: 1.22–1.63). These results suggested that some of the herds that were not notified in exposed areas probably had suffered from BTV-8 infection. In our study, the fertility decrease in non-reported herds was relatively greater, in term of magnitude of effect, than the excess of mortality found in non-reported herds

in the study of Santman-Berends [12]. An explanation could be that cow mortality lead more easily to the suspicion of BTV-8 exposure than a decrease of fertility. Moreover, the delay between virus exposure and the reproductive event observed made it difficult to associate them. There were probably less infected herds not reported that experienced an excess of mortality due to BTV-8 exposure than those which experienced a decrease of fertility for some cows.

Fertility could vary among regions due to differences in herd management and/or local weather conditions. The unexposed population considered in this study was composed of herds located in regions unexposed to the virus in 2007. A difference of fertility – independently of the exposure – between exposed and unexposed regions could bias the quantification of the effect of BTV-8 exposure. To check whether such a difference existed, the fertility before the beginning of BTV-8 epizootic, in 2005, was compared between the 2 regions exposed and unexposed. To do so, the same Cox model using the adjustment variables previously described was considered. No difference was shown, indicating that fertility was comparable before the exposure between the 2 regions. Therefore, the decreased fertility evidenced can be attributable to BTV-8 exposure and not to differences in herd management and/or local weather conditions. Finally, it was also check that there was no difference when comparing fertility between 2005 and 2007 in the exposed region.

The evidence of under-reporting of cases during an epizootic in the case of BTV-8 outbreak could be generalized to pathogens that affect cattle's performance. In cattle, most pathogens, including zoonotic agents such as Coxiella burnetii [13,14] or Rift Valley fever virus [15], have detrimental effects on cow's performance. These effects can either be due to the tropism in genital tracts or indirectly due to the decreasing food intake associated with clinical signs.

Author Contributions

Analyzed the data: SN PM. Contributed reagents/materials/analysis tools: SN PM. Wrote the paper: SN CF HS FB PM.

References

1. Durand B, Zanella G, Biteau-Coroller F, Locatelli C, Baurier F et al. (2010) Anatomy of Bluetongue Virus Serotype 8 Epizootic Wave, France, 2007–2008. Emerging Infect Dis. 16(12): 1861–8.
2. Saegerman C, Mellor P, Uyttenhoef A, Hanon JB, Kirschvink N et al. (2010) The most likely time and place of introduction of BTV8 into Belgian ruminants. PloS one. 5(2): e9405.
3. Elbers ARW, Backx A, Meroc E, Gerbier G, Staubach C et al. (2008) Field observations during the bluetongue serotype 8 epidemic in 2006: I. Detection of first outbreaks and clinical signs in sheep and cattle in Belgium, France and the Netherlands. Prev Vet Med. 87(1–2): 21–30.
4. Santman-Berends IM, Hage JJ, Rijn PA, Stegeman JA, Schaik GV (2010) Bluetongue virus serotype 8 (BTV-8) infection reduces fertility of Dutch dairy cattle and is vertically transmitted to offspring. Theriogenology. 74(8): 1377–84.
5. Nusinovici S, Seegers H, Joly A, Beaudeau F, Fourichon C (2012) Quantification and at-risk period of decreased fertility associated with exposure to Bluetongue virus serotype 8 in naïve dairy cattle herds. J Dairy Sci. 95(6): 3008–20.
6. Robert A, Beaudeau F, Seegers H, Joly A, Philipot JM (2004) Large scale assessment of the effect associated with bovine viral diarrhoea virus infection on fertility of dairy cows in 6149 dairy herds in Brittany (Western France). Theriogenology. 61(1): 117–27.
7. Malher X, Beaudeau F, Philipot JM (2006) Effects of sire and dam genotype for complex vertebral malformation (CVM) on risk of return-to-service in Holstein dairy cows and heifers. Theriogenology. 65(6): 1215–25.
8. Marce C, Beaudeau F, Bareille N, Seegers H, Fourichon C (2009) Higher non-return rate associated with Mycobacterium avium subspecies paratuberculosis infection at early stage in Holstein dairy cows. Theriogenology. 71(5): 807–16.
9. Hillers JK, Senger PL, Darlington RL, Fleming WN (1984) Effects of production, season, age of cow, days dry, and days in milk on conception to first service in large commercial dairy herds. J Dairy Sci. 67(4): 861–7.
10. Seegers H (1998) Performances de reproduction du troupeau bovin laitier: variations dues aux facteurs zootechniques autres que ceux liés à l'alimentation. J Natl GTV. 57–66.
11. R Core Team. R: A language and environment for statistical computing. R Foundation for Statistical Computing, Vienna, Austria. ISBN 3–900051–07–0.
12. Santman-Berends IM, van Schaik G, Bartels CJ, Stegeman JA, Vellema P (2011) Mortality attributable to bluetongue virus serotype 8 infection in Dutch dairy cows. Vet Microbiol. 148(2–4): 183–8.
13. Saegerman C, Speybroeck N, Dal Pozzo F, Czaplicki G (2013) Clinical Indicators of Exposure to Coxiella burnetii in Dairy Herds. Transbound Emerg Dis. doi: 10.1111/tbed.12070.
14. Agerholm JS (2013) Coxiella burnetii associated reproductive disorders in domestic animals–a critical review. Acta Vet Scand 55: 13.
15. Coetzer JA (1982) The pathology of Rift Valley fever. II. Lesions occurring in field cases in adult cattle, calves and aborted fetuses. Onderstepoort J Vet Res. 49(1): 11–7.

7

Using Hormones to Manage Dairy Cow Fertility: The Clinical and Ethical Beliefs of Veterinary Practitioners

Helen M. Higgins[1]*, Eamonn Ferguson[2], Robert F. Smith[3], Martin J. Green[1]

1 Population Health and Welfare Group, School of Veterinary Medicine and Science, University of Nottingham, Sutton Bonington, United Kingdom, **2** Personality, Social Psychology, and Health Research Group, School of Psychology, University of Nottingham, Nottingham, United Kingdom, **3** Division of Livestock Health and Welfare, School of Veterinary Science, University of Liverpool, Neston, United Kingdom

Abstract

In the face of a steady decline in dairy cow fertility over several decades, using hormones to assist reproduction has become common. In the European Union, hormones are prescription-only medicines, giving veterinary practitioners a central role in their deployment. This study explored the clinical and ethical beliefs of practitioners, and provides data on their current prescribing practices. During 2011, 93 practitioners working in England completed a questionnaire (95% response rate). Of the 714 non-organic farms they attended, only 4 farms (0.6%) never used hormones to assist the insemination of lactating dairy cows. Practitioners agreed (>80%) that hormones improve fertility and farm businesses profitability. They also agreed (>80%) that if farmers are able to tackle management issues contributing to poor oestrus expression, then over a five year period these outcomes would both improve, relative to using hormones instead. If management issues are addressed instead of prescribing hormones, practitioners envisaged a less favourable outcome for veterinary practices profitability (p<0.01), but an improvement in genetic selection for fertility (p<0.01) and overall cow welfare (p<0.01). On farms making no efforts to address underlying management problems, long-term routine use at the start of breeding for timing artificial insemination or inducing oestrus was judged "unacceptable" by 69% and 48% of practitioners, respectively. In contrast, practitioners agreed (≥90%) that both these types of use are acceptable, provided a period of time has been allowed to elapse during which the cow is observed for natural oestrus. Issues discussed include: weighing quality versus length of cow life, fiscal factors, legal obligations, and balancing the interests of all stakeholders, including the increasing societal demand for food. This research fosters debate and critical appraisal, contributes to veterinary ethics, and encourages the pro-active development of professional codes of conduct.

Editor: Bernhard Kaltenboeck, Auburn University, United States of America

Funding: This research was funded by the Wellcome Trust[087797/Z/08/Z], www.wellcome.ac.uk. The funder had no role in study design, data collection and analysis, decision to publish, or preparation of the manuscript.

Competing Interests: The authors have declared that no competing interests exist.

* E-mail: helen.higgins@nottingham.ac.uk.

Introduction

Post World War II, scientific and technological advances enabled the industrialization and intensification of agriculture. Concurrently, this has generated a multitude of ethical issues concerning the use of technologies in food production and how farm animals *ought* to be cared for [1,2]. It is perhaps surprizing, therefore, that veterinary ethics has only recently emerged as an academic discipline; the paucity of literature and lack of any devoted research journal negates an important subject that presents unique challenges, inherently distinct from medical ethics [3]. To start to address this gap in the literature this research concerns the use of a reproductive technology, the prescription of synthetic hormones to manage and improve dairy cow fertility.

There has been a steady decline in the reproductive performance of dairy cows over several decades [4,5]. Over this time period market forces have driven efficiency savings and lead to genetic selection for production traits, especially higher milk yield. As a result, the specialist dairy Holstein breed is now a substantial component of the UK national herd, managed predominately in a 'high input high output' farming system [6]. It is widely accepted that the modern Holstein cow displays less

overt signs of oestrus behaviour and for a reduced period of time relative to her lower yielding predecessors [7]. Hence todays farming and veterinary communities are challenged with managing the fertility of an animal that inherently has poorer reproductive performance. Currently in the UK, the annual culling rate for dairy herds is 23% and poor fertility is the commonest reason for culling [8]. In the face of this decline in fertility performance, hormones have been advocated [9] and increasingly been deployed to assist breeding, although to the authors' knowledge there are no data quantifying the scale of such use currently, nor that has charted this use over time. Hormones, along with all veterinary medicines, are paid for by the farmer.

This study concerned three hormones (progesterone, prostaglandin and gonadotrophin releasing hormone), when prescribed to adult lactating dairy cows, *without* reproductive pathology. Two types of use were considered. Firstly, using hormones to induce oestrus - if the farmer knows when to expect to see the cow in oestrus he will observe her more closely and this increases the probability of the cow being served either by the bull or by artificial insemination (AI); this is subsequently referred to as 'oestrus induction'. Secondly, using hormones over a period of time (often referred to as a synchronization programme) to enable

AI on a known date and time; this is subsequently referred to as 'fixed-time AI'. Oestrus induction requires less hormonal treatments but the farmer must observe the cows several times per day for oestrus (oestrus detection); fixed-time AI involves more hormonal treatments but removes the need for oestrus detection completely. In both cases, hormones can either be used as soon as the cow becomes eligible for breeding after calving, or alternatively, they may only be used if the cow has not been inseminated by the end of a certain period of time, during which she is observed for natural oestrus by the farmer. There are therefore four main ways to assist breeding, as summarised in Figure 1, with (a) involving the greatest quantities of hormones, decreasing in order to (d) with the least. The entire eligible cow population would receive hormones in (a) and (c) but a smaller proportion, depending on the success of natural oestrus detection, in (b) and (d). We focused on the acceptability of use in these four contexts when management problems exist. The acceptability in other scenarios was not explored, such as when unpredictable events occur (e.g. crop failures due to poor weather) which can have a major and unavoidable impact on fertility.

Importantly, in the public eye, the word 'hormone' in the context of food production may have negative connotations; historically there has been considerable societal controversy over the prescription of certain hormones to cattle [10]. However 'hormone' is a term that classifies a very diverse group of physiological signalling compounds, and the effect and acceptability of use rests entirely on the specific drug and prescribing context. Moreover, in the European Union, all hormones are legally categorised as 'Prescription Only Medicines Veterinarian' (POM-V) [11], making them subject to stringent control under legislation contained within Directive 2001/82/EC (as amended) [12]. In the UK this legislation is enforced by the Veterinary Medicines Directorate (VMD), an executive government agency [13,14]. In particular, manufacturers must prove that any medicine residues in edible tissues are below the statutory 'maximum residue limits' and hence safe for consumers health [15,16]. The VMD monitors on-going safety by continually testing produce for residues [13,17].

Several stakeholders have vested interests in the debate over the use of this reproductive technology in the context described. This paper explores the issue primarily from the perspective of veterinary practitioners working in private practice in England. As POM-V medicines, administration legally requires prescription from a veterinarian, giving them a central and influential role with respect to how and when these medicines are deployed. Understanding the clinical and ethical beliefs of a range of veterinary practitioners, and any divergence, is important. However to our knowledge, there are no published data on this, or their current prescribing practices. The main aims of this study

were therefore: (i) to report the current prescription of hormones to assist breeding by a sample of veterinary practitioners in England, (ii) to explore their clinical beliefs and ethical stance.

Methods

Instrument Design

Purposive sampling was used to select two veterinary academics from the University of Nottingham, one veterinary academic from the University of Liverpool and two private veterinary practitioners. Individual semi-structured interviews were conducted by the first author, and the information gathered (see Figure 2) was used to inform and design a questionnaire that was subsequently piloted on two veterinary academics, one psychologist and three veterinary practitioners. The final document comprised a mixture of question formats, and was delivered to a sample of veterinary practitioners (see next section). The questionnaire is available in Appendix S1 and subsequent references to question numbers relate to this Appendix.

Recruitment of Veterinary Practitioners

Eligible practitioners were those providing healthcare to dairy cattle in England during their normal working hours, and working within a veterinary practice that contained at least one practitioner possessing post-graduate cattle qualifications – specifically, the Royal College of Veterinary Surgeons (RCVS) post-graduate Certificate in Cattle Health and Production or the Diploma in Bovine Reproduction. A two-stage cluster design stratified by geographic location was used. Veterinary practices were selected first, using a 'without-replacement systematic method' [19], that involved randomly selecting a starting point and then systematically selecting practices with probability proportional to the number of practitioners they contained. Once 20 practices had consented to take part, five practitioners were then randomly selected from within each practice by using the random number generator function in the software programme 'R' version 2.13.1 [18] to pick numerical identifiers; all praciioners were recuirted in practices that contained less than five eligible practitioners. With this sampling strategy, every individual had approximately the same probability of being selected, irrespective of the size of the practice they worked in. The online database (http://www.rcvs.org.uk/) supplied by RCVS provided a sampling frame of veterinary practices. Practitioners were provided with an inconvenience allowance of £100 per hour (pro-rata). Data were collected from the 8th June to 1st September 2011.

Data Analysis

The data was initially entered into Excel (Version 2010, Microsoft Corporation). To compare how practitioners' opinions

a) Immediate fixed-time AI. Artificial insemination on a known date and time to be used immediately a cow becomes eligible for breeding, post-calving

b) Delayed fixed-time AI. Artificial insemination on a known date and time to be used if a cow is not inseminated by some defined point after calving, but not as soon as she is eligible for breeding

c) Immediate oestrus induction. Inducing oestrus immediately a cow becomes eligible for breeding, post-calving

d) Delayed oestrus induction. Inducing oestrus to be used if a cow is not inseminated by some defined point after calving, but not as soon as she is eligible for breeding

Figure 1. The four main ways to assist breeding in lactating dairy cattle using hormones.

Potential Advantages

- Facilitates regular veterinary visits to farms.
- Strengthens veterinary-farmer relationship.
- Generates opportunities for vets to identify and address other health/welfare issues on farm.
- Quick and practical to implement.
- Fertility may rapidly improve for relatively low investment; fewer cattle may be culled.
- May reduce future health/welfare problems related to prolonged calving intervals.
- The improved fertility is easily attributable to the action taken (i.e. the use of hormones).
- Provides vets with revenue.
- Farmers may be unable to afford the labour/time for oestrus detection.
- Farmers may be unable to make the capital investment needed to address any underlying causes of poor fertility.
- Improved job satisfaction for vets.
- Positive perception of the veterinary profession as providers of 'innovative technical solutions'.

Potential Disadvantages

- May mask underlying management and health/welfare problems.
- May diminish the need/urgency to tackle the underlying cause(s) of the problem
- May be over-prescribed; alternative (and possibly cheaper) approaches may be over-looked.
- Efficacy/cost-effectiveness may be falsely assumed if outcomes are not monitored.
- Potential for misuse exists.
- Economic benefits have not been proven against alternative approaches.
- Long-term use involves on-going costs to farmers.
- Widespread use may mean that genetic selection for improved fertility may be more difficult in the long term.
- There is a welfare cost to cows from administration
- Negative perception of the veterinary profession as providers of 'hormones' not 'expertise'.

Figure 2. Potential advantages/disadvantages of prescribing hormones from a veterinary perspective. The context relates to the use of hormones to assist breeding in lactating dairy cattle without reproductive pathology. The lists provide a summary of interviews with three veterinary academics and two veterinary practitioners. There is no significance attached to the vertical order of items.

changed between related categorical questions, two-sided marginal tests of homogeneity were performed [20] (an extension of McNemar's test for categorical variables) using the software programme SPSS Statistics (Version, 20, IBM); the significance level was <0.05.

Factor analysis was performed using the 'fa' function in the 'psych' package in the software programme R [10]. The number of factors to extract was based on a combination of: (i) Cattell's scree plot [21] (ii) eigenvalues greater than 1.0 [22] (iii) interpretability of extracted factors [23] and (iv) chi squared goodness of fit statistic for the maximum likelihood extraction (for a good fit p>0.05) [24]. Sensitivity of the results to the method of analysis was assessed with respect to two different extraction methods (maximum likelihood and principal axes) combined with two different rotations, varimax [25] and promax [26]. A final check on goodness of fit was assessed by the Root Mean Square Error of Approximation (RMSEA); an RMSEA ≤0.06 indicated acceptable fit [27]. Only variables with absolute loading values of ≥0.3 were included in the interpretation of a factor [28]. Variables with little or no variance were excluded from the interpretation. Factor scores (based on all items) for each practitioner were estimated using regression; the distribution of factor scores was assessed to establish majority views across survey questions.

Three logistic regression models were fitted to identify factors associated with responses to three questions in the questionnaire:

i. Practitioners reporting concern (yes/no) over the prescription of hormones to assist breeding (question 5).

ii. Practitioner judgement regarding the acceptability (yes/no) of the long term routine use of immediate fixed-time AI as a substitute for good management i.e. in herds with underlying management problems that are not being addressed (question 16a).

iii. Practitioner judgement regarding the acceptability (yes/no) of the long term routine use of immediate oestrus induction as a substitute for good management (question 16c).

Questions 16a and 16c carried a 'don't know' option and observations falling in this category were omitted from the analysis. MLwiN software [29] was used and veterinary practice was included as a normally distributed random effect to account for the clustered nature of the data. All models used a logit link function and a penalized quasi-likelihood method for estimation [30]. There were 30 (level 1) covariates available (see Appendix S2). For questions 16a and 16c, factors identified from the factor analysis were also included as covariates. Univariate analysis was conducted and covariates with a P-value of ≤0.05 are reported. Covariates that achieved P≤0.1 were carried forward for model building, and were retained in the final model if they achieved P≤0.05, having adjusted for the other covariates.

The study was approved in full by the Research and Ethics committee, School of Veterinary Medicine and Science, University of Nottingham.

Results

Response Rates and Characteristics of Participants

Veterinary practice response rate was 95% (19/20). Non-participation of one practice was due to a failure for all eligible practitioners within it to agree to participate. Another practice was selected and consented, from the same region. These 20 practices contained 95 eligible practitioners, 93 of whom replied, giving a practitioner response rate of 98% (93/95).

Table 1. Characteristics of veterinary practitioners (n = 94).

Characteristic	Result	
Gender	Male: 59 (63%)	Female: 34 (37%)
Employment status	Partner: 37 (40%)	Assistant: 56 (60%)
Post-graduate cattle qualifications	Yes: 23 (25%)	No: 70 (75%)
Years qualified	Median: 7	Range: 0–37

Of the 20 practices, 6 were located in the North, 3 in the Midlands, and 11 in the South of England. Table 1 summarises practitioner characteristics.

Current Prescribing Practices of Veterinary Practitioners in England

Of the 93 respondents, 81 conducted dairy cow fertility work at least once per month on one or more farms; between these practitioners this tallied to 753 farms in total, 39 (5.2%) of which operated under organic regulations that prohibit the use of hormones to assist breeding. Of the 714 non-organic farms, 4 (0.6%) never used hormones to assist breeding, 56 (7.8%) used hormones for immediate fixed-time AI on the majority of cows, 193 (27.0%) used hormones for delayed fixed-time AI on the majority of cows. The remaining 461 farms (64.6%) used hormones to induce oestrus to varying extents, and/or for occasional fixed-time AI.

Practitioners' Clinical Beliefs

A key clinical question was whether prescribing hormones contributes to making any underlying causes of poor oestrus expression, better or worse (Q11). Responses by category were: better 9 (9.8%), no effect 32 (34.7%), worse 33 (35.9%), don't know 18 (19.6%). With respect to underlying causes, practitioners were asked to list the three most important issues that they believed contributed most often to the problem of poor oestrus expression on dairy farms, see Figure 3.

Practitioners also answered a pair of questions, each concerning five key outcomes. The first question asked what effect prescribing hormones would have on each outcome (Q8), and the second question asked what effect tackling the root causes of poor oestrus

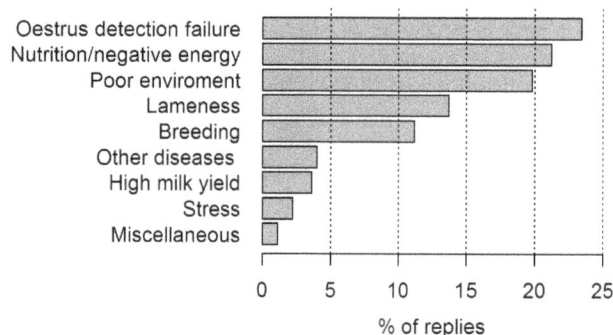

Figure 3. Factors believed to contribute to poor oestrus expression on dairy farms (n = 278 replies). Practitioners' replies to question 13a were categorized to reflect the answers given, but overlap existed in terms of concepts (e.g. high yield, breeding and lameness are related). The raw data are available in Appendix S3.

expression would have after a five year period, if this approach was taken instead of using hormones (13b); the latter was conditional on a crucial assumption, namely that farmers were in a position to make the necessary management changes, including any capital investments required. Responses to the two questions are compared in Figure 4. A two-sided marginal test of homogeneity on this data showed that if underlying management issues are addressed instead of prescribing hormones, practitioners envisaged a less favourable outcome for veterinary practices profitability (p<0.01), but an improvement in genetic selection for fertility (p<0.01) and overall dairy cow welfare (p<0.01).

Practitioners' responses to the remaining clinical questions are given in Figure 5, whilst their perceptions of other stakeholders are illustrated in Figure 6. With regard to decision-making, the main influence over practitioners' decision to prescribe (Q12) was: veterinarians 46 (51%), farmers 32 (35%), both 13 (14%). Theoretically speaking, if practitioners only had to please themselves and the dairy cow (Q10), then 55 (60%) would use hormones, versus 37 (40%) who would not.

Practitioners' Ethical Beliefs

Practitioners' responses to the question "Does the use of fertility drugs to get dairy cows served give you any cause for concern?" were divided: 48 (52%) yes, 45 (48%) no. Positive respondents were asked to describe their concerns. Their answers have been categorised in Figure 7, the raw data are available in Appendix S4. The logistic regression results for factors associated with practitioners reporting concern are reported in Table 2.

Practitioners' ethical beliefs regarding the acceptability in the different prescribing contexts are provided in Table 3. Acceptability was subject in each case to two important conditions: (i) long term routine use, i.e. involving the majority of cows, (ii) prescribing when underlying problems definitely exist that are causing the problem but are *not* being addressed.

Factor analysis identified two factors accounting for 30% of the variance. Technical details of this analysis, including the rotated factor matrix are included in Appendix S5. Factor 1 was interpreted as a 'positive attitude towards the outcomes of prescribing hormones to assist breeding'. Factor 2 was interpreted as a 'positive attitude towards outcomes if underlying causes of poor oestrus expression are tackled'. Distribution of factor scores suggested that for those variables where there was diversity in opinion, the majority of practitioners tended overall towards both a negative attitude towards the outcomes of using pharmaceutical intervention and a positive attitude towards outcomes that could be achieved if the underlying causes of poor oestrus expression can be addressed.

Logistic regression revealed that only one covariate, years qualified, was positively associated with practitioners judging long term routine use of immediate fixed-time AI acceptable in the face of unaddressed management issues (p = 0.03, OR = 1.05 per extra year, 95% CI 1.04 to 1.11).

Practitioner acceptability of long term routine use of immediate oestrus induction in the face of unaddressed management issues was positively associated with two covariates: (i) the number of farms for which the practitioner was personally currently prescribing hormones for the purpose of any form of oestrus induction (p = 0.02, OR = 1.10 per extra farm, 95% CI 1.02 to 1.24), and (ii) practitioners scores for factor 1 i.e. a positive attitude towards using hormones to assist breeding (p = 0.02, OR = 2.1 per unit increase in score, 95% CI 1.1 to 3.7). It was also negatively associated with one covariate: practitioners score for factor 2 i.e. a positive attitude towards outcomes if underlying causes of poor oestrus expression are tackled (p = 0.02, OR = 0.54 per unit

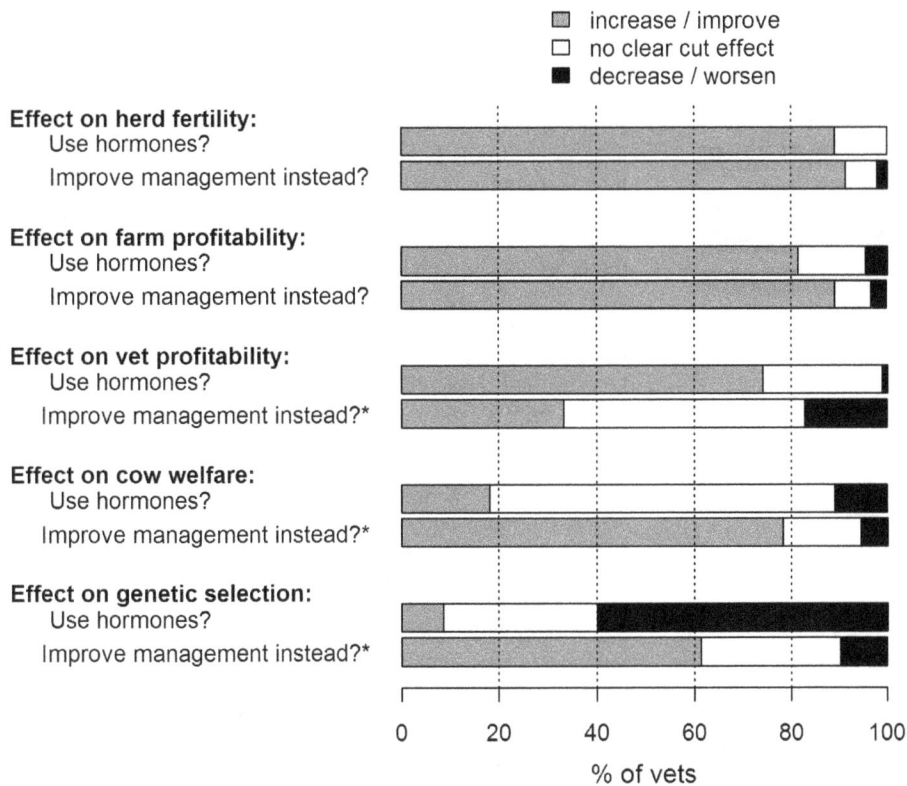

Figure 4. The effect of prescribing hormones versus addressing underlying causes instead over 5 years (n = 93 vets). *denotes a statistically significant change in the distribution of responses between categories, from the outcome if hormones are used to the outcome if management issues are improved instead (p<0.01).

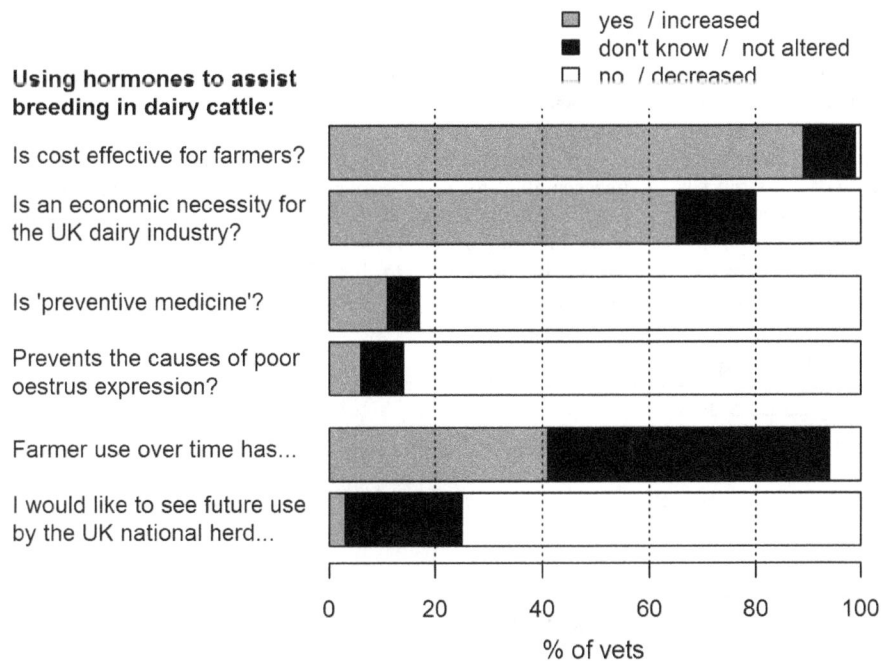

Figure 5. Practitioners' responses to clinical questions (n = 93). All questions relate to use in lactating dairy cattle, without reproductive pathology. As listed in the figure, these relate to questions 2, 17, 7, 9, 6, and 14 of the questionnaire.

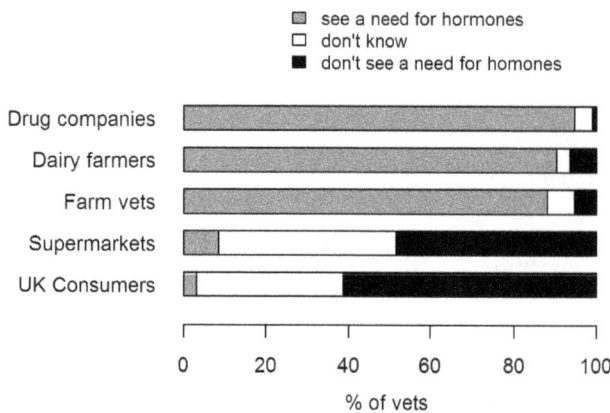

Figure 6. Practitioners' perceptions of other stakeholders (n = 93). Question 15(a-e) asked practitioners to state whether they believe other stakeholders see a need to prescribe hormones to assist breeding in lactating dairy cattle.

increase in score, 95% CI 0.31 to 0.92). The final multivariate model contained all three covariates with negligible alterations to their parameter estimates or standard errors.

Finally, participants were invited to make additional comments; 25/93 (27%) did so, and some practitioners wrote additional comments throughout the questionnaire (see Appendix S6).

Discussion

With regard to the acceptability of using hormones to assist breeding in lactating dairy cattle, our results show that even when management problems exist that are causing poor fertility and are not being addressed, the majority of veterinary practitioners judged any type of long term routine use acceptable, provided it was not straight after the start of the breeding period. This may reflect a deontological stance, related to the economic necessity for cows to become pregnant quickly after calving to avoid culling; practitioners' may consider it wrong to let animals be culled that could be saved, especially given they have a sworn an oath to 'ensure the health and welfare of animals committed to my care' [31]. There is also a clinical argument to re-breed cows quickly, since this may reduce the risk of future health problems [32]. Hormonal treatments are quick and easy to implement, however if routine use diminishes the need to tackle root causes, this may have health and welfare implications for the herd. Clinically, there

is also the question of whether using hormones contributes towards making any underlying causes of poor oestrus expression better or worse. Veterinary opinion here was ambiguous and divided but not positive, and it is worth noting that time devoted to oestrus detection is also time devoted to disease detection. A utilitarian analysis of 'do the greatest good for the greatest number' over a long period may be less supportive of use, although importantly, tackling the root causes may require large capital investment, sustained changes in human behaviour, and take time to resolve; the latter also has implications for sustaining farmer motivation. Two veterinary ethical issues reside here that need advancement. First, how to define and measure a cow's quality of life, and second how to weigh length versus quality of cow life. In human medicine, the quandary of weighing length versus quality of life has seen 'quality adjusted life years' (QALY) used for healthcare resource allocation by organizations such as The National Institute for Health and Clinical Excellence; although QALY is controversial [33] and in need of further research [34]. No equivalent practical decision making tool exists for veterinary practitioners, and the issues involved in developing any such measure are different and arguably even more complex.

Although this survey did not specifically explore how practitioners arrived at their answers with regards to the acceptability of using hormones, some insight can be gained from the additional comments they made. In particular, one practitioner commented "it is [acceptable] in humans", however there are difficulties with attempting to make reference to seemingly analogous prescribing contexts in the humans. In women the decision to undergo hormonal fertility treatment is a conscious choice, based on knowledge of the advantages and disadvantages of doing so. It is impossible to know if a cow, given the same knowledge (which we cannot impart to them) would make a similar choice to the one that we make for them - and this is assuming that cows can reason. Moreover, the reasons for use and outcomes are very different. Hormones are used to facilitate pregnancy in both fertile and non-fertile animals for reasons related, at least in part, to profitability and human convenience, and non-pregnancy results in culling for human management reasons. In contrast, hormones are only used to facilitate pregnancy in infertile humans, for the sole reason of improving fertility per se, and within a guaranteed non-fatal outcome.

Our results showed that some practitioners did consider it unacceptable to use hormones routinely when management problems are not addressed, especially if conducted at the start of the breeding period. However in reality, the line that separates 'reasonable assistance to breed' from 'a substitute for good management' may not always be clear-cut. This raises the

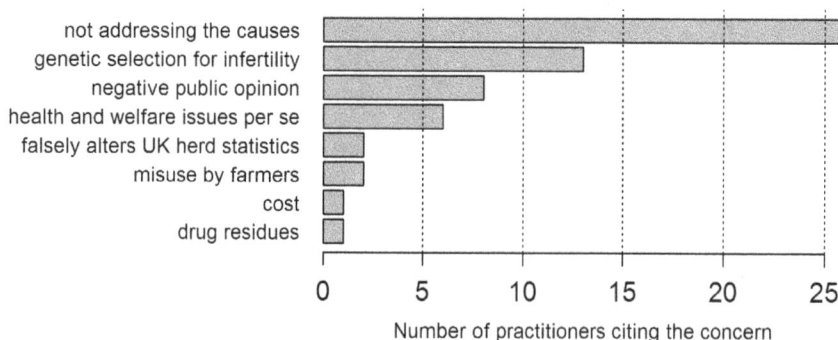

Figure 7. Practitioners' concerns regarding the use of hormones to assist breeding in lactating dairy cattle (n = 48). Note: some practitioners cited more than one concern.

Table 2. Logistic regression results for practitioner characteristics associated with reporting concern over the prescription of hormones to assist breeding.

Practitioner characteristic+	Univariable analysis		Multivariable analysis	
	Odds Ratio(95% CI)	P-value	Odds Ratio(95% CI)	P-value
Currently prescribes hormones for delayed fixed-time AI*?	3.66(1.4–10.3)	0.01		
Attended professional training event on dairy cattle fertility within 2 years?	3.89(1.52–9.94)	<0.01	3.72(1.41–9.83)	<0.01
Reports reading the journal 'UK Vet'?	3.41(1.31–8.85)	0.01		
Number of journals read (odds ratio per additional journal).	1.54(1.09–2.17)	0.01	1.47(1.04–2.08)	0.03

+ The full list of covariates available is provided in Appendix S2.
*fixed-time artificial insemination to be used if a cow has not been inseminated by some defined point after calving, but not as soon as she is eligible to be bred from.

question of whether veterinary practitioners with a business contract to provide services to a farmer, have a legal obligation to prescribe if requested by a paying client. Legally, as POM-V medicines, the decision to prescribe is the practitioners alone [35]. A farmer who disagreed could attest to a breach of business contact and claim for loss of earnings through a civil court, or in the UK, they could claim professional misconduct to the RCVS. However no precedent has been set and speculating on the outcome is difficult; ordinarily a farmer would terminate the business contract and employ the services of another. By demonstrating the diversity in clinical beliefs and ethical acceptability amongst practitioners, our results suggest that finding someone else to prescribe would not be difficult. Furthermore, veterinarians have professional obligations not only to the animals under their care, but also to farmers and to themselves. Indeed it is postulated that some of the diversity in practitioners' beliefs related to their empathy towards the various stakeholders which was not directly captured in our survey; this may partly explain why the factor analysis accounted for only one third of the observed variation. In this regard, in the Code of Professional Conduct for Veterinary Surgeons [36], produced by the RCVS, it states: "…veterinary surgeons should balance the professional responsibilities, having regard first to animal welfare." However, taking an ethical stance as an individual working in private veterinary practice is complicated by the conflicting interests - there is the potential for a substantial loss in revenue. Practitioners have both a

need and a right to earn a living, and there are consequences not only for themselves, but also for the support staff that they employ.

Our results suggest that the use of hormones to assist breeding in England is widespread, and the majority of practitioners we surveyed wanted to see future national use decreased. However this represents a challenge for the profession, especially given the conflicting interests described in the previous paragraph. Thus, our results lend support to the *pro-active* development of professional ethical codes of conduct by the RCVS that all veterinarians should abide to. Pursuing a reactive approach is unlikely to be sufficient in the future; the challenge for the 21st century is to provide the rapidly rising world population with a sustainable supply of food, in the context of an increasing demand for animal products, global climate change and declining resources. One practitioner justified their replies in the context of the wider perspective: "all my acceptable answers are making the assumption that the Holstein and its genetics and increased yield and decreased fertility is here to stay to satisfy the need for dairy produce to feed the population." How to weigh the interests of all stakeholders in the wider context is a crucial question, but currently it is consumers who have the defining influence; in a market-driven playing field it is consumers who collectively, although perhaps unwittingly, drive the efficiency savings and set the economic boundaries within which farmers and veterinary surgeons work. Furthermore, few would argue that it is important for the UK to be able to compete on global market.

With regard to consumers and the public, some practitioners had concerns over negative public perception and the majority believed that UK consumers would not see a need for hormones. It is speculated that these concerns may in part be based on beliefs that the public are not well informed on the issue and that prima facie they would perceive it negatively because it involves hormones, a word that already holds negative connotations for many in the context of food production. However, the actual view of the well informed public is unknown, and needs to be quantified so that the veterinary profession can respond accordingly. In this respect, it is worth noting that in the UK the VMD has a strong track record for ensuring the responsible and safe use of POM-V veterinary medicines and enforcing the legislation contained within the EU Directive [17]. Furthermore there are numerous examples were financial remuneration by doctors has been perceived negatively by the public and adversely affected the level of trust between the public and the medical profession [37]. The inherent financial conflict of interests that inevitably arise from exclusively private veterinary practice will always have the

Table 3. Practitioner acceptability of long-term routine prescription of hormones to assist breeding when management problems are not addressed (questions 16 and 18).

Prescribing context	Number of practitioners		
	Acceptable	Unacceptable	Don't know
Immediate fixed-time AI	25(31%*)	56(69%)	12
Delayed fixed-time AI	81(90%)	9(10%)	3
Immediate oestrus induction	44(52%)	41(48%)	8
Delayed oestrus induction	87(98%)	2(2%)	4
In general	75(82%)	8(9%)	9

*Percentages relate to the definitive replies.

potential to serve as a basis for undermining faith in veterinary expertise. This highlights the importance of studies such as these, which aim in part to inform stakeholders, as well as professional codes of conduct which provide reassurance to the public.

This study has explored some of the issues surrounding the use of one reproductive technology in a given context, but it is not difficult to envisage that veterinary ethical and clinical issues of the type debated here will become more numerous in the future. A key UK government policy for livestock production is 'sustainable intensification' [38], and it is proposed that this will be achieved through new scientific and technological advances; thus it is highly probable that, as occurred post World War II, these will bring with them an upsurge in new ethical challenges. Indeed several, such as cloning, are already upon us [3,4]. There is an urgent need to advance veterinary ethics as a subject and to ensure that it is firmly embedded in undergraduate veterinary curricula. Society has bestowed a considerable responsibility to the veterinary profession for both farm animals and their keepers. In return, society expects us to be acutely aware of the major ethical issues we are part of, to be pro-active and consistent in our approach to tackling them, and to keep the public informed; failure to do so runs the serious risk of loss of autonomy [1,3].

Supporting Information

Appendix S1 The questionnaire. This file contains the three page questionnaire which was delivered to a sample of veterinary practitioners working in England, UK.

Appendix S2 Covariate definitions and descriptions. This file contains details of all the covariates used in the statistical analysis.

Appendix S3 Factors believed to contribute to poor oestrus expression on dairy farms. This file contains the free text relies from the 93 practitioners in response to the question: Please list the 3 most important areas that you believe contribute most often to the problem of poor heat expression on dairy farms.

Appendix S4 Practitioners' concerns regarding the prescription of hormones to assist breeding in lactating dairy cattle. This file contains the free text replies detailing the concerns raised by 48 (of 93) practitioners who responded yes to the question: Does the use of fertility drugs to get dairy cows served give you any cause for concern?

Appendix S5 Factor analysis. This file contains technical details of the factor analysis.

Appendix S6 Veterinary practitioners' additional comments. This file contains (i) the free text relies detailing the additional comments made by 25 (of the 93) practitioners, in response to the question: If you have other comments about any aspect of the use of fertility drugs to get dairy cows served, or this questionnaire in general, please write them below or overleaf. (ii) additional comments made for any question posed in the questionnaire.

Acknowledgments

Thanks go to the practitioners and academics who participated, and the three reviewers for their helpful comments.

Author Contributions

Critically appraised the paper: EF RFS MJG. Conceived and designed the experiments: HMH EF RFS MJG. Performed the experiments: HMH. Analyzed the data: HMH EF MJG. Wrote the paper: HMH.

References

1. Rollin BE (2006) An introduction to veterinary medical ethics: theory and cases. Hoboken, NJ: Wiley-Blackwell.
2. Thompson PB (2007) Food biotechnology in ethical perspective. Berlin: Springer.
3. Legood G (2000) An introduction to veterinary ethics. London: Continuum.
4. Moore K, Thatcher WW (2006) Major advances associated with reproduction in dairy cattle. J Dairy Sci 89: 1254–1266.
5. Royal MD, Darwash AO, Flint APE, Webb R, Woolliams JA (2000) Declining fertility in dairy cattle: changes in traditional and endocrine parameters of fertility. Animal Science 70: 487–501.
6. van Arendonk JAM, Liinamo A (2003) Dairy cattle production in Europe. Theriogenology 59: 563–569.
7. Dobson H, Walker SL, Morris MJ, Routly JE, Smith RF (2008) Why is it getting more difficult to successfully artificially inseminate dairy cows? Animal 2: 1104–1111.
8. Orpin PG, Esslemont RJ (2010) Culling and wastage in dairy herds: an update on incidence and economic impact in dairy herds in the UK. Cattle Pract 18: 163–172.
9. Thatcher WW, Drost M, Savio JD, Macmillan KL, Entwistle KW, et al. (1993) New clinical uses of GnRH and its analogues in cattle. Anim Reprod Sci 33: 27–49.
10. Johnson R, Hanrahan CE (2010) The U.S.-EU beef hormone dispute. Congressional Research Service Report for Congress. Available: http://www.nationalaglawcenter.org/assets/crs/R40449.pdf. Accessed 30 November 2012.
11. Veterinary Medicines Directorate (2011) Controls of veterinary medicines. Available: http://www.vmd.defra.gov.uk/pdf/vmgn/VMGNote01.pdf. Accessed 30 November 2012.
12. Directive 2001/82/EC of the European parliament and of the council (2001) The community code relating to veterinary medicinal products. Available: http://ec.europa.eu/health/files/eudralex/vol-5/dir_2001_82_cons2009/dir_2001_82_cons2009_en.pdf. Accessed 30 November 2012.
13. Veterinary Medicines Directorate (2012) The work of the VMD. Available: http://www.vmd.defra.gov.uk/pdf/leaflet_workVMD.pdf. Accessed 30 November 2012.
14. The Veterinary Medicines Regulations (2011) No.2159. Available: http://www.legislation.gov.uk/uksi/2011/2159/pdfs/uksi_20112159_en.pdf. Accessed 30 November 2012.
15. Veterinary Medicines Directorate (2009) How to determine withdrawal periods. Available: http://www.vmd.defra.gov.uk/pdf/leaflet_withdrawalperiod.pdf. Accessed 30 November 2012.
16. Veterinary Medicines Directorate (2009) Avoiding veterinary residues in food-maintaining consumer confidence. Available: http://www.vmd.defra.gov.uk/pdf/leaflet_residues.pdf. Accessed 30 November 2012.
17. Dyer F, Diesel G, Cooles S, Tait A (2012) Suspected adverse reaction surveillance scheme: suspected adverse events, 2011. Vet Rec 170: 640–643.
18. R Development Core Team (2011) R: A language and environment for statistical computing. R foundation for statistical computing, Vienna, Austria. Available: http://www.R-project.org/. Accessed 4 April 2013.
19. Kalton G (1987) Introduction to survey sampling. Thousand Oaks, CA: Sage Publications.
20. Agresti A (2002) Categorical data analysis. New York: Wiley-Interscience.
21. Cattell RB (1966) The scree test for the number of factors. Multivariate Behav Res 1: 245–276.
22. Nunnally JC (1978) Psychometric theory. New York: McGraw-Hill.
23. Thompson B (2004) Exploratory and confirmatory factor analysis: understanding concepts and applications. Washington, DC: American Psychological Association.
24. Kim J, Mueller CW (1978) Factor Analysis: Statistical methods and practical issues. Thousand Oaks, CA: Sage Publications.
25. Kaiser HK (1958) The varimax criterion for analytic rotation in factor analysis. Psychometrika 23: 187–200.
26. Hendrickson AE, White PO (1964) Promax: A quick method for rotation to oblique simple structure. Br J Math Stat Psychol 17: 65–70.
27. Hu L, Bentler PM (1999) Cutoff criteria for fit indexes in covariance structure analysis: conventional criteria versus new alternatives. Struct Equ Modeling 6: 1–55.
28. Kline P (1994) An easy guide to factor analysis. London: Routledge.

29. Rasbash J, Charlton C, Browne WJ, Healy M, Cameron B (2011) MLwiN version 2.24. Centre for multilevel modelling, University of Bristol.
30. Goldstein H (2010) Multilevel statistical models. Hoboken, NJ: Wiley-Blackwell.
31. RCVS (2012) Guide to Profesional Conduct. Available: http://www.rcvs.org.uk/advice-and-guidance/code-of-professional-conduct-for-veterinary-surgeons/#declaration. Accessed 30 November 2012.
32. Green MJ, editor (2012) Dairy Herd Health. Wallingford, UK: CABI Publishers.
33. Hoey R (2007) Experts disagree over NICE's approach for assessing drugs. Lancet 370: 643–644.
34. Longworth L, Sculpher MJ, Bojke L, Tosh JC (2011) Bridging the gap between methods research and the needs of policy makers: A review of the research priorities of the National Institute for Health and Clinical Excellence. Int J Technol Assess Health Care 27: 180–187.
35. Veterinary Medicines Directorate (2011) Guidance for retailers. Available: http://www.vmd.defra.gov.uk/pdf/vmgn/VMGNote03.pdf. Accessed 30 November 2012.
36. RCVS (2012) Code of profesional conduct for veterinary surgeons. Available:http://www.rcvs.org.uk/advice-and-guidance/code-of-professional-conduct-for-veterinary-surgeons/#declaration. Accessed 30 November 2012.
37. Hobson-West P (2007) Trusting blindly can be the biggest risk of all: organised resistance to childhood vaccination in the UK. Sociol Health Illn 29: 198–215.
38. Foresight (2011) The future of food and farming executive summary. The Government Office for Science, London. Available: http://www.bis.gov.uk/assets/foresight/docs/food-and-farming/11-547-future-of-food-and-farming-summary. Accessed 30 November 2012.

8

Factors Associated with Pleurisy in Pigs: A Case-Control Analysis of Slaughter Pig Data for England and Wales

Henrike C. Jäger[1¤], Trevelyan J. McKinley[1], James L. N. Wood[1], Gareth P. Pearce[1], Susanna Williamson[2], Benjamin Strugnell[3], Stanley Done[3], Henrike Habernoll[4], Andreas Palzer[5], Alexander W. Tucker[1]*

1 Department of Veterinary Medicine, University of Cambridge, Cambridge, United Kingdom, 2 Veterinary Laboratories Agency (AHVLA), Bury St Edmunds, Suffolk, United Kingdom, 3 Veterinary Laboratories Agency (AHVLA), West House, Thirsk, North Yorkshire, United Kingdom, 4 BQP Ltd, Stradbroke Business Centre, Stradbroke, Suffolk, United Kingdom, 5 Ludwig-Maximilians-Universität München, Clinic for Swine, Sonnenstrasse, Oberschleissheim, Germany

Abstract

A case-control investigation was undertaken to determine management and health related factors associated with pleurisy in slaughter pigs in England and Wales.

Methods: The British Pig Executive Pig Health Scheme database of abattoir pathology was used to identify 121 case (>10% prevalence of pleurisy on 3 or more assessment dates in the preceding 24 months) and 121 control units (≤5% prevalence of pleurisy on 3 or more assessment dates in the preceding 24 months). Farm data were collected by postal questionnaire. Data from respondents (70 cases and 51 controls) were analysed using simple logistic regression models with Bonferroni corrections. Limited multivariate analyses were also performed to check the robustness of the overall conclusions.

Results and Conclusions: Management factors associated with increased odds of pleurisy included no all-in all-out pig flow (OR 9.3, 95% confidence interval [CI]: 3.3–29), rearing of pigs with an age difference of >1 month in the same airspace (OR 6.5 [2.8–17]) and repeated mixing (OR 2.2 [1.4–3.8]) or moving (OR 2.2 [1.5–3.4]) of pigs during the rearing phase. Those associated with decreased odds of pleurisy included filling wean-to-finish or grower-to-finish systems with piglets from ≤3 sources (OR 0.18 [0.07–0.41]) compared to farrow-to-finish systems, cleaning and disinfecting of grower (ORs 0.28 [0.13–0.61] and 0.29 [0.13–0.61]) and finisher (ORs 0.24 [0.11–0.51] and 0.2 [0.09–0.44]) accommodation between groups, and extended down time of grower and finisher accommodation (OR 0.84 [0.75–0.93] and 0.86 [0.77–0.94] respectively for each additional day of downtime). This study demonstrated the value of national-level abattoir pathology data collection systems for case control analyses and generated guidance for on-farm interventions to help reduce the prevalence of pleurisy in slaughter pigs.

Editor: Todd Davis, Centers for Disease Control and Prevention, United States of America

Funding: The authors thank the British Pig Executive (BPEX - a part of the UK's Agricultural and Horticultural Development Board) for funding this project and providing the BPHS data base. The funders had no role in study design, data collection and analysis, decision to publish, or preparation of the manuscript.

Competing Interests: Dr H. Habernoll worked, until June 2011, as a veterinarian for BQP Ltd - a commercial pig production company. She contributed time (paid by BQP) to the design and testing of a questionnaire, but was not involved in the analysis of data.

* E-mail: awt1000@cam.ac.uk

¤ Current address: Garth Partnership, Straight Lane, Beeford, East Yorkshire, United Kingdom

Introduction

Pleurisy is defined as inflammation of the pleural membranes, the serosal surfaces of the lung and chest cavity that facilitates smooth inflation of the lung. It is a particular problem in the pig industry [1] and is evident at necropsy or slaughter as fibrinous or fibrous adhesions between the lung lobes (visceral pleurisy) and/or the lungs and chest wall (parietal pleurisy). Interest in the economic and welfare impacts of pleurisy has increased since the high prevalence of this condition in finisher pigs has become apparent [1]. The economic impacts require further investigation, but chronic pleurisy is associated with increased time to slaughter [2]. It also causes problems in abattoirs because carcases require trimming causing extra labour, slower production line speeds, and result in increased waste. Respiratory disease is known to have significant negative impacts on indicators of pig welfare [3].

Pleurisy is a common finding in slaughter pigs in the UK, as evidenced by data from the systematic abattoir pathology recording under the British Pig Executive's (BPEX) Pig Health Scheme (BPHS); data provided to us from 14 abattoirs showed that of 15,237 slaughter consignments between July 2005 and October 2008, 80% were affected by pleurisy. Within these consignments, at the individual pig level 12.5% of 641,763 pigs were affected. Studies in other countries have found similar and even increasing pleurisy prevalence over the last 20 years (Table 1). Pleurisy is a multifactorial syndrome that can be caused by a number of different infections and which is predisposed to by a range of different management factors.

Previous studies of management factors associated with pleurisy in pigs have identified some common management factors, as well as some regional differences. The most important risk factors found in previous studies were related to transmission of infections at herd or pig level such as pig density in neighbourhood [4,5], poor biosecurity [5], increased herd size [6] or number of pigs per pen [7], lack of complete all-in/all-out practice [4,8], and mixing of pigs

Table 1. Pleurisy prevalence, presented as percentage of individual affected pigs, in EU countries.

Country	Period	Prevalence
Belgium	2000	16% [5]
	2009	20.8% [7]
Denmark	1987	14 [9]
	1998	24% [29]
	2000	25% [4]
Netherlands	1990	12% [14]
	2004	22.5% [14]
Norway	1991	41% [12]
Spain	2009	26.8% [8]
UK	1988	16% [1]

in the finishing stage [4]. But whereas Maes (2001) detected a higher prevalence of pleurisy in slaughter pigs in January/February in Belgium, with more severe lesions in March/April, in the Netherlands Elbers (1992) found highest prevalence in June/August.

The presence of antibodies to *Actinobacillus pleuropneumoniae* (APP) is associated with pleurisy either alone [6,7,9,10] or in combination with Porcine Reproductive and Respiratory Syndromevirus (PRRSV) [8]. Also *Mycoplasma hyopneumoniae* (M. hyo) [7,11], *Mycoplasma hyorhinis* [12] and Swine Influenza virus (SIV) [6] have been shown to be associated with higher frequency of pleurisy. More recently PCV2 has also been suggested to be associated with increased levels of pleurisy [13], and in addition porcine atrophic rhinitis (PAR) has been associated with pleurisy in Denmark [6,9].

Understanding the health associated factors and clinical signs in live pigs with pleurisy would permit more effective and timely targeting of control measures, since often the disease is only apparent at slaughter. However, work in this area has been limited—coughing and lethargy are considered to be indicative, but not specific for pleurisy, but attempts to identify pigs suffering from pleurisy pre-mortem based on pyrexia and dyspnoea have not been successful [14].

The present analysis focused on management and health-related associative factors for pleurisy and took into account the three main types of slaughter pig production systems relevant in the European Union (farrow-to-finish, wean-to-finish, grow-to-finish). Most previous studies looked at only one [5] or two types of production systems [8,9]. A case-control analysis was conducted, using retrospective abattoir pathology data collected at national level within the BPHS over the previous two years. Due to the ubiquity of pleurisy in the UK, pig units were defined as cases or controls based on underlined consistently high or low pleurisy prevalence at unit level. One goal was to demonstrate the value of a nation-wide abattoir pathology database in identifying these consistent case and control units since it provided objective data representing around 80% of the farm assurance accredited English and Welsh production base. Herd specific information on management practices and health observations were gathered by a postal questionnaire from units that met the criteria for case or control.

Materials and Methods

Selection of target units based on pre-existing abattoir pathology data

The British Pig Executive (BPEX), representing English and Welsh levy paying pig producers, launched the BPHS abattoir

pathology monitoring scheme database in 2005 [15]. BPHS is considered a comprehensive representation of the slaughter pig population in England and Wales since it captures data from approximately 75% of all commercial slaughter herds (1036 of a total 1400 herds, based on 2010 data) [16]. For a given consignment of slaughter pigs, each containing from 10 to >200 pigs, assessments are recorded from every second pig on the slaughter-line up to a maximum sample size of 50 pigs per consignment. The scheme operates at the 14 largest pig abattoirs in England and Wales using 37 specialist veterinarian assessors to collect on-line pathology data on 1 to 4 assessment days per month depending on the size of the abattoir. Assessment days rotate ensuring each day of the week is represented allowing every herd to be assessed at least once a quarter. Standardisation of assessment data between abattoirs and assessors is monitored by the scheme and includes regular training and rotation of assessors [15,16].

Criteria for case and control definitions were developed from this pre-existing database, taking into account the distribution of the data, and aiming to avoid data collected from small sample populations or from producers that recorded highly variable pleurisy prevalence over time. The database was used to identify all producers that had 50 slaughter pigs assessed on at least three occasions in the 24 months prior to October 2008 (778 (56%) producers of a total of approximately 1400 commercial herds) (Table 2). Fifty nine percent of consignments assessed for these producers had at least a 5% prevalence of pleurisy during the 24 month period but the prevalence was highly variable on some units. As such it was felt important to define a case-control measure based on *consistency* of prevalence of pleurisy over time, in order to attempt to separate units with endemic pleurisy problems from those that exhibited more transient occurrences. *Cases* were defined as those that had >10% of pleurisy-affected pigs in each of the three most recent consignments in the 24 month period prior to October 2008, and *controls* were those that had ≤5% of pleurisy-affected pigs in each of the three most recent consignments in that same period. Selection of these cut-offs was based on examining the distribution of the full dataset while attempting to balance study power and maximum discrimination of case and control groups. Indicative sample size calculations were done on the basis of a single factor analysis and indicated that data would be needed from 105 case units and 105 control units to detect statistical significance ($p<0.05$) of a risk factor found in 20% of the control units that had an odds ratio of 2.5, with a desired study power of 80%.

Questionnaire to collect farm-level information

Herd health and management data were gathered by a closed-question postal questionnaire sent to 242 units (121 cases, 121 controls) followed up by telephone liaison with the farm manager and the appropriate private veterinarian. Respondents were not informed of their case/control categorisation in order to minimise selection bias. A pilot questionnaire was validated at three units before dispatch. The questions were composed to ensure clarity for producers and sufficient detail for statistical analysis. An outline of investigated variable factors is presented in Table 3.

Processing and statistical analysis of data

Data were stored and manipulated in Microsoft Access and Excel (Microsoft 2007). All statistical analyses were conducted in the R statistical language (R Core Development Team 2008).

The questionnaire was stratified into a series of categories, representing different characteristics of a unit. These were: general farm information (including production type), mortality and productivity, health status, herd environment and herd management. To explore the data in a systematic manner we stratified the

Table 2. The number (%) of herds at each level of the sampling strategy.

Herds (cases and controls)	Number (%)
Commercial slaughter-pig holdings in England and Wales	1400 (100%) [16]
Herds sampled by BPHS scheme (data for 2010)	1036 (74% of 1400) [16]
Herds with 50 pigs sampled by BPHS on at least 3 occasions prior to October 2008	778 (56% of 1400)
Number of eligible cases	121(16% of 778)
Number of eligible controls	306 (39% of 778)
Total number of eligible herds	427 herds (55% of 778; 31% of 1400)
Number of dispatched questionnaires	242 (121 cases, 121 controls)
Number of completed questionnaires	121 (50% of 242; 16% of 778; 9% of 1400)
	51 cases (7% of 778)
	70 controls (9% of 778)
Number of herds included in univariable model	121
Number of herds included in multivariable model	121

The number (%) of herds at each level of the sampling strategy, including the number of eligible case and control herds, as a proportion of the total number of commercial slaughter-pig herds in England and Wales.

Table 3. Outline of variables included in a questionnaire addressed to pig farms.

Variable	Levels (if applicable)
Production unit type (and number of sources where applicable)	Farrow-finish/wean-finish/grow-finish
All-in/All-out pig flow	By unit/room/pen
Number of finisher places	value
Distance to next pig unit (km)	value
Experience of senior stockman (years)	value
Ongoing training of stockmen	Yes/No
Accommodation systems (for weaning −30 kg, and 30 kg – slaughter)	Fully slatted/part slatted/straw yards/assisted ventilation
Number of times pigs moved after weaning	value
Number of times pigs mixed after weaning	value
Is airspace shared by pigs of >1 month age gap?	Yes/no
Maximum number of pigs in shared airspace	value
Feeding regime (for 7–30 kg, for 30–50 kg, and for 50 kg – slaughter)	Meal/pellets/wet feed
	Home-mixed/purchased compound/by-product
	Ad libitum/restrict fed
Medication: number at group level	Product/duration/in feed or water/reason
Medication: individual treatments:	Number in past week/reason
Farmer observations of disease (main effect: none, few, many; where an age effect requested this is 7–30 kg & >30 kg; data requested for 2008 & 2007)	Scours (by age)/sneezing (by age)/coughing (by age)/dyspnoea (by age)/meningitis/wasting (by age)/sudden deaths (by age)/porcine dermatitis and nephropathy syndrome (PDNS)/other
Farmer or herd vet knowledge of specific disease status (believed present, confirmed by vet, believed absent, not known)	porcine reproductive and respiratory syndrome (PRRS))/A. pleuropneumoniae (APP)/Glasser's Disease/enzootic pneumonia (EP)/post-weaning multisystemic wasting syndrome (PMWS)
Vaccination of finisher pigs	Absence of any vaccination/EP (one or 2 dose regime)/Porcine circovirus type 2 (PCV2)/PRRS/Glasser's Disease/Ileitis/Other
Post-weaning mortality	Values for 2008, 2007, 2006
Mortality recording system type	Computer/other
Vet health plan in place on unit	Yes/No

Outline of variables included in a questionnaire addressed to pig farms defined as case (pleurisy prevalence consistently >10%) or control (pleurisy prevalence consistently <5%) to seek relationships between pleurisy and production unit type, key indicators of general management, and health observations.

variables into two main groups: those that corresponded to farm management characteristics (for which the influence is possibly independent of the disease status), and disease associated factors (those factors that were directly dependent on the disease status of the farm).

It was necessary to re-categorise some of the categorical variables to ensure that there were >5 observations in any level of the factor and also to aid interpretation. Variables having large numbers of missing values (>60) were removed at the outset, as were those categorical variables that had <5 samples in a group and could not be easily re-categorised. Within each group of variables (e.g. management characteristics and disease associated characteristics) the data were screened by applying a simple logistic regression model to each variable in turn, using a chi-squared likelihood ratio test (LRT) [17], and correcting for multiple comparisons using Bonferroni step-down procedures. The extent and distribution of missing values precluded the development of a comprehensive multivariable regression model. However, it was possible to produce a limited multivariable model examining relationships between pleurisy and some of the more important management related factors obtained from the univariate analyses (see results sections for further discussion). Variable selection was conducted using forwards stepwise selection routines and Akaike Information Criterion (AIC) (using the MASS package in R [18]), including only those variables where p = 0.05 or less in the Bonferroni corrected LRT results. Collinearity between variables was assessed by examining the standard errors. As such, in addition to the univariable results we also present some further discussion regarding associations between some of the explanatory variables based on the constrained multivariable models. As a result of the aforementioned limitations, we did not explore interaction effects in this instance. Goodness-of-fit was assessed using the le Cessie-van Houwelingen normal test statistic for the unweighted sum of squared errors [19,20], as implemented in the "Design" package in R [21]. Discriminatory power was assessed using the Area Under the Receiver Operating Characteristic Curve (AUC), using the "verification" package [22]. Each observation with a standardised Pearson residual of >2 was removed from the final model in turn to check for undue influence due to outliers.

Results

Recruitment of respondent farms

Overall there were 126 respondent farms from the original 242 targeted: 51 cases, 70 controls, with 2 questionnaires unusable due to incorrect herd identification. Three had ceased business. Hence the overall usable response rate was 50%. The mean, minimum and maximum pleurisy prevalences across case producers were 29.5%, 12% and 76.7%. Across control producers the mean pleurisy prevalence was 1.6%, ranging from a minimum of 0% to a maximum of 3.3%.

Management factors

The univariable results for management related risk factor analysis are shown in Table 4. Absence of all-in/all-out (AIAO) pig herd management was an important factor associated with increased pleurisy (OR 9.3) compared to complete AIAO. All-in/all-out by room was similar to no all-in/all-out practice (OR 0.96). Keeping pigs of more than one month age difference in the same airspace was associated with increased pleurisy prevalence (OR 6.5). In addition there was an association between moving and mixing of pigs on farms and higher levels of pleurisy (OR 2.2 and 2.2 per move/mix respectively). Partial slatted flooring for weaners

was a strongly associated factor (OR 21.4), but had a very wide confidence interval (3.7–400).

Factors associated with reduced prevalence of pleurisy included wean-to-finish and grow-to-finish production systems compared to farrow-to-finish systems (OR 0.10 and 0.45 respectively), cleaning and disinfection on finishing batches (ORs 0.24 and 0.20 for cleaning and disinfecting respectively), and on grower batches (ORs 0.28 and 0.29 respectively). Also associated was purchasing feed for growers as compared to home-mixing of feed (OR 0.22). Farrow-to-finish production was associated with higher levels of pleurisy than multisite operations that sourced pigs from other breeding units. However, the protective effect became less strong (and statistically insignificant) when these grow-outs sourced from >3 units (ORs 0.18 for ≤3 sources compared to 0.69 for >3 sources). Finally, longer periods of downtime between grower and finisher batches were associated with reduced pleurisy prevalence (ORs 0.84 and 0.86 for each additional day of downtime respectively).

Due to the stratified nature of some of the variables (e.g. grow-to-finish units do not have weaner accommodation), and the within-unit heterogeneity (particularly with regards to some of the accommodation types), it was difficult to design a sensible multivariable model that included all of the variables, such that there were sufficient samples to produce reasonable statistical power. Instead, we restricted attention to some of the more important variables identified in Table 4. Since we needed complete data in order to use stepwise selection, we excluded variables that had more than 5 missing values (leaving 10/15 variables). Then we excluded all batches that had any missing values across these 10 remaining variables (leaving 110 batches). We then fitted a forward stepwise selection model and report the results in Table 5.

Interestingly, the strongest variable from the univariable analysis (herd management) was the first to be added, and remained in the model until the final step, where it seems that the combination of cleaning between batches (growers), air-space shared by multiple age groups, and number of moves rendered herd management unnecessary to remain in the model. There was a strong association between shared air and herd management (only 2/30 herds with shared air = true practiced AIAO, compared to 57/80 herds with shared air = false), and also between the number of moves and herd management (median of 1 move for AIAO systems and 3 moves for non-AIAO systems). The association with cleaning between batches and herd management was less pronounced. This final model showed no statistically significant lack-of-fit (p = 0.15) and showed a relatively good discriminatory power (AUC = 0.83). Overall, three observations had an absolute standardised Pearson residual of >2 and <2.5, and three more of >2.5. Removing these in turn made negligible difference to the parameter estimates.

Disease associated factors

Case units had an increased post-weaning mortality, dyspnoea (both<30 kg and >30 kg in weight), coughing (>30 kg) and increased odds of farmer declared positive status for APP. Also, increased frequency of group medication was associated with pleurisy (Table 6).

The median post-weaning mortality rate between 2006 and 2008 (Figure 1) was consistently higher in case units (by 3.3%) (2006: case = 7.7%, control = 5%; 2007: case = 7.7%, control = 4%; 2008: case = 6%, control = 4%. All figures are median values).

Discussion

The BPHS database, which represents approximately 74% of slaughter pig production in England and Wales, proved suitable

Table 4. Analysis of management related factors related to pleurisy in slaughter pigs.

Variable	Adj. LRT p-value	n	Type	Levels	OR	Lower 95% CI	Upper 95% CI
Herd management	0.00	117	-	AIAO	-	-	-
			-	By room	0.96	0.05	7.2
			-	Mixed	8.2	3.0	24
			-	None	9.3	3.3	29
Shared air	0.00	121	-	False	-	-	-
			-	True	6.5	2.8	17
Number moves (per move)	0.00	119	-	-	2.2	1.5	3.4
Production type	0.00	121	-	Farrow-to-finish	-	-	-
			-	Wean-to-finish	0.10	0.03	0.28
			-	Grow-to-finish	0.45	0.18	1.1
Disinfect between batches	0.00	121	Finisher	False	-	-	-
				True	0.20	0.09	0.44
Downtime (per add. day)	0.00	81	Grower	-	0.84	0.75	0.93
Partial slatted	0.01	80	Weaner	False	-	-	-
				True	21	3.7	400
Number source units	0.01	116	-	0	-	-	-
			-	<=3	0.18	0.07	0.41
			-	>3	0.69	0.13	4.0
Clean between batches	0.01	121	Finisher	False	-	-	-
				True	0.24	0.11	0.51
Downtime (per add. day)	0.01	83	Finisher	-	0.86	0.77	0.94
Feed origin	0.02	104	Grower	Homemix	-	-	-
				Purchased	0.22	0.09	0.52
Number mixes (per mix)	0.03	120	-	-	2.2	1.4	3.8
Disinfect between batches	0.04	121	Grower	False	-	-	-
				True	0.29	0.13	0.61
Clean between batches	0.04	121	Grower	False	-	-	-
				True	0.28	0.13	0.61

Results of independent logistic regression models fitted to each management variable in turn, showing odds ratios (OR) and 95% confidence intervals for the variables shown to be statistically significant at the 5% level from univariable logistic regression models using likelihood ratio tests (LRT) with Bonferroni adjustments. Continuous and discrete variables are shown with a dash in the "Levels" column, with the OR corresponding to the OR per unit increase; for the categorical variables the OR is relative to the referent level, which is always shown first.

Table 5. Results from a constrained multiple regression model.

Variable	Type	Level	OR	Lower 95% CI	Upper 95% CI
Clean between batches	Grower	False	-	-	-
		True	0.33	0.11	0.89
Number of moves (per move)	-	-	2.3	1.5	3.8
Shared air	-	False	-	-	-
	-	True	4.0	1.4	12

Results from a constrained multiple regression model fitted to ten variables across 110 batches to further investigate the relationship between management factors and pleurisy in slaughter pigs. Continuous (or discrete) variables are shown with a dash in the "Levels" column, with the OR corresponding to the OR per unit increase; for the categorical variables the OR is relative to the referent level, which is always shown first.

for the purpose of identifying case and control units. However, many units within it had a large variation in pleurisy prevalence over the 24 month period studied. Because of this we imposed a strict definition of *consistency* in pleurisy levels over time in our case/control definitions. Hartley (1988) made the same observation regarding pleurisy variability and concluded that this was due to disease dynamics and variation in susceptibility of disease influenced by the environment and management. This may also be impacted by differences from batch to batch in sourcing and mixing of pigs that comprise a batch on entry to a given wean- or grow-to-finish system such that the same unit could have a history of highly variable pleurisy prevalence over time. Chance variation in the infections introduced with different pig batches could be important. The case/control definitions used here provided a metric for distinguishing between *consistently* higher or lower risk units, and must be interpreted as such.

Within responding units there were varying degrees of missing data. This was partly to do with unforeseen heterogeneity in management practices. For example, many units used multiple

Table 6. Analysis of health related factors related to pleurisy in slaughter pigs.

Variable	Adj. LRT p-value	n	Levels	OR	Lower 95% CI	Upper 95% CI
Mortality 2007	0.00	117	-	1.5	1.3	1.9
APP(farmer or vet declared)	0.00	92	Absent	-	-	-
			Present	8.8	3.4	25
Mortality 2008	0.00	114	-	1.3	1.1	1.6
Mortality 2006	0.00	111	-	1.3	1.1	1.5
Dyspnoea (>30 kg) 2007	0.00	121	Absent	-	-	-
			Present	4.8	2.2	11
Dyspnoea (>30 kg) 2008	0.01	121	Absent	-	-	-
			Present	4.1	1.9	9.0
Cough (>30 kg) 2007	0.03	121	Absent	-	-	-
			Present	4.4	1.8	12
Number of group medications	0.04	117	0	-	-	-
			1–2	3.6	1.5	10
			>=3	9.6	2.7	40
Cough (>30 kg) 2008	0.05	121	Absent	-	-	-
			Present	4.0	1.7	10.4
Dyspnoea (<30 kg) 2007	0.05	80	Absent	-	-	-
			Present	4.9	1.9	14

Results of independent logistic regression models fitted to each disease associated variable in turn, showing odds ratios (OR) and 95% confidence intervals for the variables shown to be statistically significant at the 5% level from likelihood ratio tests (p-value) with Bonferroni adjustments. Continuous (or discrete) variables are shown with a dash in the "Levels" column, with the OR corresponding to the OR per unit increase; for the categorical variables the OR is relative to the referent level, which is always shown first.

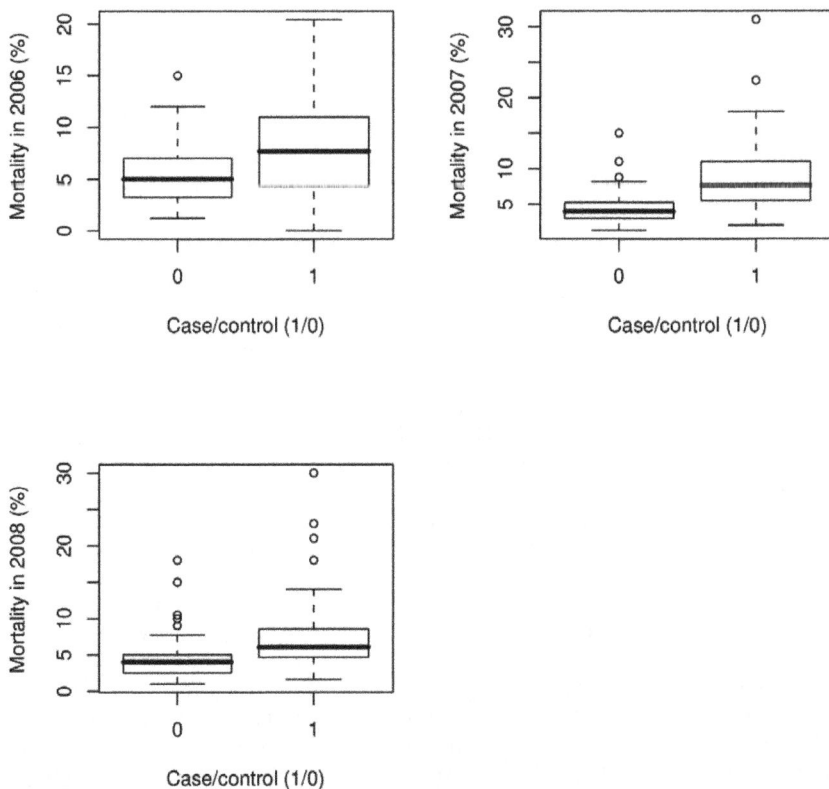

Figure 1. Post-weaning mortality distributions, shown as percentages, for pig farms categorised as pleurisy affected (case) or less affected (control) for 2006–2008.

accommodation types, sometimes for different age groups. These relationships were not clear before the study, but meant that it was difficult to stratify these variables in a sensible manner without incorporating missing information (e.g. stratifying accommodation by age group meant that grow-to-finish units would have missing values for weaning-age variables). Furthermore, there was also a tendency for respondents not to complete all questions. These limitations emphasise the importance of designing data capture questionnaires in a way that maximises the collection of relevant data but minimises the potential for missing data.

Since the definition of cases and controls was determined before recruitment, and the classification was unknown to the respondent, this should reduce the impact of selection bias. Nonetheless, more control farms replied than cases (59% and 41% respectively). We were unable to identify any systematic bias in terms of explanatory variables since we had no data from non-responders. However, the differing response rates suggest that there may be a relationship between producers' 'attitudes' to communication about this on-farm health issue and the prevalence of pleurisy. Similar future studies should take account of these differing response rates and factor in the need for follow-up phone calls to responders. Finally, the analysis only included units that had 50 pigs assessed (i.e. 100 or more pigs submitted) on each of 3 successive occasions and, although this means that the results might not extrapolate to small-scale producers, it nevertheless provides information about farm management and health characteristics that are associated with consistently high or low levels of pleurisy in larger, more economically significant, units.

We used a series of univariable logistic regression models using a conservative Bonferroni step-down multiple adjustment procedure [23]. One limitation of this approach is that it is difficult to assess the impact of confounding and effect interactions. As such the individual factors obtained from the univariable analyses that were associated with increased or decreased odds of pleurisy must be viewed in terms of providing information about potential foci for control and intervention that could be tested, and are discussed in the context of other studies and/or prior knowledge. Due to the stratified nature of some of the variables, and the degree-of-missing data, it was only possible to fit a multivariable model to a subset of the data to explore limited associations. However, caution must be used in the interpretation of these results, due to the limited scope of the variables included in the analysis. Nonetheless they further highlight the importance of the variables that were also identified in the univariable analysis.

The results of univariable analysis indicated that failure to implement strict AIAO (by unit or building) was strongly associated with increased pleurisy and this was in line with previous studies [4]. In contrast, the final multivariable model contained cleaning between batches (growers), air-space shared by multiple age-groups, and number of moves but not AIAO. Interestingly AIAO remained in the multivariable analysis until the final step of the procedure before dropping out. Cleaning between batches and avoidance of sharing airspace by pigs of different ages, factors that are both present in the final multivariable model, are important contributory elements of effective AIAO management. Not practising AIAO potentially allows diseases to circulate because susceptible pigs are continuously introduced and older pigs can pass on infections to the younger generation [2]. The univariable analysis findings that repeated mixing, moving, the co-existence of pigs of >1 month age difference in the same air space, and failures in cleaning or disinfection were also factors associated with increased pleurisy reinforced the biological relevance of this observation since these are key practical components of an AIAO management system.

Conversely, implementing AIAO by room, as opposed to by building or unit, was associated with increased pleurisy in the univariable analysis. It seems that there is sometimes confusion about the definition of AIAO – a management system that segregates pigs of a defined age span (e.g. 3 weeks) in an airspace that is separate from groups of other aged pigs throughout their life. A key part of AIAO is that the segregated airspace or accommodation is fully emptied before repopulation occurs. AIAO can break disease cycles, but only if the entire population is included in the process. Our data suggested that AIAO by room cannot be regarded as effective AIAO. In most cases, although the situation varies from farm to farm, a room is not separated enough from other pigs to allow calling the process of emptying a room 'all-out' or filling a room 'all-in'.

The odds of pleurisy increased each time pigs were mixed (univariable analysis) or moved (univariable and multivariable models). Moving and mixing are stressors for pigs which may impact on immunity [24], and are opportunities for pathogens such as APP to spread to susceptible pigs [25]. Although identifying the role of specific infections in causing pleurisy was not a central aim of the current work, vet or farmer-declared presence of clinical APP on the farm was associated with higher levels of pleurisy. APP status might have been determined by clinical or serological status. Vaccination against APP might have impacted on the serological status, or masked clinical disease, but vaccination against this organism is very uncommon in England and Wales. The role of APP in pleurisy is supported by several serological studies [6,7,8,9,10].

A number of previously undescribed protective factors were identified in this analysis. Firstly, cleaning and disinfection of grower and finisher accommodation between batches was identified in the univariable model, with cleaning of grower pens remaining in the final multivariable model. Secondly, increased "down time" between batches for finisher and grower accommodation was identified in the univariable model. These are issues that have previously been identified as important associative factors relating to enteric disease [26] but less so in the context of respiratory disease. Nevertheless, cleaning might be expected to contribute to respiratory health through reduced levels of dust, environmental bacteria and fungal spores. Resting buildings allows complete drying after disinfection and would be expected to optimise killing of important respiratory pathogens. This has been demonstrated in pig transport trailers for PRRSV [27] but studies of total aerobic bacterial counts were unable to show an effect of down time (Amass 2007). This is nevertheless an important area for future investigation since the presence of organic matter can significantly affect environmental survival of respiratory pathogens such as APP (Gottschalk 2006).

Compared to farrow-to-finish (FF) operations, grow-to-finish (GF) but especially wean-to-finish (WF) systems showed lower levels of pleurisy (GF OR = 0.45; WF OR = 0.1) according to the univariable analysis. The continuous presence of breeding and growing pigs on FF units may be responsible for continuous circulation of infections. Strict AIAO production, at building level, on FF units in the UK is extremely unlikely to occur and pigs must progress through what is often a closely located set of buildings. On the other hand, WF and GF units are more suited to strict AIAO, in spite of the fact that their population usually involves the mixing of pigs from different breeding sources. The observed additional protective effect of WF units over GF units is worthy of further investigation. Of potential importance might be the residual colostrally derived passive immunity at mixing during population in WF units. Population (and mixing of sources) on GF units takes place after the decline of passive immunity with, potentially, a consequential increase in the effective population of susceptible pigs. Also, or alternatively, if infections causing pleurisy spread soon after mixing on AIAO WF units, pigs have a longer period until slaughter during which lesions may resolve.

Another apparently protective factor identified in the univariable analysis was sourcing of piglets to WF or GF sites from ≤3 units in comparison to the single sourcing associated with farrow-finish (no external sources). This association was weaker when a batch was sourced from >3 breeding units. The protective effect over FF may be in part a proxy for the management conditions of WF and GF farms, although the reduced protective effect when more than 3 sources are taken is consistent with the notion that an increase in the likelihood of introduction of disease occurs when sourcing piglets from higher numbers of different units. The use of purchased grower feed versus home mixed feed was found to be associated with lower prevalence of pleurisy (OR = 0.2) but the absence of associations relating to feed at the finisher or weaner stages suggests that this finding may be an artefact, or may be correlated to other factors such as production type (home mixing is more common on FF units in the UK) but this could not be ascertained in the current project.

Regarding associations between pleurisy prevalence and disease related factors, the univariable study differentiated clinical signs by age group (< and >30 kg) and year (2007 and 2008). Similar to previous studies where observable respiratory disease in late finishing was associated with the presence of pleurisy [8], the present study found dyspnoea and coughing in pigs >30 kg were associated with pleurisy in 2007 and 2008. In 2007 dyspnoea in pigs <30 kg could also be related to increased pleurisy in slaughter pigs, but this effect was not observed in 2008. However, these clinical observations are not specific for pleurisy and may indicate other, co-existent, respiratory diseases. Previous research has indicated a link between pleurisy prevalence and prevalence of pneumonia [28], but more recent work suggests this relationship may not be straightforward since lesions of pneumonia were negatively associated with pleurisy lesions [5,10]. Much opportunity remains to understand how pleurisy relates to pneumonia in pigs and how it might be detected ante mortem.

Increased mortality was consistently and strongly associated with the units being defined as cases in each of the 3 years for which data was requested. This basis of this association is worthy of further

investigation because, on one hand, it is another indication that pleurisy is a disease of generally lower health status units and, on the other, an indication of the economic consequences of pleurisy on units where it is a consistent problem. As a proxy for the overall health of a unit, increased numbers of group level medication periods in the post-weaning period were associated with units with consistent pleurisy. While this observation would be consistent with a tendency for pleurisy to occur on units of generally lower health status and with higher consequent production costs, it is probable that some of these additional medications would have been a direct consequence of pleurisy.

In conclusion, this study identified management and health related factors associated with pleurisy based on a questionnaire across 121 respondent units producing slaughter pigs and a national abattoir pathology surveillance database – demonstrating the value of this national disease surveillance system. The identified factors were mostly related to transmission of infectious diseases and the analyses highlighted the importance of AIAO but also a group of management factors associated with it. In addition, farrow-finish management systems were shown to be particularly at risk of consistent pleurisy, in part likely due to the difficulty in implementing strict AIAO in these systems in the UK. Since implementation of complete AIAO management, for example at the building or unit level, has significant cost implications a better understanding of the relative importance of specific management factors that contribute to AIAO and which can be implemented in any production system, is of value to the industry.

Acknowledgments

The authors thank Dr Barbara Wieland and Dr Pablo Alarcon Lopez, both of the Royal Veterinary College, UK, for their assistance with design and review of the postal questionnaire and the sharing of relevant data.

Author Contributions

Conceived and designed the experiments: HCJ TJM JLNW GPP SW BS SD HH AP AWT. Performed the experiments: HCJ TJM AWT. Analyzed the data: HCJ TJM JLNW AWT. Contributed reagents/materials/analysis tools: GPP SW BS SD HH AP. Wrote the paper: HCJ TJM JLNW AWT. Obtained BPHS dataset: HCJ TJM. Designed questionnaire: HCJ TJM JLNW GPP SW BS SD HH AP AWT. Tested questionnaire: HCJ HH.

References

1. Rubies X, Kielstein P, Costa L, Riera P, Artigas C, et al. (1999) Prevalence of Haemophilus parasuis serovars isolated in Spain from 1993 to 1997. Vet Microbiol 66: 245–248.
2. Sorensen V, Jorsal SE, Mousing J (2006) Diseases of the respiratory tract. In: Straw B, Zimmermann J, D'Allaire S, Taylor D, eds. Diseases of Swine. 9 ed. Oxford: Blackwell Scientific. pp 149–177.
3. Schimmel D, Kielstein P, Hass R (1985) [Serological typing of Haemophilus parasuis]. Arch Exp Veterinarmed 39: 944–947.
4. Cleveland-Nielsen A, Nielsen EO, Ersboll AK (2002) Chronic pleuritis in Danish slaughter pig herds. Prev Vet Med 55: 121–135.
5. Maes DG, Deluyker H, Verdonck M, F C, Miry C, et al. (2001) Non-infectious factors associated with macroscopic and microscopic lung lesions in slaughter pigs from farrow-to-finish herds. Vet Record 148: 41–46.
6. Mousing J, Lybye H, Barfod K, Meyling A, Rønsholt L, et al. (1990) Chronic pleuritis in pigs for slaughter: an epidemiological study of infcetious and rearing system-related risk factors. Prev Vet Med 9: 107–119.
7. Meyns T, Van Steelant J, Rolly E, Dewulf J, Haesebrouck F, et al. (2011) A cross-sectional study of risk factors associated with pulmonary lesions in pigs at slaughter. Vet J 187: 388–392.
8. Fraile L, Alegre A, Lopez-Jimenez R, Nofrarias M, Segales J (2010) Risk factors associated with pleuritis and cranio-ventral pulmonary consolidation in slaughter-aged pigs. Vet J 184(3): 326–33.
9. Enøe C, Mousing J, Schirmer AL, Willeberg P (2002) Infectious and rearing-system related risk fcators for chronic pleuritis in slaughter pigs. Prev Vet Med 54: 337–349.
10. Wiegand M, Kielstein P, Pohle D, Rassbach A (1997) [Examination of primary SPF swine after experimental infection with Haemophilus parasuis. Clinical symptoms, changes in hematological parameters and in the parameters of the cerebrospinal fluid]. Tierarztl Prax 25: 226–232.
11. Sørensen V, Jorsal SE, Mousing J (2006) Diseases of the Respiratory System. In: Straw BE, Zimmermann JJ, D'Allaire S, Taylor DJ, eds. Diseases of Swine: Blackwell Publishing. pp 149–177.
12. Falk K, Hoie S, Lium BM (1991) An abattoir survey of pneumonia and pleuritis in slaughter weight swine from 9 selected herds. II. Enzootic pneumonia of pigs: microbiological findings and their relationship to pathomorphology. Acta Vet Scand 32: 67–77.
13. Kielstein P, Rapp-Gabrielson VJ (1992) Designation of 15 serovars of Haemophilus parasuis on the basis of immunodiffusion using heat-stable antigen extracts. J Clin Microbiol 30: 862–865.
14. Augustijn M, Stockhofe-Zurwieden N, Nielen M, Jirawattanapong P, Cruijsen A, et al. (2008) The etiology of chronic pleuritis is pigs: a clinical, pathological and serological study. Proceedings of the 20th Congress of the International Pig Veterinary Society, Durban. OR.05.12.
15. Anon (2008) The British Pig Health Scheme 2003–2008.: British Pig executive.
16. Sanchez-Vazquez MJ, Strachan WD, Armstrong D, Nielen M, Gunn GJ (2011) The British pig health schemes: integrated systems for large-scale pig abattoir lesion monitoring. Vet Rec 169: 413.
17. Hosmer D, Lemeshow S Applied Logistic Regression: John Wiley and Sons.
18. Venables WN, Ripley BD (2002) Modern Applied Statistics with S. New York: Springer.
19. le Cessie S, JC vH (1991) Biometrics 47: 1267–1282.
20. Hosmer D, Hosmer T, Lemeshow S, le Cessie S (1997) A comparison of goodness-of-fit tests for the logistic regression model. Stat in Med 16: 965–980.
21. Harrell F Design Package in R Package. 2.3-0 ed.

22. Program N-RA (2010) verification: Forecast. Verification utilities. R package. 1.31 ed.

23. Martin J, Gunther H, Janetschke P, Schonherr W, Kielstein P (1977) [Contribution to the experimental hemophilus infection (Haemophilus para-haemolyticus, Haemophilus parasuis) in SPF piglets. 2. Comparative pathology and histology]. Arch Exp Veterinarmed 31: 347–357.

24. Salak-Johnson JL, McGlone JJ (2007) Making sense of apparently conflicting data: stress and immunity in swine and cattle. J Anim Sci 85: E81–88.

25. Gottschalk M, Taylor DJ (2006) Actinobacillus pleuropneumoniae. In: Straw B, Zimmermann JJ, D'Allaire S, Taylor DJ, eds. Diseases Of Swine 9 ed: Blackwell Publishing. pp 563–576.

26. Janetschke P, Kielstein P, Schonherr W, Martin J, Gunther H (1977) [Contribution to the experimental haemophilus infection (haemophilus parahemolyticus, haemophilus parasuis) in specific pathogen-free piglets. 1. microbiology, experimental arrangement, results]. Arch Exp Veterinarmed 31: 129–137.

27. Zimmermann J, Benfield DA, Murthaugh MP, Osorio F, Stevenson GW, et al. (2006) Porcine Reproductive and Respiratory Syndrome Virus (Porcine Arterivirus). In: Straw B, Zimmermann JJ, D'Allaire S, Taylor DJ, eds. Diseases Of Swine 9 ed: Blackwell Publishing. pp 387–417.

28. Elbers ARW, Tielen MJM, Snijders JMA, Cromwijk WAJ, Hunneman WA (1992) Epidemiological studies on lesions in finishing pigs in the Netherlands. I. Prevalence, seasonality and interrelationship. Prev Vet Med 14: 217–231.

29. Christensen G, Enoe C (1999) The prevalence of pneumonia, pleuritis, pericarditis, and liver spots in Danish slaughter pigs in 1998, including comparison with 1994. Danish Veterinary Journal 82: 1006–1015.

9

Parasite Co-Infections and Their Impact on Survival of Indigenous Cattle

Samuel M. Thumbi[1*¤a¤b], Barend Mark de Clare Bronsvoort[2], Elizabeth Jane Poole[3], Henry Kiara[3], Philip G. Toye[3], Mary Ndila Mbole-Kariuki[3], Ilana Conradie[5], Amy Jennings[2], Ian Graham Handel[2], Jacobus Andries Wynand Coetzer[5], Johan C. A. Steyl[6], Olivier Hanotte[4], Mark E. J. Woolhouse[1]

1 Centre for Immunology, Infection and Evolution, University of Edinburgh, Edinburgh, United Kingdom, 2 The Roslin Institute and Royal (Dick) School of Veterinary Studies, University of Edinburgh, Roslin, United Kingdom, 3 International Livestock Research Institute, Nairobi, Kenya, 4 School of Life Science, University of Nottingham, University Park, Nottingham, United Kingdom, 5 Department of Veterinary Tropical Diseases, Faculty of Veterinary Science, University of Pretoria, Onderstepoort, South Africa, 6 Department of Paraclinical Sciences, Faculty of Veterinary Science, University of Pretoria, Onderstepoort, South Africa

Abstract

In natural populations, individuals may be infected with multiple distinct pathogens at a time. These pathogens may act independently or interact with each other and the host through various mechanisms, with resultant varying outcomes on host health and survival. To study effects of pathogens and their interactions on host survival, we followed 548 zebu cattle during their first year of life, determining their infection and clinical status every 5 weeks. Using a combination of clinical signs observed before death, laboratory diagnostic test results, gross-lesions on post-mortem examination, histo-pathology results and survival analysis statistical techniques, cause-specific aetiology for each death case were determined, and effect of co-infections in observed mortality patterns. East Coast fever (ECF) caused by protozoan parasite *Theileria parva* and haemonchosis were the most important diseases associated with calf mortality, together accounting for over half (52%) of all deaths due to infectious diseases. Co-infection with *Trypanosoma* species increased the hazard for ECF death by 6 times (1.4–25; 95% CI). In addition, the hazard for ECF death was increased in the presence of *Strongyle* eggs, and this was burden dependent. An increase by 1000 *Strongyle* eggs per gram of faeces count was associated with a 1.5 times (1.4–1.6; 95% CI) increase in the hazard for ECF mortality. Deaths due to haemonchosis were burden dependent, with a 70% increase in hazard for death for every increase in strongyle eggs per gram count of 1000. These findings have important implications for disease control strategies, suggesting a need to consider co-infections in epidemiological studies as opposed to single-pathogen focus, and benefits of an integrated approach to helminths and East Coast fever disease control.

Editor: Thomas A. Smith, Swiss Tropical & Public Health Institute, Switzerland

Funding: The authors would like to thank the Wellcome Trust (grant No. 079445) for the financial support for this work. The funders had no role in study design, data collection and analysis, decision to publish, or preparation of the manuscript.

Competing Interests: The authors have declared that no competing interests exist.

* E-mail: samthumbi@gmail.com

¤a Current address: Paul G. Allen School for Global Animal Health, Washington State University, Pullman, Washington, United States of America
¤b Current address: KEMRI/CDC Research and Public Health Collaboration, Kisumu, Kenya

Introduction

Natural populations living under wild or field conditions are constantly exposed to a large diversity of parasites. As a result individual hosts, including humans and animals, are frequently co-infected with multiple pathogens either concurrently or in sequence [1]. These multispecies co-infections may result in pathogen-pathogen interactions which may influence the epidemiology of co-infecting parasites [2–4] or the consequent effects of infection on host health and performance [5–7].

Although co-infections are common in the field and important epidemiologically, most epidemiology studies have focused on single-pathogen infections, and fewer have considered co-infections while assessing the burden of infectious diseases. The last decade has seen increased attention paid to co-infections, with reported studies on animals [3,7–10] and on humans, for example malaria and helminth infections [11] or co-infections involving HIV [12,13]. From these studies and others, it is evident that

pathogen-pathogen interactions frequently occur and that their effect will differ both in strength and direction.

Dependent on the mechanisms by which pathogen-pathogen interactions occur, co-infections may cause a) more harm on the host than the combined effect of the component infections, b) less harm than the combined effect of the component infections [14,15]. The possible mechanisms by which pathogen-pathogen interactions occur modifying host outcomes have been reviewed in detail [2,16,17].

Disease-induced mortality will depend on many factors including characteristics of the host, environmental conditions under which the animals are raised, characteristics of infecting pathogens and the pathogen-pathogen interactions in situations where hosts are co-infected. Although most studies on mortality generate useful data on risk factors and mortality rates, the role of co-infections is rarely examined, even in populations where co-infections are known to frequently occur. Knowledge of pathogen-pathogen interactions is limited and we do not know which co-infections are

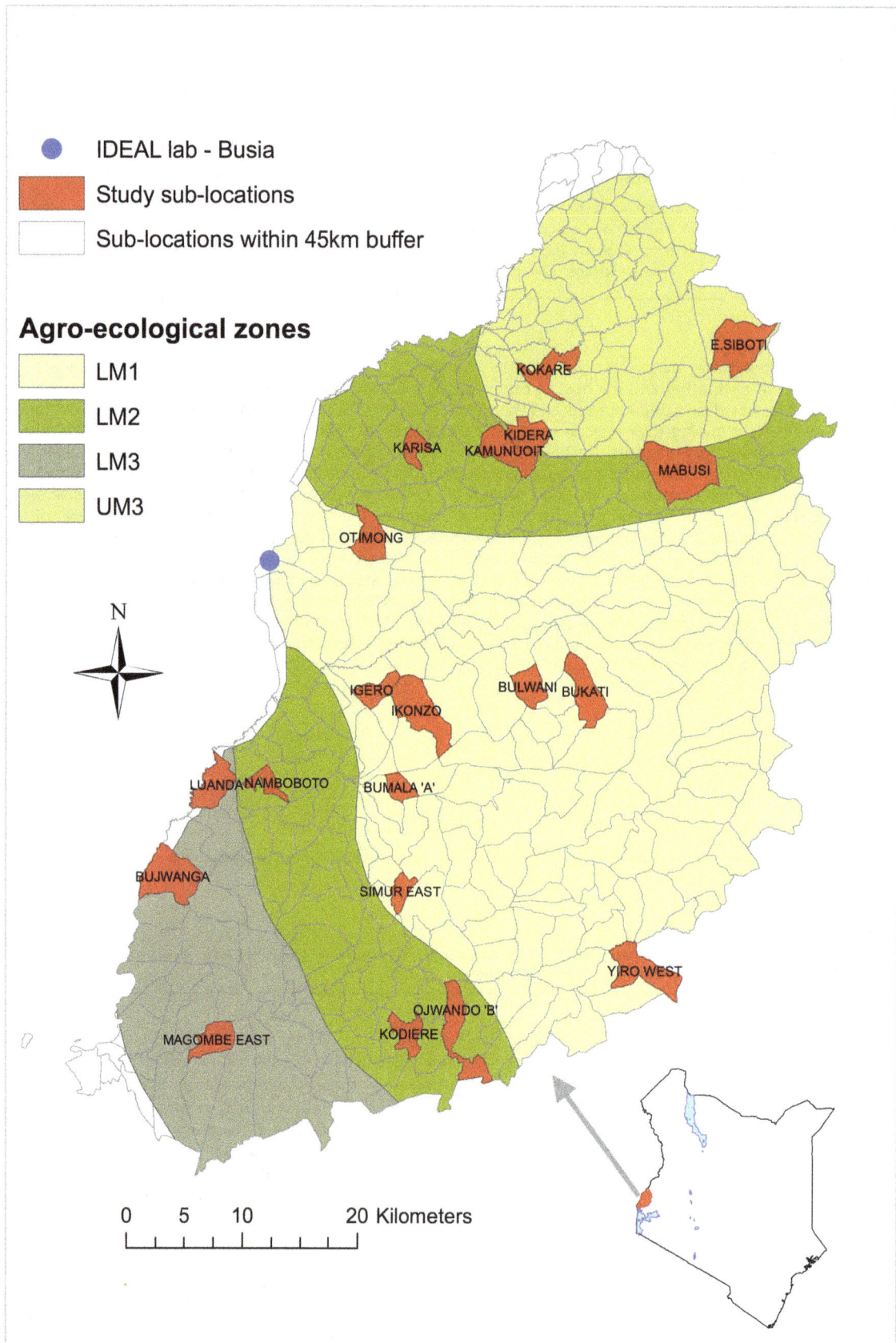

Figure 1. Map of Western Kenya showing the 4 agro-ecological zones and the 20 study sub-locations (in red). The study area comprised sub-locations falling within a 45 km radius from Busia town where the IDEAL project laboratory was located.

important among domestic animals, and how these influence their survival probabilities. If our understanding on pathogen-pathogen interactions is improved, cost-effective control programs that make use of multispecies approach to the control of morbidity and mortality attributable to infectious diseases may be applied [18,19]. Our work on mortality of indigenous zebu cattle has identified East Coast fever (ECF), and haemonchosis as the most common definitive aetiological causes of death during the calves' the first year of life, together accounting for over half (52%) of the observed infectious disease mortalities [20].

This paper investigates the specific risk factors for deaths due to the two main causes of calf mortality in indigenous zebu cattle; ECF and haemonchosis, and tests for the effect size and direction of co-infections on the risk of cause-specific calf mortality. Information on synergistic or antagonistic pathogen-pathogen interactions influencing survival probabilities provide better estimates of the impact of diseases, potentially improving the design of disease control strategies, and ultimately their effectiveness in reducing host mortality.

Materials and Methods

Ethics Statement

The study was reviewed and approved by the University of Edinburgh Ethics Committee (reference number OS 03–06), and by the Animal Care and Use Committee (AUCUC) of the International Livestock Research Institute, Nairobi. Standard techniques were used to collect blood and faecal samples for diagnosis and identification of disease and infecting pathogens. The calves were restrained by professional animal health assistants, and by veterinarians. A veterinary surgeon was available to examine any calf falling sick during the course of the study. Any calves in severe distress due to trauma or disease were humanely euthanised by intravenous injection of sodium pentobarbital, administered by a veterinary surgeon. All participating farmers gave informed consent in their native language before recruiting of their animals into the study.

Study Population

The data used in this paper are from the Infectious Disease of East Africa Livestock (IDEAL) cohort study. This study, conducted between October 2007 and September 2010, followed 548 indigenous zebu calves from birth until one year old. The animals came from an area in Western Kenya falling within a 45 km radius of Busia town at the Kenya-Uganda border and covering 4 agro-ecological zones. The study's field laboratory was located in Busia town, Kenya. Using a stratified (by agro-ecological zone) random cluster sampling approach, study animals were selected from smallholder farms in 20 sub-locations (smallest administrative unit in Kenya). Figure 1 shows the map for the study site. The inclusion criteria required that the calves were recruited into the study within 7 days of birth, be born to a dam that had been on the farm for at least one year, and the calf should have been conceived through natural insemination as opposed to artificial insemination. Additionally, only one calf per farm would be in the study at any one time, and the herd should not be under stall-feeding. The exclusion of herds under stall-feeding and calves from dams artificially inseminated was meant to lower the probability of recruiting crossbred animals. The main production system practiced in the farms was smallholder mixed crop-livestock system. An average farm is 2 hectares in size, grows food crops and keeps approximately 5 cattle among other livestock species. Following recruitment into the study, animals were routinely monitored at 5-week intervals until leaving the study at one year,

or until death. The IDEAL cohort study has been described in detail elsewhere, see [21].

Data Collection

A complete clinical examination was conducted on each study calf at the recruitment visit and during each of the 5-week routine visits. Clinical samples including blood smears, whole blood, serum samples, and faecal samples were collected for screening of pathogens, and measurement of clinical parameters such as total serum proteins and packed cell volume. Live body weight measures (in kilograms) and girth measurements (in centimeters) of the study calves were recorded during the routine visits. Pre-tested questionnaires capturing data on farm characteristics, management practices, herd structure changes, herd health and veterinary treatments were administered at each calf visit. The general body health, udder health, girth measurements and body condition score for each of the study dams were recorded, at each corresponding calf visit. These data on the dam were collected until the study calf was weaned or until leaving the study at one year.

For the study animals that died or that were euthanised during the study, a complete post-mortem (PM) examination was carried out following a standard body system by body system veterinary PM routine [22]. A team of experts reviewed results from parasitological, and histological examination of samples collected at PM, and gross-lesions observed at PM, and determined the specific aetiological cause of death for each case [20].

For the serology data on *Theileria parva*, *Theileria mutans*, *Anaplasma marginale* and *Babesia bigemina*, a sero-conversion event was assumed if there was evidence of a rising titre between two consecutive calf visits, and that the titre level was >20 percent positivity (pp).

Outcome Variable

Two outcome variables were used in this analysis; ECF deaths and haemonchosis deaths. These were defined as deaths in the study animals during the study observation time whose main aetiological cause of death was ECF or haemonchosis respectively. All deaths by cause other than that under investigation were right censored in the analysis.

Data Analysis

Survival time was defined as the age at which a calf died from the specific aetiological cause under investigation. Cox proportional hazard models as described in Equation 1 were used.

$$h_i(t) = h_0(t)e^{\beta X + \varepsilon_i} \tag{1}$$

It expresses the *hazard* at time t (i.e the probability of a calf dying from ECF or from haemonchosis at time t) as a function of; a) baseline hazard $h_0(t)$ which is the unspecified baseline hazard when the predictors are 0 or absent, b) linear combination of predictors βX which is an exponential function of a series of variables, and c) cluster term ε_i - a random effect accounting for the correlated measurements for study animals from the same study site.

Univariable analysis was carried out with each of the potential non-infectious and infection risk factors listed in Table 1. Factors with a p value ≤ 0.2 were retained and incorporated in the subsequent multivariable model. A backward selection model simplification method was used until only factors significant at a p

Table 1. List of covariates tested for their relationship with mortality due to ECF and haemonchosis.

Farm factors	**Farmer's age, gender, education level, main occupation, herd size, land size**
Management factors	Tick control, worm control, trypanosome control, vaccine use, grazing practices, watering practices, housing
Maternal status	Heart girth measurement, body condition score, suckling, health condition, dam antibody titres against *Theileria parva*, *Theileria mutans*, *Anaplasma marginale*, *Babesia bigemina*
Environmental variables	Normalised difference vegetation index (NDVI), farm altitude (elevation)
Calf factors	Calf sex, birth weight, heterozygosity, European introgression, clinical episodes, total serum protein, packed cell volume, white blood cell counts
Infectious factors	**ELISA tests (serology):** *Theileria parva*, *Theileria mutans*, *Anaplasma marginale*, *Babesia bigemina*, **Microscopy:** *Trypanosoma spp.*, *Coccidia spp.*, *Theileria spp.*, *Trichophyton spp.*, **McMaster microscopy:** *Strongyloides* eggs, *Strongyle* eggs, *Trichuris spp.*, *Toxocara vitulorum*, **Sedimentation technique:** *Calicophoron spp.*, *Fasciola spp.*, **Direct Baermann's technique:** *Dictyocaulus viviparous*, **Faecal larval cultures:** *Haemonchus placei*, *Microfilaria spp.*, *Oesophagostomum radiatum*, *Trichostrongylus axei*, *Cooperia spp.*

For infectious factors, the diagnostic tests (in bold) used are recorded against pathogens identified.

value <0.05 remained in the model. The dropped variables were then added back to the model one at a time to test if there was significant improvement in model fit. The model diagnostics were carried out through graphical evaluation of scaled Schoenfeld residuals plotted against time to test violations of proportional hazards assumption.

The statistical analysis was done using the *survival* statistical package [23], on the R platform [24]. The raw data used in this study is available from the authors on request.

Results

A total of 548 calves were recruited and followed up to 51 weeks or until they died, contributing a total of 25,104 calf weeks (481.1 calf years) of life to the study. Five animals were lost to follow due to non-compliance to study protocol or were stolen from the study farms. A total of 88 calves died before reaching 51 weeks of age, giving a crude mortality rate of 16.1 (13.0–19.2; 95% CI) per 100 calves in their first year of life. Of the 88 animals that died, 33 deaths were attributed to East Coast fever, 10 to haemonchosis, and 6 to heartwater. In addition, one death was attributed to each of the following; babesiosis, rabies, salmonellosis, trypanosomiasis, black quarter, viral pneumonia, multifocal abcessation due to *Actinomyces pyogenes*, and *Arcanobacterium* infection. Due to logistical reasons, post mortems were not carried out on 6 of the study calves and the cause of death remained unknown. Seven animals died from known non-infectious causes including trauma, starvation and plant poisoning. The remaining calves were treated as having died from infectious diseases, most with clinical signs indicative of infectious cause but the definitive cause remained unidentified.

The main aetiological causes of calf mortality among the indigenous zebu cattle were ECF and haemonchosis, accounting for 40% and 12% of all infectious disease deaths respectively. About 80% of deaths attributable to ECF occurred before calves were 6 months old, with only a few ECF deaths recorded in older calves, whereas deaths due to haemonchosis occurred in older calves, mostly greater than 6 months of age, see Figure 2. ECF deaths were observed across the study region, although Magombe East (in the south) and Bumala A recorded higher numbers of ECF deaths (6 and 4 respectively) compared to the other study sub-locations, see Figure 3. Deaths attributed to haemonchosis were observed in a number of the study sub-locations in low numbers (one death per sub-location), except in East Siboti sub-location located in the north where 4 deaths attributed to haemonchosis were recorded, Figure 4.

Predictors for ECF Deaths

Putative non-infectious and infectious risk factors were initially run as univariable analyses to test their association with ECF deaths, see results in Table S1. Presence of a clinical episode and blood parameters such as packed cell volume, white blood cell count and total serum proteins were significantly associated with ECF-mortality. These variables were however not included in the multivariable analysis since they were considered a consequence rather than a cause of infection. High intensity (level 3– more than one infected cells per microscopy field) infection with *Theileria* spp. was associated with increased risk for ECF-mortality. This variable was left out in the multivariable analysis since these data had been used as part of the ECF-death case definition.

After controlling for other significant covariates in the model, co-infection with *Trypanosoma* spp. was estimated to increase the hazard for ECF death by 6 times (1.4, 25.8; 95% CI). In addition, the hazard for ECF death was increased by presence of strongyle eggs and this was burden dependent. An increase in strongyle eggs of 1000 was associated with a 1.5 times (1.4, 1.6; 95% CI) increase in the hazard for ECF mortality.

Sero-positivity to *T.parva* was identified to be associated with a protective effect against ECF-mortality. The risk hazard for ECF-mortality was reduced by 88% (78, 93; 95% CI) in animals that were sero-positive for *T.parva* compared to sero-negative animals.

Controlling for ticks within the farm in the rest of the herd was identified as the main husbandry practice associated with a protective effect against ECF-mortality. Farms that carried out tick control were associated with lowered hazard for ECF deaths by 54% (19, 75; 95% CI) compared to farms that did not control for ticks in the rest of the herd. The results of the minimum adequate model showing the predictors with significant association with ECF-mortality are provided in Table 2. Model diagnostics did not show evidence of violation of the proportional hazards assumption.

Predictors for Haemonchosis Deaths

The association between haemonchosis deaths and putative risk factors was initially tested through univariable analyses, see Table S2. While controlling for other covariates, results from the multivariable model revealed that calves from farms providing supplementary feeding had a 90% (48, 98; 95% CI) lower hazard for haemonchosis death compared to calves in farms that did not provide supplements. The main supplements provided to the calves were crop residues offered to the calves left at the homestead when adult cattle go grazing in the fields.

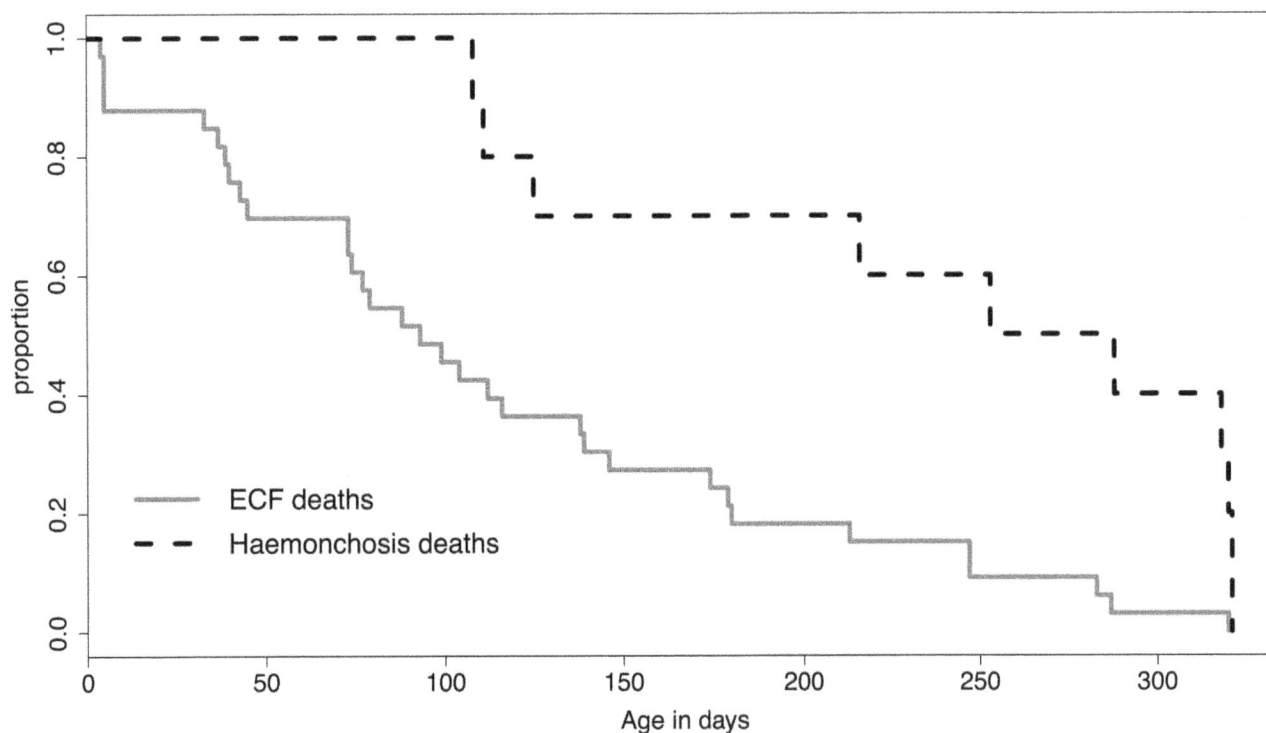

Figure 2. Plot of time to death for ECF and haemonchus deaths, the two main causes of calf mortality causing 33 and 10 deaths respectively. More than 80% of ECF deaths were observed in calves below 6 months of age, whereas most deaths attributed to haemonchosis were in calves older than 6 months.

High worm burdens as measured by strongyle epg were associated with increased hazard for haemonchosis deaths with an estimated increase of 1.7 times (1.5, 2; 95% CI) in the hazard for every 1000 strongyle epg count increase. This finding indicates that the risk for haemonchosis death is burden-dependent. Since *H.placei* is a strongyle egg-producing helminth, the variable was omitted from the final model to test if the association of haemonchus deaths with the other covariates remained. The covariates remained significant in the absence of strongyle epg count in the model.

The results of the final model containing the significant predictors for haemonchosis deaths are provided in Table 3. Model diagnostics did not show evidence of violation of the proportional hazards assumption.

Discussion

The findings presented here show that co-infections, which are common in areas endemic with diverse parasites, has important implications on host outcomes, in this study - calf survival. The study has investigated the risk factors for the two main causes of calf mortality in the study (ECF and haemonchosis) and tested the role co-infections play in determining the survival probabilities of zebu calves under one year.

East Coast fever, a disease caused by the protozoan parasite *Theileria parva* and transmitted by the tick *Rhipicephalus appendiculatus*, was identified as the main aetiological cause of death, accounting for 40% of all infectious disease calf mortality. Deaths due to ECF occurred mainly in young calves with up to 80% of deaths attributed to ECF occurring in calves below 6 months of age.

The risk of ECF death was itself significantly increased by high helminth burden (measured as strongyle epg) and by co-infection with *Trypanosoma* spp., evidence of co-infecting pathogens exacerbating the effect of infection with *T.parva*. An increase in strongyle egg per gram count of 1000 was associated with a 50% increase in hazard for ECF death, whereas co-infection with *Trypanosoma* spp. was associated with a 6 fold increase in the risk of dying from ECF. This is the first time such a result has been demonstrated and quantified in cattle, and underlines the importance of considering multiple infections in quantifying disease burden in conditions where polyparasitism is a rule rather than the exception.

The mechanisms by which *T.parva* and helminth infections interact to result in increased hazards for ECF deaths are unclear, and have not been described before. However, a similar co-infection profile involving *Plasmodium* spp., also a protozoan parasite, and helminth infections (including hookworms) has been the subject of many studies in humans, and in animal models. *Plasmodium* parasites are frequently occurring as co-infections with geohelminths, particularly hookworms with which they are co-distributed sharing extensive geographical overlaps in most of Africa [6]. Although the literature has conflicting results with reports of synergistic (increasing severity and incidence of malaria) and antagonistic (decreasing malaria cases) interactions [25–28] and reviewed by Nacher [29], most studies point to high helminth burden being associated with increased incidences and severity of malaria cases. More recently, a review by Adegnika and Kremsner [11] on the epidemiology of malaria and helminth interactions based on studies published in the last decade has concluded a general trend towards a worsening effect on the pathogenesis and incidence of malaria by hookworms and *Schistosoma mansoni*, and a protective effect by *Schistosoma hematobium* and *Ascaris lumbricoides*.

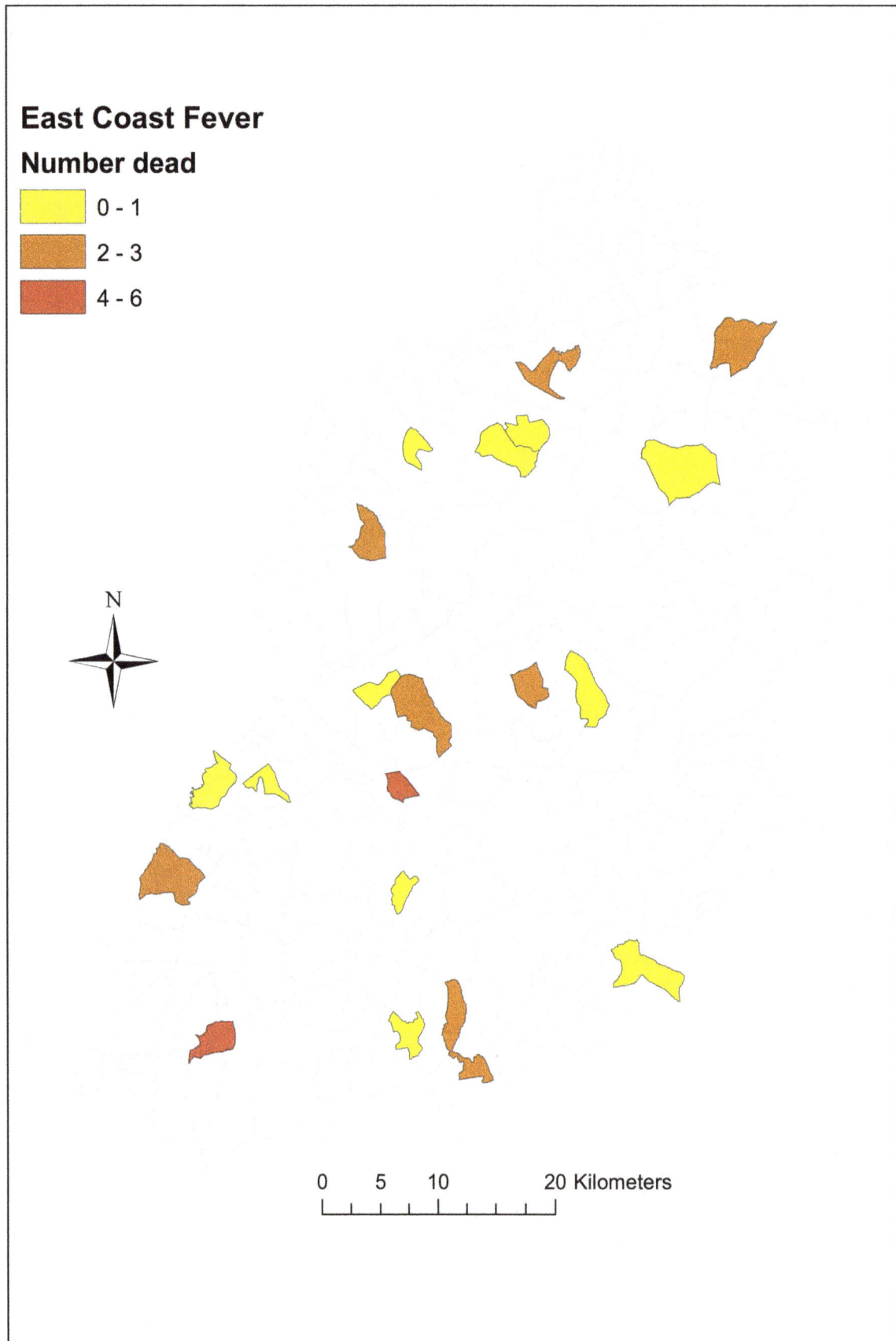

Figure 3. Map showing number of deaths attributable to ECF by sub-location. In total 33 of 88 deaths were attributed to ECF.

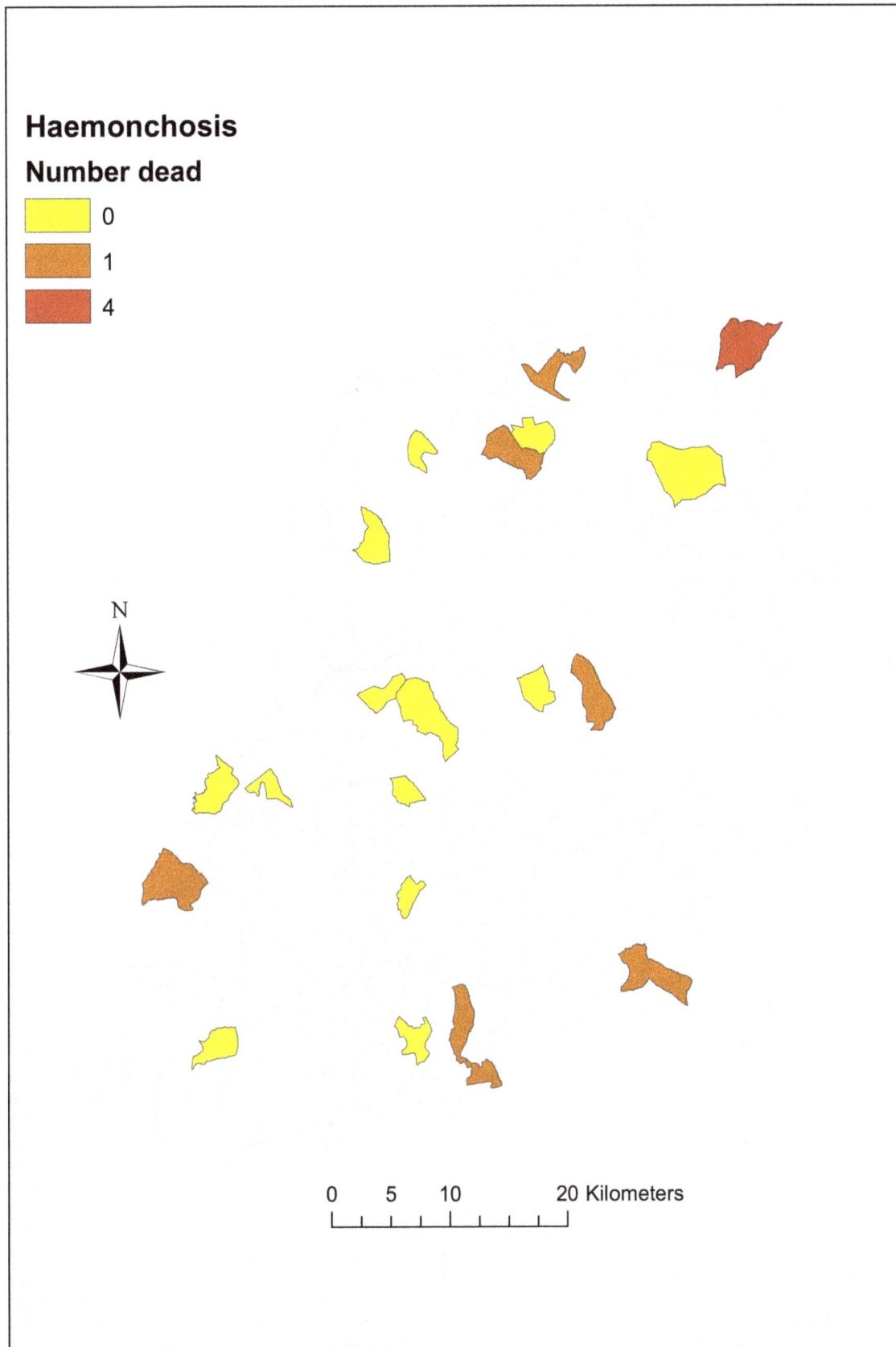

Figure 4. Map showing number of deaths attributable to haemonchosis by sub-location. In total, 10 of 88 deaths were attributed to haemonchosis.

Table 2. Results of significant predictors of East Coast Fever deaths.

	Hazard Ratio	lower CI	upper CI	p-value
Fixed effects				
Tick control	0.46	0.25	0.81	0.007
T.parva seroconversion	0.12	0.07	0.22	<0.001
Trypanosoma spp.	5.98	1.39	25.75	0.007
Strongyle eggs (per 1000 eggs)	1.48	1.37	1.61	<0.001
Group	Std Dev	Variance		
Sub-location random effect	0.47	0.22		

Table 3. Results of significant predictors of haemonchosis deaths.

	Hazard Ratio	lower CI	upper CI	p-value
Fixed effects				
Supplements use	0.19	0.04	0.85	0.03
Strongyle eggs (per 1000 eggs)	1.67	1.43	1.94	<0.001
Group	Std Dev	Variance		
Sub-location random effect	0.02	0.0004		

The interactions are thought to occur chiefly through immuno-regulation by helminth infections in two possible ways. First, the immune response becomes skewed to T-helper cell type 2 (Th2), required for fighting extracellular invaders, at the expense of T-helper cell type 1 (Th1) responses which are required for the control of microparasite infections including malaria parasitemia [30]. The second mechanism is through helminth induced immunomodulation that down-regulates both Th1 and Th2 responses, a strategy thought to be employed by helminths to avoid host immunity and possibly explaining why helminth infections even with known pathogenic species are often asymptomatic [31].

If similar mechanisms are at work with these study calves, a helminth skewed Th2 response and a dampened Th1 response would render a host co-infected with *T.parva* more susceptible to developing disease and affecting survival outcomes. Th1 responses are important for the generation for cytotoxic T lymphocytes (CTL), and if the helminth infections are skewing the response away from Th1 responses they may adversely affect the animal's ability to generate CTL and thus its ability to control a *T.parva* infection. Here the risk for ECF death increases with helminth burden (measured by strongyle epg), which from larval cultures and identification of L3 show *Haemonchus placei* to be the main helminth producing strongyle eggs.

These results suggest co-infections with the hookworm *H.placei* may be playing a role in reducing the host's ability to fight off *T.parva* infections. It is also possible that hookworms, which attach to the abomasal wall and suck whole blood, may be causing significant damage on their own weakening the calf more and increasing the risk of death with additional pathology from other co-infecting pathogens.

Trypanosomosis was not identified as a major cause of death in these cattle but the presence of trypanosome infections (mostly *T.vivax* – data not shown) increased the risk of death from ECF by up to 6 times. Like *T.parva*, infection with *Trypanosoma* spp. is known to lead to immuno-suppression. In addition, animals infected with trypanosomes have fever, lowered appetite, considerable weight loss, and anaemia. These effects coupled with immunosuppresion may lead to increased susceptibility and pathology in the host co-infected with *T.parva*.

Seropositivity to *T.parva* was associated with a protective effect against ECF-mortality. This result suggests that animals dying from ECF either die acutely before an antibody response that can be detected as a rising titre has occurred, or simply that the animals that do not mount an antibody response strong enough to

be detected as sero-conversion are at a high risk of succumbing to an ECF infection. As naturally acquired antibodies are thought to play no role in resolving *T.parva* infections, seropositivity may reflect prior exposure rather than being a direct indicator of immune status. If ECF death is acute it would be interesting to know why some animals survive first exposure (evidence by seropositivity) and others die on first infection. The intensity of *Theileria* spp. infection, specifically level 3 infection - multiple infected cells in multiple microscopy fields, was identified to be associated with a high risk for mortality. The risk for death, it appears, is related to the intensity of infection which may be the result of a high dose of infection or an indication of a host unable to control the within host multiplication of the infecting pathogen.

Results of the analysis of risk factors associated with ECF deaths revealed controlling for ticks in a farm was associated with a protective effect. The risk of ECF-death in farms carrying out tick control was 80% lower than in farms not controlling for ticks. Tick control was not done on the study calves and the observed protective effect is a benefit associated with control in the rest of the herd.

Infections with *Haemonchus placei* were themselves identified as the second most important aetiological cause of mortality in zebu calves. A high burden of strongyle eggs was identified as a significant predictor for deaths due to haemonchosis, pointing to their impact being burden-dependent. *H.placei* accounted for more that 80% of all larvae hatched following incubation of the strongyle eggs.

Farms that reported providing supplements (mainly crop residue) to the animals had significantly lower hazards for haemonchosis deaths than those that did not provide supplements. Calves in such farms are fed mainly while within the homesteads, and as a result will visit grazing pastures less frequently or take longer before starting to access communal grazing fields. These factors reduce the exposure to helminths, and may explain the association between supplement feeding and risk for deaths due to haemonchosis. It is also possible that animals receiving supplementation have improved nutrition reducing the effects of helminthosis.

The findings of this study suggest reduction in calf mortality would be attained through improved husbandry practices to reduce levels of exposure to pathogens to calves. Reducing the burden of livestock diseases, including exacerbated burden associated with pathogen-pathogen interactions during co-infections, is crucial if livestock are to be a viable pathway out of poverty. This is especially important in protecting livestock assets belonging to people living in poverty against mortality, and reducing losses in production associated with these diseases [32,33]. The results suggest that integrated tick, trypanosomes and worm-control programs would likely have large benefits in not just reducing mortality due to individual diseases, but also excess co-infection exacerbated mortality. Such integrated control programs have been suggested for example in the control of anaemia-related burden of malaria in humans, which is worsened by high hookworm burden [6].

Supporting Information

Table S1 Results of survival analysis univariable screening for infectious and non-infectious predictors of ECF mortality (33 cases). The table contains all risk factors with a p-value ≤ 0.2 and that were offered to the multivariable analysis.

Table S2 Results of survival analysis univariable screening for infectious and non-infectious predictors of deaths attributable to haemonchosis (10 cases). The table contains all risk factors with a p-value ≤ 0.2 and that were offered to the multivariable analysis.

Acknowledgments

This work was done as part of the Infectious Diseases of East African Livestock (IDEAL) project, a collaborative project between the University of Edinburgh, University of Pretoria, University of Nottingham and the International Livestock Research Institute (ILRI), Nairobi, Kenya. We would like to thank the Kenyan Department of Veterinary Services for their logistical support, participating farmers, and the animal health and laboratory technicians who participated in running of the project. We are grateful to Olga Tosas-Auguet and Maia Lesosky for their contribution in the designing and management of the databases.

Author Contributions

Conceived and designed the experiments: MEJW BMdCB JAWC OH HK EJP PGT. Performed the experiments: SMT HK EJP MNMK IC AJ. Analyzed the data: SMT MNMK JCAS IC IGH AJ BMdCB MEJW. Contributed reagents/materials/analysis tools: JCAS JAWC. Wrote the paper: SMT MEJW BMdCB JAWC OH HK EJP PGT MNMK JCAS IC IGH AJ.

References

1. Petney TN, Andrews RH (1998) Multiparasite communities in animals and humans: frequency, structure and pathogenic significance. International Journal for Parasitology 28: 377–393.
2. Pedersen AB, Fenton A (2007) Emphasizing the ecology in parasite community ecology. Trends in Ecology & Evolution 22: 133–139.
3. Telfer S, Lambin X, Birtles R, Beldomenico P, Burthe S, et al. (2010) Species interactions in a parasite community drive infection risk in a wildlife population. Science (New York, NY) 330: 243–246.
4. Ezenwa VO, Jolles AE (2011) From host immunity to pathogen invasion: the effects of helminth coinfection on the dynamics of microparasites. Integrative and Comparative Biology 51: 540–551.
5. Mwangi TW, Bethony JM, Brooker S (2006) Malaria and helminth interactions in humans: an epidemiological viewpoint. Annals of Tropical Medicine and Parasitology 100: 551–570.
6. Brooker S, Akhwale W, Pullan R, Estambale B, Clarke SE, et al. (2007) Epidemiology of plasmodium-helminth co-infection in Africa: populations at risk, potential impact on anemia, and prospects for combining control. The American Journal of Tropical Medicine and Hygiene 77: 88–98.
7. Craig BH, Tempest LJ, Pilkington JG, Pemberton JM (2008) Metazoan-protozoan parasite co-infections and host body weight in St Kilda Soay sheep. Parasitology 135: 433–441.
8. Lello J, Boag B, Fenton A, Stevenson IR, Hudson PJ (2004) Competition and mutualism among the gut helminths of a mammalian host. Nature 428: 840–844.
9. Behnke JM (2008) Structure in parasite component communities in wild rodents: predictability, stability, associations and interactions .... or pure randomness? Parasitology 135: 751–766.
10. Telfer S, Birtles R, Bennett M, Lambin X, Paterson S, et al. (2008) Parasite interactions in natural populations: insights from longitudinal data. Parasitology 135: 767–781.
11. Adegnika AA, Kremsner PG (2012) Epidemiology of malaria and helminth interaction: a review from 2001 to 2011. Current Opinion in HIV and AIDS 7: 221–224.
12. Harms G, Feldmeier H (2002) Review: HIV infection and tropical parasitic diseases–deleterious interactions in both directions? Tropical Medicine & International Health 7: 479–488.
13. Abu-Raddad LJ, Patnaik P, Kublin JG (2006) Dual infection with HIV and malaria fuels the spread of both diseases in Sub-Saharan Africa. Science (New York, NY) 314: 1603–1606.
14. Cox FE (2001) Concomitant infections, parasites and immune responses. Parasitology 122 Suppl: S23–38.
15. Alizon S, van Baalen M (2008) Multiple infections, immune dynamics, and the evolution of virulence. The American Naturalist 172: E150–68.
16. Graham AL (2008) Ecological rules governing helminth-microparasite coinfection. Proceedings of the National Academy of Sciences of the United States of America 105: 566–570.
17. Supali T, Verweij JJ, Wiria AE, Djuardi Y, Hamid F, et al. (2010) Polyparasitism and its impact on the immune system. International journal for parasitology 40: 1171–1176.
18. Drake LJ, Bundy DA (2001) Multiple helminth infections in children: impact and control. Parasitology 122 Suppl: S73–81.
19. Molyneux DH, Hotez PJ, Fenwick A (2005) "Rapid-impact interventions": how a policy of integrated control for Africa's neglected tropical diseases could benefit the poor. PLoS Medicine 2: e336.
20. Thumbi SM, Bronsvoort BM de C, Kiara H, Toye PG, Poole J, et al. (2013) Mortality in East African shorthorn zebu cattle under one year: predictors of infectious-disease mortality. BMC Veterinary Research 9: 175.
21. Bronsvoort BM de C, Thumbi SM, Poole EJ, Kiara H, Tosas Auguet O, et al. (2013) Design and descriptive epidemiology of the Infectious Diseases of East African Livestock (IDEAL) project, a longitudinal calf cohort study in western Kenya. BMC Veterinary Research 9: 171.
22. King J, Dodd D, Roth L (2006) The Necropsy Book: A guide for veterinary students, residents, clinicians, pathologists, and biological researchers. 4th ed. Illinois: Charles Davis DVM Foundation.
23. Therneau T (2012) A Package for Survival Analysis in S. R package version 2.36–14. Available: http://cran.r-project.org/package=survival. Accessed 15 February 2012.
24. R Development Core Team (2011) R: A language and environment for statistical computing. R Foundation for Statistical Computing. Available: http://www.r-project.org. Accessed 9 July 2011.
25. Spiegel A, Tall A, Raphenon G, Trape JF, Druilhe P (2003) Increased frequency of malaria attacks in subjects co-infected by intestinal worms and Plasmodium falciparum malaria. Transactions of the Royal Society of Tropical Medicine and Hygiene 97: 198–199.
26. Druilhe P, Tall A, Sokhna C (2005) Worms can worsen malaria: towards a new means to roll back malaria? Trends in Parasitology 21: 359–362.
27. Brutus L, Watier L, Briand V, Hanitrasoamampionona V, Razanatsoarilala H, et al. (2006) Parasitic co-infections: does Ascaris lumbricoides protect against Plasmodium falciparum infection? The American Journal of Tropical Medicine and Hygiene 75: 194–198.
28. Ezeamama AE, McGarvey ST, Acosta LP, Zierler S, Manalo DL, et al. (2008) The synergistic effect of concomitant schistosomiasis, hookworm, and trichuris infections on children's anemia burden. PLoS Neglected Tropical Diseases 2: e245.
29. Nacher M (2011) Interactions between worms and malaria: good worms or bad worms? Malaria Journal 10: 259.
30. Hartgers FC, Yazdanbakhsh M (2006) Co-infection of helminths and malaria: modulation of the immune responses to malaria. Parasite Immunology 28: 497–506.
31. Maizels RM, Balic A, Gomez-Escobar N, Nair M, Taylor MD, et al. (2004) Helminth parasites–masters of regulation. Immunological Reviews 201: 89–116.
32. Perry B, Sones K (2007) Science for development. Poverty reduction through animal health. Science (New York, NY) 315: 333–334.
33. Rich KM, Perry BD (2011) The economic and poverty impacts of animal diseases in developing countries: new roles, new demands for economics and epidemiology. Preventive veterinary medicine 101: 133–147.

10

The Spread of Fecally Transmitted Parasites in Socially-Structured Populations

Charles L. Nunn[1]*, Peter H. Thrall[2], Fabian H. Leendertz[3], Christophe Boesch[4]

1 Department of Human Evolutionary Biology, Harvard University, Cambridge, Massachusetts, United States of America, **2** CSIRO Plant Industry, Canberra, Australia, **3** Research Group Emerging Zoonoses, Robert Koch-Institute, Berlin, Germany, **4** Max Planck Institute for Evolutionary Anthropology, Leipzig, Germany

Abstract

Mammals are infected by a wide array of gastrointestinal parasites, including parasites that also infect humans and domesticated animals. Many of these parasites are acquired through contact with infectious stages present in soil, feces or vegetation, suggesting that ranging behavior will have a major impact on their spread. We developed an individual-based spatial simulation model to investigate how range use intensity, home range overlap, and defecation rate impact the spread of fecally transmitted parasites in a population composed of social groups (i.e., a socially structured population). We also investigated the effects of epidemiological parameters involving host and parasite mortality rates, transmissibility, disease–related mortality, and group size. The model was spatially explicit and involved the spillover of a gastrointestinal parasite from a reservoir population along the edge of a simulated reserve, which was designed to mimic the introduction pathogens into protected areas. Animals ranged randomly within a "core" area, with biased movement toward the range center when outside the core. We systematically varied model parameters using a Latin hypercube sampling design. Analyses of simulation output revealed a strong positive association between range use intensity and the prevalence of infection. Moreover, the effects of range use intensity were similar in magnitude to effects of group size, mortality rates, and the per-contact probability of transmission. Defecation rate covaried positively with gastrointestinal parasite prevalence. Greater home range overlap had no positive effects on prevalence, with a smaller core resulting in less range overlap yet more intensive use of the home range and higher prevalence. Collectively, our results reveal that parasites with fecal-oral transmission spread effectively in socially structured populations. Future application should focus on parameterizing the model with empirically derived ranging behavior for different species or populations and data on transmission characteristics of different infectious organisms.

Editor: Brock Fenton, University of Western Ontario, Canada

Funding: This research was supported by the Max Planck Society and Harvard University. The funders had no role in study design, data collection and analysis, decision to publish, or preparation of the manuscript.

Competing Interests: The authors have declared that no competing interests exist.

* E-mail: cnunn@oeb.harvard.edu.

Introduction

Mammals are host to a wide diversity of infectious agents [1,2]. Many of these parasites and pathogens are gastrointestinal and spread through fecal-oral transmission routes which involves fecal contamination of the soil, food items or other substrates and subsequent consumption of infectious stages of the parasite by other hosts. Examples of fecally transmitted micro- and macro-parasitic organisms found in wild mammals include protozoa such as *Giardia* and *Cryptosporidium* [3,4], intestinal nematodes such as *Ascaris*, *Enterobius* and their close relatives [5], many species of fungi [6], bacteria such as pathogenic *Escherichia coli* [7], and viruses such as adenoviruses [8]. In wild primates, the prevalence of gastrointestinal macroparasites can exceed 50% [9,10]. A variety of gastrointestinal infectious agents are also well known in human populations, including Norwalk virus, pathogenic *E. coli*, cholera, and *Cryptosporidium*. Many of these infectious organisms – hereafter also referred to simply as parasites – are harmful to wild animals, for example by increasing mortality and reducing fecundity [11,12,13,14].

Despite growing knowledge of the parasites that cause wildlife infections, the dynamics of fecally transmitted infectious agents in natural animal populations are still not well understood. An individual mammalian host harboring a gastrointestinal parasite may shed large numbers of infectious agents to the environment, potentially infecting other animals in close proximity or those that come into contact with excreted material at a later time. This contact may occur, for example, when individuals from different groups overlap at food or water resources (i.e., home range overlap), suggesting that heterogeneity in resource distribution could play a major role in the dynamics and persistence of fecally transmitted infectious agents. In addition, some gut pathogens such as cholera result in diarrhea, which could benefit the pathogen by disseminating infectious stages more widely, especially when host movement is not impaired or when fecal material can contaminate water sources. Thus, a number of important epidemiological questions arise concerning interactions among factors involving host sociality, ranging patterns and parasite transmission mechanisms [15,16,17].

Parasites are of increasing concern in the conservation of biodiversity [18,19,20,21], including the decline of animals that typically live in socially structured populations, such as primates [22,23,24,25]. At an applied level, understanding the dynamics of infectious disease in relation to anthropogenic impacts and population structure – and how these might influence subsequent ecological and evolutionary trajectories of parasites in terms of virulence and transmissibility – is critical for making informed conservation management decisions [21,26]. Of relevance in this context, domesticated animals and humans along habitat edges may introduce new parasites into wild populations, which can then spread based on social, ecological and infection characteristics of the system [7,27]. Given that wild animals, domesticated animals and humans often overlap along the edges of nature reserves, it is critically important to improve our understanding of the ecological factors that enable some parasites to penetrate and persist in host populations of wild animals [20,28,29].

Several studies have investigated how range use behavior might influence the spread of fecally transmitted parasites. For example, territoriality could reduce home range overlap and contact between groups, resulting in fewer opportunities for the spread of parasites [the "territoriality benefits" hypothesis, 30]. Conversely, more intensive use of a home range could increase exposure to fecal material in the home range, resulting in higher levels of infection [the "fecal exposure" hypothesis, 16]. In a comparative test of parasite richness aimed at investigating these possibilities, Nunn and Dokey [15] found that helminth richness covaried positively with the intensity of range use in primates, thus providing support for the fecal exposure hypothesis over the territoriality benefits hypothesis. They also investigated whether home range overlap influenced parasite diversity across host species, but found no significant effects. In ungulates, Ezenwa [16] found that territorial species have higher prevalence of parasitic nematodes (strongyles) than non-territorial species and, among gregarious hosts, territorial species were found to have higher richness than non-territorial species. Similarly, amongst two groups of mantled howler monkeys (*Alouatta palliata*), Stoner [31] found that parasitism was higher in a group that used a narrow forest corridor between two blocks of forest (rather than a more cohesive block of forest for the other group). The more intensive use of habitat in the corridor was one of several factors that may have increased parasitism in the more heavily infected group [see also 28].

Here, we developed an individual based model to investigate how social, ecological and parasitological factors influence the spread of fecally transmitted infectious agents in socially structured populations (i.e., where individuals live in spatially distributed social groups and disperse among groups). In socially structured populations, parasites face a major challenge in spreading from one group to another; groups are in effect "islands" for parasites, and this effect might be strengthened if territorial behavior and social structure further restrict movement of parasites [29,32,33,34]. For fecally-transmitted parasites, three major routes of group-to-group transmission seem most likely: through movement of infected individuals among groups, resulting in the introduction of the parasite to the home range of a new group; through shared resources and resulting home range overlap among groups; and through direct social interactions between groups, including mating and territorial interactions. We focused on the first two of these mechanisms by investigating whether the rate of movement between groups (dispersal) or range overlap has a bigger impact on the spread of parasites in socially structured populations. We did not explicitly model intergroup encounters, and thus we do not directly consider how territoriality could reduce infection risk by limiting home range overlap or social interactions. To investigate the "fecal exposure" hypothesis, we varied the intensity of home range use (i.e., day range relative to home range).

In addition to dispersal and ranging, our model incorporated several other factors expected to play key roles in gastrointestinal

parasite dynamics. Group size may be important if larger groups produce more fecal contamination per unit area of the environment, both within the group's home range (causing more individuals to become infected) and outside the range (causing other groups to become infected). Some gut parasites may increase fecal output (e.g., diarrhea), which could lead to increased spread of infectious agents among individuals in social groups. To study whether increasing fecal output might influence infectious disease dynamics, we varied the rate at which infected individuals defecated. In addition, a variety of standard epidemiological parameters should influence the dynamics of gastrointestinal parasites. Thus, a higher background mortality rate or death rate due to disease should reduce the ability of a parasite to become established in a host population. Similarly, the spread of infectious organisms will be enhanced by a higher transmission rate and longer infectious period in the soil or in the host (provided that the benefits of longer infectious periods are not offset by higher disease-related mortality). A longer latent period in the soil, however, may reduce parasitism rates, because with longer latency, groups will on average be farther from the site of defecation when the parasites become infectious.

Several studies have documented the potential for infections to spread from humans and their domesticated animals into wildlife [e.g., nonhuman primates, 7,27,35,36]. Thus, we explicitly investigated the conservation implications for fecally transmitted parasites by modeling the introduction of infectious organisms along one edge of a simulated "reserve" and quantifying the spread of infections across the reserve.

In our simulation model, individual hosts are part of social groups that range on a landscape composed of 81 distinct social groups, where individuals of the same social group range as a cohesive unit on the landscape. The hosts are exposed to fecal contamination from a hypothetical population of domesticated animals that border one edge of the landscape; the possibility for infection occurs when individuals come into contact with feces from this domesticated animal reservoir. Newly infected individuals then spread the infection to other individuals in their groups, and to individuals in different groups through dispersal or in areas of home range overlap. We use the model to evaluate the relative importance of social, ecological and parasitological factors likely to influence the spread of fecally transmitted infections.

Results

We conducted 1000 simulations that varied the 12 parameters according to the minima and maxima shown in Table 1. As output, we focused on prevalence of infection with the parasite and population loss at various points in the simulation (prevalence related terminology is summarized in Table 2). Both population dynamics and prevalence of infection varied greatly across simulation runs, with mean population prevalence ranging from 0 to 98.7% (calculated over the last one-tenth of time steps for each of 1000 simulations, at which point infection dynamics had stabilized). In most simulations, however, population prevalence was low (Figure 1, median prevalence = 0.4%, mean = 22.4% over the last one-tenth of time steps).

Total population loss over the simulation showed a bimodal distribution (Figure 2). For many parameter combinations, changes in population size were characterized by only slight losses or gains (expected due to the stochastic effects of births and deaths, shown as the highest peak around zero in Figure 2). However, 41.9% of the simulations resulted in losses of more than 10% of the population. Maximum population loss was 58.8%.

Table 1. Simulation parameters and range of values used (Latin Hypercube Sample).

Parameter	Units	Minimum	Maximum	Midpoint	Upper Quartile
Group size (g)	Individuals	4	40	22	31
Mortality rate[1] (m_b)	Probability per time step (day)	0.000055	0.0055	0.0028	0.0014
Disease mortality (m_d)	Probability per time step (day)	1	100	50.5	25.75
Day range[2] (D)	Range matrix grid cells	2	30	Variable	Variable
Core area[3] (c)	Proportion of a group's range matrix	0	0.5	0.25	0.375
Latency – soil[4] (b_s)	Time steps (days)	1	15	8	11.5
Infectious – soil[4] (f_s)	Time steps (days)	1	50	25.5	37.75
Latency – host[4] (b_h)	Time steps (days)	3	14	8.5	11.25
Infectious – host[4] (f_h)	Time steps (days)	4	365	184.5	274.75
Defecation rate[5] (d)	Probability per time step (day)	0.5	3	1.75	2.375
Transmission (β)	Probability per time step (day)	0.00001	0.001	0.00051	0.00075
Dispersal rate (i)	Probability per time step (day)	0.001	0.01	0.0055	0.0078

[1]Based on life span range of 0.5–50 years and time step of one day.
[2]Number of movement steps per simulated time step. Range was based on values of the D-index from Mitani and Rodman [37], i.e. 0.2 to 3 when converted to the D-index.
[3]Rounded down to increments of 0, 0.1, 0.2, 0.3, and 0.4.
[4]Integer values.
[5]For infected hosts only, and used as a rate per day calculated as d / D.

Along the edge where infections were introduced, mean group prevalence was 22.8% (maximum of 98.9%), and group prevalence was greater than zero in 72.7% of simulations. A similar pattern was found at the far edge of the reserve (i.e., furthest from the source of new infections), with mean group prevalence of 21.5% (maximum = 98.7%). At the far edge, however, fewer simulations showed group prevalence greater than zero (43.3% of simulations), probably due to the continual introduction of parasites at the near edge resulting in a constant inflow of infections.

In a general linear model of the 1000 simulations using the Latin hypercube sample of input parameters, we found that average population prevalence (recorded at the last time step of simulations) was best explained by group size, parasite infectious period in the soil, and transmission probability (Table 3, $R^2 = 0.60$, $F_{12,987} = 127.4$). Prevalence also increased with day range and the rate of defecation. Increases in both intrinsic mortality and disease-related mortality had negative effects on prevalence. Importantly, the size of the core area had an effect on population prevalence that was opposite to predictions of the territory benefit hypothesis.

A smaller core area reduced home range overlap, but tended to increase population prevalence (Table 3), probably because a smaller core area resulted in greater re-use of cells in the core area. Thus, counter to expectations under the territory benefits hypothesis (and across a wide range of parameter values), reduced overlap with neighboring groups failed to result in lower prevalence at the population level.

Another finding of interest is that dispersal rate did not have strong effects on population prevalence (Table 3). One possibility is that dispersal (and possibly home range overlap) has a greater impact on pathogen spread early in an epidemic, as compared to effects on prevalence when dynamics reached a steady state. We therefore examined population prevalence at an earlier stage in the simulations, over the first 1/10 of the simulation run (time steps 1 to 730, representing units of single days and thus equivalent to 2 years of transmission dynamics). Average population prevalence was 9.2% during this initial phase, which as expected was much less than average prevalence of 22.4% at the end of the simulation. A GLM of the predictors of population prevalence early in the simulations accounted for 52% of the variation in

Table 2. Output Measures.

Measure	Description	Timeframe Used for Calculation
Population prevalence	Prevalence based on all individuals in the population	Mean or median over the last 730 time steps (last 1/10 of the simulation) or in final time step
Total population loss	Change in population size as a percentage of the starting population	Time step 1 to time step 7300
Group prevalence	Prevalence of individuals in groups, averaged across groups, and useful for assessing what proportion of groups are infected	Last time step
Group prevalence at edges	Prevalence of infection among individuals along particular segments of the reserve, measured relative to the spillover population	Last time step
Maximum prevalence	Maximum recorded population prevalence over the course of the simulation	Time step 1 to time step 7300
Number of groups infected	Number of groups that were infected when a simulation ended	Time step 7300

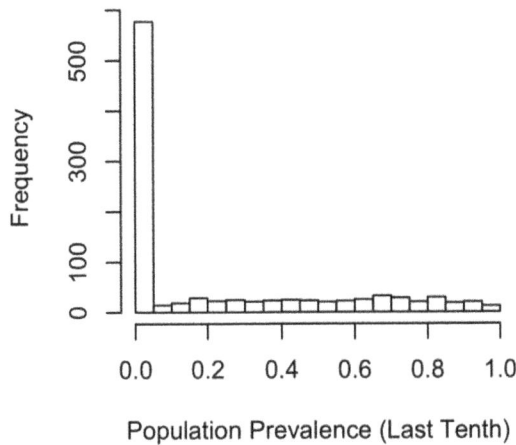

Figure 1. Proportion of the population infected. The histogram shows the frequency in which particular proportions of the population were infected. Results are based on average prevalence over the last one-tenth of time steps (730 steps in total) across 1000 simulations.

prevalence. Relative to the results at the end of the simulation (see Table 3), the standardized coefficient for the rate of dispersal increased three-fold (coefficient = 0.018, t_{987} = 4.84), while the effect of core area became substantially weaker but remained positive (coefficient = 0.008, t_{987} = 2.27, indicating that less overlap increases prevalence). These findings suggest that shortly after introduction, the rate of dispersal influenced the rate at which a gastrointestinal parasite spreads through a host population. Other results were similar to those presented in Table 3, with group size, infectious period in the soil, transmission probability and day range having the largest effects on prevalence (although with smaller standardized coefficients on average).

We also generated linear models to examine the predictors of maximum prevalence, group prevalence, number of groups infected, and population loss due to infectious disease. These analyses produced remarkably similar results, with the ranking of effects identical (or nearly so) to the results in Table 3 (see Supporting Information Tables S1 to S4). Of particular interest for

conservation effort is population loss, with population loss increasing with increases in the following key variables: infectious period in the soil, group size, probability of transmission, and day range (see Table S4). A higher mortality rate (and higher disease related mortality) tended to depress the degree to which populations declined due to disease.

To illustrate the effects of ranging intensity, we re-ran the simulations holding all parameters constant except for day range, which we varied from 2 to 30. Setting all other variables to their midpoint values (Table 1), we found a positive association between ranging intensity and parasite prevalence (Figure 3 shows results for maximum recorded prevalence). In addition, the plot reveals a clear threshold around 12 movements per time step, with the infectious disease generally unable to persist at lower movement rates. However, the average population prevalence at the end of these simulations was fairly low (12.6%). We repeated the analysis with the upper quartile of values (or lower quartile for variables that show a negative association with prevalence, Table 3). We again found a strong association between ranging intensity and prevalence (Figure 4 for maximum prevalence), with much higher average population prevalence, as expected, at the end of simulations (84.2%).

Our results may be sensitive to the underlying ranging model that we used. To investigate this possibility, we implemented a different model of exposure in the home range for a focused set of parameters. Specifically, we altered the model to hold constant the number of exposure steps, as described in the Methods. Holding other variables constant at their midpoints, we found that day range had a positive effect on prevalence (Figure 5), albeit a weaker overall effect than in the general model (cf. Figures 3 and 4).

Discussion

The general results from our model suggest that gastrointestinal parasites can be of significant conservation concern in socially structured populations of wild hosts by exhibiting high prevalence, causing significant population declines, and spreading effectively from one side of a simulated reserve to the other side across

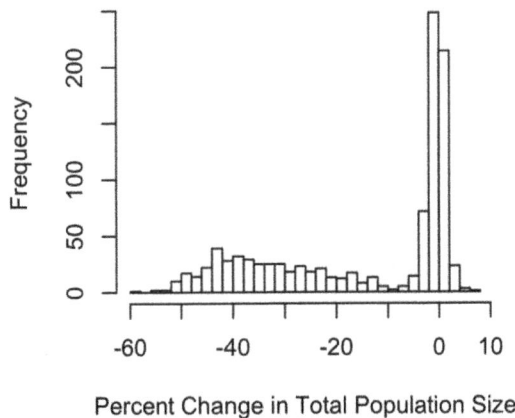

Figure 2. Proportion of the population lost. The histogram shows a bimodal distribution of changes in population size. In most simulations, population changes were slightly negative or positive, reflecting stochastic variation related to births and deaths (indicated by the tall bars around zero). In a sizable number of simulations, however, population losses exceeded 10%.

Table 3. General linear modeling of average population prevalence.

Predictor	Estimate	t-statistic
Intercept	0.224	36.4
Group size (g)	0.105	17.0
Infectious – soil (f_s)	0.105	17.0
Transmission (β)	0.100	16.1
Day range (D)	0.087	14.1
Disease mortality (m_d)	−0.083	−13.4
Mortality rate (m_b)	−0.066	−10.7
Defecation rate (d)	0.062	10.0
Smaller core area (c)[1]	0.051	8.19
Latency in host (b_h)	0.030	4.77
Infectious – host (f_h)	0.018	2.98
Dispersal rate (i)	0.006	1.00
Latency in soil (b_s)	−0.003	−0.471

[1]In the model, core area was parameterized as the difference from the edge of a ranging matrix to the edge of the core area. Thus, higher values of this difference indicate a smaller core area.

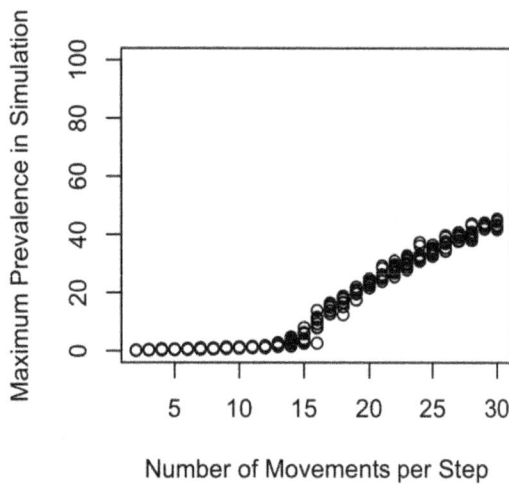

Figure 3. Maximum population prevalence in relation to day range: midpoint values. Plot shows how maximum prevalence increases with day range (movements per time step) when using the midpoint of the range of values in Table 1. Day range is the number of steps that a group moved on the ranging matrix per time step. Given a home range diameter of 10, values of the D-index can be obtained by dividing number of range movements by 10. Prevalence was taken as the maximum recorded prevalence across each simulation. Use of averages (rather than maxima) produced similar patterns.

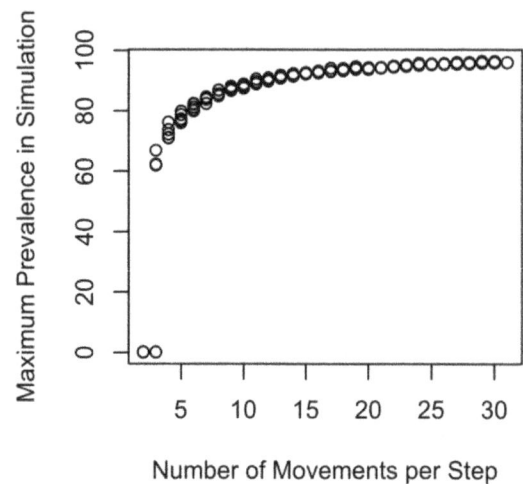

Figure 4. Maximum population prevalence in relation to day range: "upper" values. Plot shows how maximum prevalence increases with day range (movements per time step) when using the upper quartile of the range of values, where upper refers to the direction for the parameter that would be expected to increase prevalence. Day range is the number of steps that a group moved on the ranging matrix per time step. Given a home range diameter of 10, values of the D-index can be obtained by dividing number of range movements by 10. Prevalence was taken as the maximum recorded prevalence across each simulation. Use of averages (rather than maxima) produced similar patterns.

multiple home ranges. Although disease-related mortality should slow the spread of infectious agents, for the environmentally transmitted parasites in our simulated populations, it appears that even virulent parasites can spread widely. Partly this reflects the buildup of material in the soil that can remain infectious for many time steps, and partly it reflects that newly susceptible individuals are born into the population in a density-dependent manner.

Social groups represent biological islands for infectious disease, and thus exclusive use of a home range (i.e. reducing among-group contacts) might be expected to reduce the risk of parasitism [30]. Previous work in primates and ungulates suggests, however, that territoriality and its correlates, such as higher intensity of range use, increase the risk of infection with fecally transmitted parasites [15,16]. One explanation for this effect is that territoriality tends to result in more intensive use of a home range [37], resulting in higher rates of re-infection. An alternative explanation is that territoriality and ranging are costly, for example in terms of physical effort and risk associated with defending the territory or elevated levels of testosterone or cortisol [16]. Thus, individuals who are defending a territory may be more susceptible to infectious disease. Similarly, parasites might spread among individuals in different groups through physical contact during inter-group encounters in a more territorial species.

Our model allowed us to assess whether greater exposure to parasites in the soil – generated from more intensive ranging – results in higher levels of infection at the group and population levels. We found strong evidence for greater range use as a driver of higher prevalence, with day range exhibiting effects that were similar to those found for fundamental epidemiological parameters involving transmission rate, mortality rate, and a combination of population size and contact rate (i.e., group size). Conversely, greater home range overlap appeared to have no effect on the spread of gastrointestinal parasites; overlap actually resulted in lower levels of infection (rather than the expected positive effect). This effect occurred because groups with greater overlap used their own core areas less intensively, suggesting again that intensity

of range use is the primary ranging parameter that impacts prevalence. Similarly, rates of dispersal appeared to be important only during the initial spread of an infectious disease. We also investigated whether higher defecation rate in infected individuals impacts transmission dynamics. As expected, defecation rate had a significant positive impact on overall prevalence. However, compared to the effects of other parameters, such as mortality rates, defecation rate was less important (see Table 3 for standardized regression coefficients).

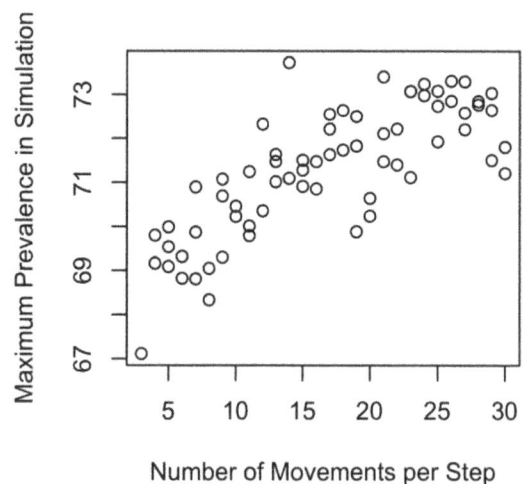

Figure 5. Maximum prevalence and movement when holding infection risk constant. Plot shows how maximum prevalence covaries with day range using the alternative ranging model. In this model, groups have the same number of opportunities for infection, regardless of day range.

In the simulation model, we assumed that animals move in a random walk within their core ranges; outside the core, they moved in a biased random walk, with a tendency to return to their core area. Such a movement pattern could lead to higher rates of infection, given that animals are more likely to cover the same ground under a random walk when compared, for example, to animals exhibiting other movement patterns [e.g., 38]. Indeed, we expect that under more realistic models of ranging, latency periods in the soil might have greater impacts on the spread of parasites because animals might be less likely to encounter feces shortly after their deposition. In addition, larger social groups may require larger ranges [39,40], which could reduce exposure to infectious stages in the soil and reduce disease risk. Individuals also could have spatial memory of resources and environmental risks, which may impact ranging patterns and thus patterns of infection [e.g., 41]. An important area for future research is to build stronger theoretical linkage between the risk of fecally-transmitted parasites and empirically derived patterns of ranging behavior and social interactions [e.g., in primates, 42,43].

We also assumed that ranging behaviors are independent of infection levels in the group. However, it is possible that groups with higher levels of infection might have shorter day ranges, for example if infected individuals show more sickness behaviors, such as resting [44]. Although not formally modeled here, our results suggest that disease-related reduction in ranging would reduce the spread of infection in the population. This could be investigated in future empirical and theoretical research, and suggests that efforts to reduce ranging by infected groups (e.g., through provisioning) could lead to reduced levels of infection at the broader population level.

Our model explicitly considered the conservation impacts of an introduced gastrointestinal parasite. To do this, we modeled the continuous spillover from a reservoir host, such as domesticated animals or humans, along one edge of a reserve containing a wild host population sub-structured into a large number of social groups. We found that a fecally-transmitted parasites penetrated the population very readily, commonly reaching the far edge of the reserve. In addition, the introduced gastrointestinal parasite could cause significant mortality, with more than 40% of the simulations resulting in loss of 10% or more of the original population.

Highly pathogenic infectious diseases have attracted much recent attention, such as Ebola in African apes [24,45,46,47]. Our model suggests, however, that in the context of conservation concerns, gastrointestinal pathogens could be as important as infectious agents that are transmitted by close contact or by vector. For example, higher disease-related mortality tended to slow the spread of infectious disease in our model, as expected given that this reduces the pool of infected individuals in the population [48], yet population declines due to disease can be great and increase with increasing infectious period in the soil, group size, probability of transmission, and day range length (see Supporting Information, Table S4). By comparison, a previous model of infectious disease dynamics involving a highly virulent introduced pathogenic infection, which was modeled after Ebola, found that the infectious agent rarely spread widely in the population and never caused extinction of the simulated host population [33]. Of course, high rates of spillover from a reservoir population could lead to severe population declines for a highly pathogenic infectious disease, and these risks should be monitored closely. Our model suggests that simultaneous with such monitoring, we should also be aware of infections with less immediate mortality effects in wild animal populations. In addition, the model serves as a call for more information on characteristics of parasites that infect wild

animals, so that latency, transmissibility and disease-related death rates can be parameterized more effectively.

In terms of applications, our model provides several new insights for the control of gastrointestinal infections in spatially and socially structured host populations. First and foremost, it appears that once such parasites enter a population, they commonly spread throughout the range, often relatively quickly. Thus, in terms of measures aimed at prevention of initial invasion and spread, it is essential to prevent the initial introduction of gastrointestinal parasites from reservoir populations. A model like ours could be used to investigate the effects of ranging behavior by the reservoir population, or to examine approaches aimed at reducing habitat sharing between reservoir and wildlife populations. Second, we cannot count on territorial behavior to reduce the risk of infectious disease establishment in a wild host population. Infectious diseases appear to spread remarkably easily through dispersal and shared range use, with day range more important than actual measures of home range overlap. Lastly, rates of dispersal appear less important to the spread of parasites than range use, but once dispersal of an infected individual into a new group occurs, infectious material can build up in the soil of the new group and result in new infections. Thus, it may be important to constrain host movements, both in terms of habitat sharing and dispersal, especially during early stages of infectious disease spread (i.e., while infection is spatially limited to a small number of social groups). However, this may only be possible for intensively managed wildlife such as those living in game ranches.

In summary, our study provides new insights into the role of ranging behavior on the spread of gastrointestinal parasites. While previous comparative and field studies have found such links, they were unable to establish that these links were caused by more intensive ranging, or by alternative mechanisms involving territoriality, such as increased susceptibility from stressors related to territorial encounters, or exposure to parasites at territorial boundaries. Our model demonstrates that ranging behavior is likely to have strong effects on parasitism that are equivalent in magnitude to other well-established epidemiological factors. Moreover, by including a spillover host, our model demonstrates the importance of gastrointestinal parasites for conservation of biodiversity. Collectively, our results highlight the need for renewed attention to reducing the flow of infections into wildlife populations, and for greater empirical effort to investigate whether ranging and other behaviors increase the spread of these parasites into wildlife.

Methods

Basic Simulation Structure

The goal of the model was to investigate the social, ecological and epidemiological parameters that influence the spread of fecally transmitted parasites in socially structured populations, specifically in the context of spillover from a neighboring population of animals on the edge of the habitat (such as domesticated animals or humans). The model was designed to simulate the spatial movement of groups of individuals relative to a "core area" of the home range, and the movement of individuals between different social groups through dispersal.

Simulations took place on a 9×9 square lattice (*social group matrix*), within which smaller square lattices of cells (*ranging matrix*) were designated that reflect a *home range* (10×10 cells) for each group on the social group matrix; collectively, the area of the range lattice that includes social groups for the focal host species was referred to as the *reserve* (Figure 6). Within each home range a *core area* was further defined as the percentage of cells away from the edge of the home range that the animals prefer to use. When this parameter equaled zero, the core area and the home range coincided (10×10, i.e. 100 cells); when the parameter equaled 0.1, the core area represented the inner 64 cells (8×8); and when this parameter equaled its maximum of 0.5, the core area was a point in the center of the range (0×0 core area, and thus agents tightly used the center of the range). Given that animals prefer to range in their core area but can move outside of it (see below), a smaller core area resulted in less home range overlap among groups, which was confirmed using data on group location recorded during the simulations.

Around the range lattice we then added a further 10 cells, which is equivalent to one home range. This *buffer* enabled groups of the *focal population* to range outside the reserve, and for a second species (the *spillover population*) to contaminate one edge of the reserve with infected feces. Parasites were introduced to the focal population from the spillover population (e.g., infected cattle), which in our simulations always ranged along the upper edge of the reserve and penetrated one-half of the home range of the nearest focal population by five cells (Figure 6). Spillover infections occurred at the rate of 10 infected feces scattered randomly in this area in each time step of the simulation.

Feces containing infectious stages of parasites accumulated in the range lattice and, following a *soil latency period* on the ground, were potentially infectious during a *soil infectious period* to individual hosts in the focal population. We thus took into account that parasites exhibit a latency period and mortality during the soil stage (i.e., they were not continuously infectious).

Individual hosts were associated with one of the 81 groups in the social structure lattice, and each group had a location in the range lattice that was typically, but not always, in the designated home range of that particular group (see "Group Social Behavior and Population Dynamics" below). Individuals were further characterized by their infection status, including number of days in a defined *host latency period* (i.e., exposed but not yet infectious) and, following host latency, number of days in a *host infectious period*. During the host infectious period, feces were produced that are infectious to other individuals after a soil latency period. The defecation rate was defined as number per day rather than per movement step in a day, and thus was comparable across

simulations with different day ranges. Infection occurred with transmission probability β for each infectious pile in the ranging grid cell, and the probability of infection was calculated for each movement step and, in a subset of simulations, holding this constant per day. We assumed that after clearing the infection, individuals have no immunity to the infectious agent and thus were susceptible to re-infection (i.e., a susceptible-exposed-infected-susceptible model). While infected, however, individuals could not become infected with another parasite; thus, the individual had to move through the infectious periods to be re-infected. Some gastrointestinal infectious agents may elicit varying degrees of immunity, but we did not consider this possibility in our current model.

We ran each simulation for 7300 time steps, which were in units of one day and thus equivalent to 20 years of infection dynamics. In initial runs under a wide variety of parameter settings, we determined that the simulation reached a steady state well before time step 7300. Specifically, we recorded key statistics, such as prevalence (see Table 2), across 10 blocks of 730 time steps each (corresponding to 2 year periods). We then confirmed empirically that prevalence had stabilized by the last 1/10 of the simulation.

Model Parameterization and Exploration

For each simulation run, groups of individuals were formed based on user-specified values for group size by drawing random numbers from a Poisson distribution. All groups had at least two individuals, and all individuals in the population were initially uninfected. Groups were then assigned a random location on the range matrix. Deaths, births and dispersal of individuals will tend to cause the initial social group structure to drift over a simulation run, especially when simulations are run for many time steps. To help maintain initial demographic conditions, we retained a matrix of the initial numbers of males and females in each group. This *initiating matrix* was used to stochastically adjust probabilities associated with demographic parameters (birth and dispersal) to help maintain initial conditions for each group throughout a simulation run (see below).

To explore how different parameters influence disease dynamics, we undertook multivariate analyses using random sampling. Random sampling was conducted using Latin hypercube sam-

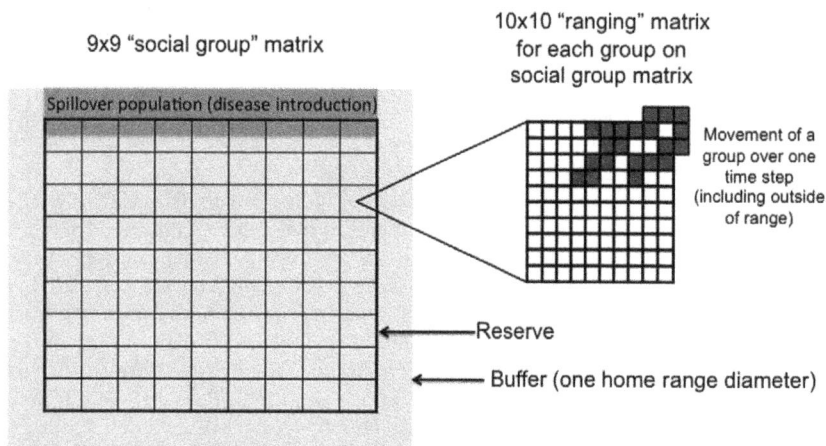

Figure 6. Social group, ranging and spillover areas. Social groups are arranged on the landscape and identified by the *social group lattice*, which was a 9×9 lattice in all simulations presented here (n = 81 social groups). Social groups range within the *ranging lattice*, which is a 10×10 lattice for each of the 81 social groups and contains a core area (see Figure 2). The 81 10×10 ranging lattices constitute the *reserve*. Around this reserve, a further 10 cell *buffer* occurs, producing a total potential ranging area of 110×110. Along the top edge of the buffer and reserve, a *spillover population* exists; it penetrates the reserve within 5 cells, thus overlapping with the uppermost social groups of the *focal population*.

pling, which is a type of stratified Monte Carlo sampling that has been used in epidemiological modeling and is more efficient in this context than random sampling regimes or those that include all possible parameter values [49,50,51,52]. Twelve parameters were varied across uniform (flat) distributions in the Latin hypercube sample: group size, transmission probability, background mortality, disease-related mortality, rate of dispersal, defecation rate, day range, core area, soil latency period, host latency period, and host infectious period. Table 1 summarizes the parameters that we investigated, along with the ranges of variation that were sampled for each parameter. Parameters that required integer or discrete values for the model (e.g., host infectious period) were represented as continuously varying traits in the Latin hypercube sample and then averaged appropriately. Using this approach, we generated 1000 Latin hypercube samples reflecting the range of variation in Table 1 (i.e., 1000 simulations).

In addition to the Latin Hypercube sample, we undertook an additional set of analyses to investigate how day range influenced prevalence while holding other parameters constant. We conducted these analyses using the midpoint of values from the Latin Hypercube sample, and then repeated the process using the upper or lower quartile as the value (selecting upper or lower quartile values to produce higher expected prevalence, based on the results from the Latin hypercube sample and epidemiological theory). The values used are given in Table 1.

Group Social Behavior And Population Dynamics

Model dynamics proceeded in discrete time steps, which represent single days in the lives of the simulated agents. In each time step four processes took place sequentially: (1) ranging and possible infection of hosts due to exposure to feces in the ranging matrix, (2) deaths due to stochastic factors and infection, (3) stochastic dispersal of individuals to neighboring groups, and (4) stochastic births to replace individuals lost to disease or other factors. These processes are explained in further detail below.

Individuals moved in their home ranges (i.e., the ranging matrix) with other members of their social group. Groups ranged in a random walk within their *core areas* on the range matrix (Figure 7), and all members of a group moved as a cohesive unit in the same ranging matrix cell (i.e., groups are cohesive). Core areas were centered inside a group's designated home range, and thus did not overlap with other groups' core areas.

Groups could range outside of their defined core areas, including into other groups' home ranges and core areas, but they did so with a "rubber-band" process that tended to pull them back towards the core area (and thus ranging is not a random walk when a group is outside the core area). More specifically, in a given time step, a random draw determined whether a group moved horizontally or vertically. Assuming that a vertical movement was selected, a group within its core area has an equal probability of moving either up or down, which is then determined by drawing a random number. Outside the core area, however, this decision to move up or down was biased by the vertical distance from the edge of the core area. Specifically, to the base probability of 1/2 for moving up or down, we added one to both numerator and denominator for each cell away from the core for the probability of moving back to the core. Thus, if the group was one cell "above" its core area, the probability of moving "down" on the next step became 2/3, if it was two cells away the probability was 3/4, if three cells away the probability was 4/5, and so on, asymptotically to a probability of 1. The same procedure was used for movements in the horizontal direction. Hence, the probability of movement toward the core area

A Group's "Ranging Matrix"

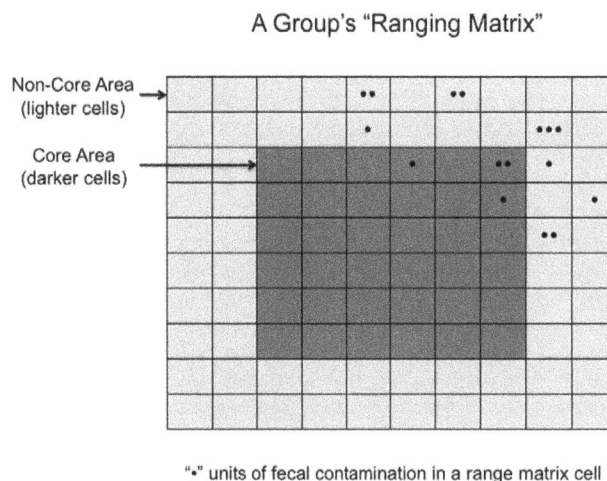

"•" units of fecal contamination in a range matrix cell

Figure 7. Core area and fecal contamination. Within each 10×10 ranging area per group, a *core area* is defined as a proportion of the range and centered in it. This core is identified as a certain number of cells in from the range. In this case, the core area is 2 cells from the edge, giving a 6×6 core area. Groups range with a random walk within the core, and exhibit a tendency to move toward the core when outside of it, where the bias toward the core is a function of how far the group is currently away from the core. This figure further shows the build-up of infectious material (fecal contamination) within and outside the group's core area. An individual cell in the range matrix can have zero, one or multiple feces that harbor infection, and risk of infection increases with increasing fecal contamination.

increased with distance outside the core area. All movements were independent of previous moves.

Two further constraints were placed on ranging behavior. First, groups were unable to move off the total matrix, which included the social group matrix plus the buffer zone equivalent to one home range diameter that surrounded the reserve (see Figure 6). Second, groups could not occupy a grid cell already occupied by another group in that step. When movement brought a group to a boundary or an already occupied cell, the ranging procedure was repeated up to 10 times, and if a suitable range cell was not located, the social group remained where it was for that time step.

The ranging component of the model has two key parameters: the core area affects the probability of overlap with other groups (relevant to the territory benefits hypothesis), while the day range impacts the intensity of range use (and thus exposure to parasites in the soil and relevant to the fecal exposure hypothesis). We consider each of these in turn.

A larger core area meant that groups tended to range closer to the boundary of their home ranges before the rubber band process biased movement back to the group's core area within its home range. In such cases, a given group could cross over into a neighboring group's range or into the buffer, including the area where the spillover population was located (Figure 6). Thus, a larger core area increased the probability that a group overlapped with the range of another group or the reservoir host. Conversely, a smaller core area (which was centered in the group's range) meant that groups were less likely to range outside of their home ranges, resulting in decreased home range overlap.

Range use intensity also was varied systematically. In primates and other mammals, researchers have used a measure known as the defensibility index (D-index) to measure range use intensity [37], and this measure was investigated in a recent comparative study of parasitism and primate ranging [15]. The D-index measures the intensity of range use by examining day journey length relative to home range size. Here, all groups had the same home range size; hence, the D-index was varied by simply changing the day range. In other words, greater range use intensity was equivalent to increased number of ranging movements per time step, as described above. We therefore refer to day range intensity simply as *day range* (*D*).

Following each movement to a new cell, three further stochastic processes took place in the following order. First, infected individuals defecated with probability *d* (adjusted for the number of movement steps per time step to make *d* comparable across simulation runs). The location of feces was recorded on the range lattice based on the location of the group, and following the soil latency period, they became infectious to individuals occupying that cell in future time steps within the soil infectious period. Uninfected individuals in the range cell were exposed to infectious fecal material and become infected with probability *β* per fecal pile in the cell. Finally, 10 feces per time step were placed randomly within the northernmost cells on the range lattice [i.e. within the area defined by coordinates (1,11), (15,11), (1,100), and (15,100), see Figure 6]. These ten fecal contaminations were assumed to come from the infected spillover population, and they underwent the same process of soil latency and infectious periods as described for parasites deposited by hosts in the focal population. We did not explicitly model the ranging behavior of the spillover population.

In our model, a larger day range corresponded to more opportunities for infection because each "movement step" during ranging (the day range) was associated with an opportunity for infection when the group was located on a ranging cell with infectious material. By doing this, we assumed that greater movement is equivalent to greater utilization of the habitat; thus, groups with larger day ranges used their habitat more intensively, resulting in more opportunities for infection as they moved. Instead of considering movement steps, infection could be based on the time available per day, and thus held constant across simulations with different day ranges. In this case, it is possible that by staying in the same grid cell, agents would be more exposed to existing parasites in that cell and might defecate, resulting in buildup of infectious material even when they are not moving. We therefore ran an additional set of simulations that kept the number of movement steps constant for each time step, with the probability of actual movement represented as a linear function of the day range. Averaged across time steps of a simulation, this procedure produced the user-defined day range, while holding time available for exposure constant across simulations.

The second step in the model dynamics involves disease-related and background mortality. Each individual experienced a baseline probability of death (m_b), and infectious individuals had an additional source of mortality due to disease (m_d), where m_d was simply a multiplier of m_b (range of values is given in Table 1). Infected individuals that died were removed from the simulation and could no longer infect other individuals.

The third step involved dispersal of individuals to neighboring groups with probability *m*. Individuals always moved to adjacent neighboring ranges, which were selected randomly. Dispersal was completed in one time step.

Lastly, births occurred for groups with at least one individual present. We recorded the initial population size and also the initial sizes of each group, and assigned a higher probability of birth if the current population size was less than the initial population size (and conversely, a lower probability if the current population was larger than its initial size). The baseline probability of birth (*b*) was set to equal the baseline probability of death (m_b) when the current population size was equal to the initial population. When the current population departed from initial conditions, the probability of birth was set to $m_b{}^f$, where *f* is the current population size as a proportion of the initial population size. We calculated the number of births for populations as a random draw from the binomial distribution with probability b^f, and then assigned births to groups. Groups that were smaller in the current time step relative to the initializing values, but that still had at least one individual in the group, were given a higher probability of receiving a birth. Specifically, they were twice as likely to be assigned a birth as other groups that matched or exceeded their group size at time step 1.

Statistical Analyses of Model Output

We used general linear models to investigate how parameters from the Latin Hypercube sample influenced average prevalence, maximum prevalence, group prevalence, number of groups infected, and population loss due to disease (i.e., total number of individuals that die). The data were continuously varying, and we checked the normality of residuals to investigate the appropriateness of the statistical models. Because significance levels are sensitive to the sample size and here we are interested in relative effects, we avoided interpreting the findings based on frequentist statistical tests of null hypotheses, such as p-values. Instead, we standardized all the predictor variables prior to analysis by subtracting, for each datum, the mean of the data for that predictor and dividing by the standard deviation. We thus estimated standardized regression coefficients and interpreted larger coefficients as corresponding to larger effects. In addition, several of the variables were expressed in the Latin Hypercube sample as continuously varying, but effectively treated in the simulation as taking specific discrete values. Thus, for core area, we used values binned into increments of 0, 0.1, 0.2, 0.3, and 0.4, and we examined the actual number of expected defecations per day, which was normalized relative to the day range. Analyses were conducted in *R* [53].

In addition to analyses of the 1000 simulations in which we used the LHS of parameter values, we provide simple graphical output for data from simulations that varied the day range while holding other variables constant, including for the variant of the model in which opportunities for infection were held constant across different simulated day ranges.

Supporting Information

Table S1 General linear model: predictors of maximum prevalence.

Table S2 General linear model: predictors of average group prevalence.

Table S3 General linear model: predictors of number of groups infected.

Table S4 General linear model: predictors of population decline due to disease.

Acknowledgments

We thank Luke Matthews, Joanna Rifkin, other members of the Comparative Primatology Lab Group at Harvard University, and two anonymous referees for their helpful comments on the manuscript.

Author Contributions

Conceived and designed the experiments: CLN PHT FHL CB. Performed the experiments: CLN. Analyzed the data: CLN. Contributed reagents/materials/analysis tools: CLN. Wrote the paper: CLN PHT FHL CB.

References

1. Samuel WM, Pybus MJ, Kocan AA (2001) Parasitic Diseases of Wild Mammals Iowa State Press. 559 p.
2. Williams ES, Barker IK (2001) Infectious diseases of wild mammals. Ames: Iowa State University Press viii, 558.
3. Appelbee A, Thompson R, Olson M (2005) Giardia and Cryptosporidium in mammalian wildlifeñcurrent status and future needs. Trends in Parasitology 21: 370–376.
4. Nizeyi JB, Mwebe R, Nanteza A, Cranfield MR, Kalema GRNN, et al. (1999) Cryptosporidium sp and Giardia sp infections in mountain gorillas (Gorilla gorilla beringei) of the Bwindi Impenetrable National Park, Uganda. Journal of Parasitology 85: 1084–1088.
5. Hugot JP, Gardner SL, Morand S (1996) The Enterobiinae subfam nov (Nematoda, Oxyurida) pinworm parasites of primates and rodents. International Journal for Parasitology 26: 147–159.
6. Al- Doory Y (1969) The mycology of the freeliving baboon. Mycopathologia et mycologia applicata 38: 7–15.
7. Goldberg TL, Gillespie TR, Rwego IB, Wheeler E, Estoff EL, et al. (2007) Patterns of gastrointestinal bacterial exchange between chimpanzees and humans involved in research and tourism in western Uganda. Biological Conservation 135: 527–533.
8. Wevers D, Leenderttz FH, Scuda N, Boesch C, Robbins MM, et al. (in review) A novel adenovirus of Western lowland gorillas (Gorilla gorilla gorilla). Virology Journal.
9. Gillespie TR, Chapman CA, Greiner EC (2005) Effects of logging on gastrointestinal parasite infections and infection risk in African primates. Journal of Applied Ecology 42: 699–707.
10. Ashford RW, Lawson H, Butynski TM, Reid GDF (1996) Patterns of intestinal parasitism in the mountain gorilla Gorilla gorilla in the Bwindi-Impenetrable Forest, Uganda. Journal of Zoology 239: 507–514.
11. Gulland FMD, Albon SD, Pemberton JM, Moorcroft PR, Clutton-Brock TH (1993) Parasite-Associated Polymorphism in a Cyclic Ungulate Population. Proceedings of the Royal Society of London Series B-Biological Sciences 254: 7–13.
12. Dunbar RIM (1980) Demographic and life history variables of a population of gelada baboons (*Theropithecus gelada*). Journal of Animal Ecology 49: 485–506.
13. Scott ME (1988) The Impact of Infection and Disease on Animal Populations: Implications for Conservation Biology. Conservation Biology 2: 40–56.
14. Nunn CL, Altizer SM (2006) Infectious Diseases in Primates: Behavior, Ecology and Evolution. Oxford: Oxford University Press.
15. Nunn CL, Dokey ATW (2006) Ranging patterns and parasitism in primates. Biology Letters 2: 351–354.
16. Ezenwa VO (2004) Host social behavior and parasitic infection: a multifactorial approach. Behavioral Ecology 15: 446–454.
17. Loehle C (1995) Social barriers to pathogen transmission in wild animal populations. Ecology 76: 326–335.
18. Daszak P, Cunningham AA, Hyatt AD (2000) Emerging infectious diseases of wildlife: Threats to biodiversity and human health. Science 287: 443–449.
19. Harvell CD, Mitchell CE, Ward JR, Altizer S, Dobson AP, et al. (2002) Climate warming and disease risks for terrestrial and marine biota. Science 296: 2158–2162.
20. Dobson A, Foufopoulos J (2001) Emerging infectious pathogens of wildlife. Philosophical Transactions of the Royal Society of London Series B-Biological Sciences 356: 1001–1012.
21. Smith K, Acevedo Whitehouse K, Pedersen A (2009) The role of infectious diseases in biological conservation. Animal Conservation 12: 1–12.
22. Gillespie T, Nunn C, Leenderttz F (2008) Integrative approaches to the study of primate infectious disease: implications for biodiversity conservation and global health. Yearbook of physical anthropology 51: 53–69.
23. Leenderttz FH, Pauli G, Maetz-Rensing K, Boardman W, Nunn CL, et al. (2006) Pathogens as Drivers of Population Declines: The Importance of Systematic Monitoring in Great Apes and Other Threatened Mammals Biological Conservation 131: 325–337.
24. Walsh PD, Abernethy KA, Bermejo M, Beyersk R, De Wachter P, et al. (2003) Catastrophic ape decline in western equatorial Africa. Nature 422: 611–614.
25. Chapman CA, Gillespie TR, Goldberg TL (2005) Primates and the ecology of their infectious diseases: How will anthropogenic change affect host-parasite interactions? Evolutionary Anthropology 14: 134–144.
26. Altizer S, Harvell D, Friedle E (2003) Rapid evolutionary dynamics and disease threats to biodiversity. Trends in Ecology and Evolution 18: 589–596.
27. Goldberg TL, Gillespie TR, Rwego IB, Estoff EL, Chapman CA (2008) Forest Fragmentation as Cause of Bacterial Transmission among Nonhuman Primates, Humans, and Livestock, Uganda. Emerg Infect Dis 14: 1375–1382.
28. Hess GR (1994) Conservation Corridors And Contagious-Disease - A Cautionary Note. Conservation Biology 8: 256–262.
29. Hess G (1996) Disease in metapopulation models: Implications for conservation. Ecology 77: 1617–1632.
30. Freeland WJ (1976) Pathogens and the evolution of primate sociality. Biotropica 8: 12–24.
31. Stoner KE (1996) Prevalence and intensity of intestinal parasites in mantled howling monkeys (Alouatta palliata) in northeastern Costa Rica: Implications for conservation biology. Conservation Biology 10: 539–546.
32. Freeland WJ (1979) Primate Social Groups as Biological Islands. Ecology 60: 719–728.
33. Nunn CL, Thrall PH, Stewart K, Harcourt AH (2008) Emerging infectious diseases and animal social systems. Evolutionary Ecology 22: 519–543.
34. Cross PC, Lloyd-Smith JO, Johnson PL, Getz WM (2005) Dueling timescales of host movement and disease recovery determine invasion of disease in structured populations. Ecology Letters 8: 587–595.
35. Nizeyi JB, Cranfield MR, Graczyk TK (2002) Cattle near the Bwindi Impenetrable National Park, Uganda, as a reservoir of Cryptosporidium parvum and Giardia duodenalis for local community and free-ranging gorillas. Parasitology Research 88: 380–385.
36. Koendgen S, Kuhl H, N'Goran PK, Walsh PD, Schenk S, et al. (2008) Pandemic Human Viruses Cause Decline of Endangered Great Apes. Current Biology 18: 260–264.
37. Mitani JC, Rodman PS (1979) Territoriality: the relation of ranging pattern and home range size to defendability, with an analysis of territoriality among primate species. Behavioral Ecology and Sociobiology 5: 241–251.
38. Smouse P, Focardi S, Moorcroft P, Kie J, Forester J, et al. (2010) Stochastic modelling of animal movement. Philosophical Transactions of the Royal Society B: Biological Sciences 365: 2201–2211.
39. Clutton-Brock TH, Harvey PH (1977) Primate ecology and social organization. Journal of Zoology 183: 1–39.
40. Nunn CL, Barton RA (2000) Allometric slopes and independent contrasts: A comparative test of Kleiber's law in primate ranging patterns. American Naturalist 156: 519–533.
41. Bonnell T, Sengupta R, Chapman C, Goldberg T (2010) An agent-based model of red colobus resources and disease dynamics implicates key resource sites as hot spots of disease transmission. Ecological Modelling 221: 2491–2500.
42. Waser PM (1976) Cercocebus albigena: Site Attachment, Avoidance, and Intergroup Spacing. American Naturalist 110: 911–935.
43. Normand E, Boesch C (2009) Sophisticated Euclidean maps in forest chimpanzees. Animal Behaviour 77: 1195–1201.
44. Hart BL (1990) Behavioral adaptations to pathogens and parasites: five strategies. Neuroscience and Biobehavioral Reviews 14: 273–294.
45. Leroy EM, Kumulungui B, Pourrut X, Rouquet P, Hassanin A, et al. (2005) Fruit bats as reservoirs of Ebola virus. Nature 438: 575–576.
46. Bermejo M, Rodriguez-Teijeiro JD, Illera G, Barroso A, Vila C, et al. (2006) Ebola outbreak killed 5000 gorillas. Science 314: 1564–1564.
47. Caillaud D, Levrero F, Cristescu R, Gatti S, Dewas M, et al. (2006) Gorilla susceptibility to ebola virus: the cost of sociality. Current Biology 16: R489–R491.
48. Anderson RM, May RM, eds (1982) Population Biology of Infectious Diseases. Berlin: Springer-Verlag.
49. Seaholm SK, Ackerman E, Wu SC (1988) Latin Hypercube Sampling and the Sensitivity Analysis of a Monte-Carlo Epidemic Model. International Journal of Bio-Medical Computing 23: 97–112.
50. Blower SM, Dowlatabadi H (1994) Sensitivity and Uncertainty Analysis of Complex-Models of Disease Transmission - an Hiv Model, as an Example. International Statistical Review 62: 229–243.
51. Rushton SP, Lurz PWW, Gurnell J, Fuller R (2000) Modelling the spatial dynamics of parapoxvirus disease in red and grey squirrels: a possible cause of the decline in the red squirrel in the UK? Journal of Applied Ecology 37: 997–1012.
52. Nunn CL, Thrall PH, Bartz K, Dasgupta T, Boesch C (2009) Do transmission mechanisms or social systems drive cultural dynamics in socially structured populations? Animal Behaviour 78: 1515–1524.
53. R, Development, Core, Team (2009) R: A language and environment for statistical computing. ViennaAustria: R Foundation for Statistical Computing.

11

Expression of Ovine Herpesvirus -2 Encoded MicroRNAs in an Immortalised Bovine – Cell Line

Katie Nightingale, Claire S. Levy¤, John Hopkins, Finn Grey, Suzanne Esper, Robert G. Dalziel*

The Roslin Institute & R(D)SVS, University of Edinburgh, Edinburgh, Midlothian, United Kingdom

Abstract

Ovine herpesvirus-2 (OvHV-2) infects most sheep, where it establishes an asymptomatic, latent infection. Infection of susceptible hosts e.g. cattle and deer results in malignant catarrhal fever, a fatal lymphoproliferative disease characterised by uncontrolled lymphocyte proliferation and non MHC restricted cytotoxicity. The same cell populations are infected in both cattle and sheep but only in cattle does virus infection cause dysregulation of cell function leading to disease. The mechanism by which OvHV-2 induces this uncontrolled proliferation is unknown. A number of herpesviruses have been shown to encode microRNAs (miRNAs) that have roles in control of both viral and cellular gene expression. We hypothesised that OvHV-2 encodes miRNAs and that these play a role in pathogenesis. Analysis of massively parallel sequencing data from an OvHV-2 persistently-infected bovine lymphoid cell line (BJ1035) identified forty-five possible virus-encoded miRNAs. We previously confirmed the expression of eight OvHV-2 miRNAs by northern hybridization. In this study we used RT-PCR to confirm the expression of an additional twenty-seven OvHV-2-encoded miRNAs. All thirty-five OvHV-2 miRNAs are expressed from the same virus genome strand and the majority (30) are encoded in an approximately 9 kb region that contains no predicted virus open reading frames. Future identification of the cellular and virus targets of these miRNAs will inform our understanding of MCF pathogenesis.

Editor: James P. Stewart, University of Liverpool, United Kingdom

Funding: KN is funded by a University of Edinburgh Principal's Career Development Scholarship and the Roslin Institute, SE was funded by Biotechnology and Biological Sciences Research Council (BBSRC) Institute Strategic Programme Grant to The Roslin Institute, FG is a Wellcome Trust Career Development Fellow. The funders had no role in study design, data collection and analysis, decision to publish, or preparation of the manuscript.

Competing Interests: The authors have declared that no competing interests exist.

* E-mail: bob.dalziel@roslin.ed.ac.uk

¤ Current address: The Scripps Research Institute, La Jolla, California, United States of America

Introduction

Malignant catarrhal fever (MCF) is a fatal disease of cattle, deer and pigs caused by one of two related gammaherpesviruses (γ-HV), ovine herpesvirus -2 (OvHV-2) or alcelaphine herpesvirus 1 (AlHV-1). MCF is characterized by sudden onset of fever followed by lymphadenopathy, leukocytosis, severe congestion, necrosis and erosion of the oral, conjutival and nasal mucosæ [1]. The disease occurs as the result of infection of susceptible hosts by contact with an asymptomatic carrier species that acts as a virus reservoir. OvHV-2 is the major cause of sheep associated MCF worldwide [1]. It infects most sheep, where it establishes a latent but asymptomatic infection. AlHV-1 is the major cause of MCF in sub-Saharan Africa where the wildebeest is the asymptomatic carrier species.

The same cell populations are infected in both cattle and sheep [2,3] but only in cattle does virus infection cause dysregulation of cell function leading to uncontrolled proliferation, cytotoxicity and disease. In both species the infected cells arise from common lymphoid progenitors [4] but interleukin 2-dependent cell lines can be cultured only from affected animals. There is currently no tissue culture system for OvHV-2 and such cell lines are the only resource for working with the virus. In affected species the infected cells have been described as large granular lymphocytes (LGLs) [5]. The immortalized cell lines have a variety of phenotypes; all express CD2 but vary in their expression of CD4 and CD8 [2,3].

The mechanism by which OvHV-2 induces MCF is unknown; virus-induced cytopathology is thought not to be involved in lesion development and it has been proposed that tissue damage arises from non-antigen specific, MHC unrestricted cytotoxicity of the LGLs. The key question in understanding OvHV-2 pathogenesis is; why infection of the same cell type in two closely related species leads to such different disease outcomes, i.e. lymphoid cell dysregulation and MCF in cattle versus asymptomatic infection in sheep.

MicroRNAs (miRNAs) constitute a large family of small, non-coding RNAs functioning in post-transcriptional regulation of mRNA in eukaryotes [6–8] as well as in a number of viruses, particularly in the members of the family *Herpesviridae* [9–11]. miRNA regulation of expression is by binding of the miRNA seed sequence (~nucleotides 2–8) to complementary sequences in target mRNAs and directing these for degradation or translational silencing; the majority of miRNAs target sequences within the 3′ UTR [6]. Herpesvirus-encoded miRNAs have been shown to be effective regulators of both cellular and virus gene expression and to influence cell processes including the cell cycle [12–17]. The pathology of the herpesviruses Epstein Barr virus (EBV) and Marek's disease virus (MDV) also involves aberrant lymphocyte proliferation, and virus-encoded miRNAs play a key role in the induction of this proliferation. Furthermore, deletion of a single (MDV) or a small cluster (EBV) of virus-encoded miRNAs

Table 1. OvHV-2-encoded microRNAs.

ovhv2-miR-	Previous name	Abundance RNA-seq	Walz et al.	5'nt	3'nt	Sequence	Validation Method
Ov2-2	miR-1	10588	✓	927	906	AAGGCUUGAUAAGUAGCACUGA	Levy et al.
Ov2-1		253	✓	1182	1161	AUGCUUGUUUAGGCCCAUGAA	Sequencing
17-30		434	✓	27722	27702	UUUGGGUGUCUCCUGUCAUCU	Sequencing
17-29	miR-2	39169	✓	27603	27881	AUCUUGGACGCAUCUGUCAGUAG	Levy et al.
17-28		6200	✓	28066	28045	UCUAGGUUGCAUUUUGCUGUAG	Sequencing
17-27		6015	✓	28209	28188	CCCACAUUUAAGGUGCUCGUGU	Sequencing
17-26		322	✓	28381	28361	AUAUUCGUUUAGACGCAAGUA	Sequencing
17-25		4717	✓	28515	28495	CAAUGCUGCUUUGUGCCUCA	Sequencing
17-24		1014	✓	28683	28661	GGGUUCCUCGAGUGGAUAUUGUU	Sequencing
17-23		21686	✓	28781	28761	AUACACACUGAAAGAGCUAGA	Sequencing
17-22		740	✓	28888	28866	AUAAGGCCAACACUAGGUGCUGU	Sequencing
17-21		31227	✓	29052	29028	AAGCACCUUGGGUGAUGUCUCUGUU	Sequencing
17-20	miR-3	14694	✓	29248	29226	UCUGUAUCAUAGGGUUGUGUGUUG	Levy et al.
17-19		6487	✓	29345	29323	AAGCAUAGCUGGGAGUGUCUAGA	Specific cDNA
17-18		9219	✓	29455	29434	UAGUAGUCCGUUAACGCAAAGU	Sequencing
17-17	miR-4	17508	✓	29637	29616	AAGGAUCCUUAAGUGACGAACG	Levy et al-
17-16		8095	✓	29745	29725	UAAACUGGUGGUAGCGGGUCU	Sequencing
17-15		2967	✓	29945	29923	UAGCAGUUAUGCAGGUAUCUGGU	Sequencing
17-14		3794	✓	30091	30067	UGGCAUUUCCAGGAGCCUGUUGUUC	Sequencing
17-13		24497	✓	30338	30316	UUGGGUCCAACAUGAGACGCGGU	Sequencing
17-12		14966	✓	30510	30489	UAUGUCAGAAGUGAAGCUGAGA	Specific cDNA
17-11		1357	✓	30632	30611	UGGUUUGCAUCUGCACCCAGUU	Sequencing
17-10	miR-5	11187	✓	30818	30796	UGAAGUUACAGCUGCACCUGGAU	Levy et al.
17-9		5457	✓	30980	30956	UAGAGUUACUAAGGAUUCCCUGGUA	Sequencing
17-8		942	✓	31085	31066	AAUCGCCGGUGCCUUCUAG	Sequencing
17-7		351	✓	31359	31340	UAUAGACGGGUAUGCUGCCG	Specific cDNA
17-6	miR-6	10378	✓	31462	31440	UAUUUUUAGCGGAGACCUCUAGG	Levy et al.
17-5		1535	✓	31603	31582	CCUUUUUGGUGAGUUGCCCUGU	Sequencing
17-4		517	✓	32075	32054	GAUUUGAUAAAGCCUGCCUGCG	Sequencing
17-3	miR-7	16574	✓	36313	36289	GAAGGCGCAUCAUAGACACCACUUC	Levy et al.
17-2		7834	✓	36462	36441	ACCCCGGGGGUAUGUGCAGGAC	Sequencing
17-1	miR-8	46048	✓	36575	36554	UGGCUCAGCGCGUGACUGCUUC	Levy et al.
24-1		1	✗	48585	48560	GAGCAGUACUACACAGCAGACAACAU	Sequencing

Table 1. Cont.

ovhv2-miR-	Previous name	Abundance RNA-seq	Walz et al.	5′nt	3′nt	Sequence	Validation Method
61-1		1	x	96435	96411	UUGGGGACGUGCUGGCUGACGACGU	Specific cDNA
73-1		6064	x	117122	117100	UAAUCUCUGCUCCAAUUGUAAAU	Specific cDNA

The 35 validated miRNAs are listed. **Previous name**: designation in Levy et al. 2012. **Abundance (RNA-seq)**: Total number of sequence tags representing the miRNA in the RNA-seq data [22]. **Walz et al.**: miRNAs predicted by Walz et al. √ = yes; X = no. **5′nt/3′nt**: the first and last nucleotides of the mature miRNA on the OvHV-2 genome (AY839756) [28]. **Sequence**: sequence of the mature miRNA. **Validation method**: Levy et al.: validated previously [22]; Sequencing: validated using the RT-PCR and subsequent sequencing; Specific cDNA: validated using the approach of Varkonyi-Gasic et al.[24].

attenuates these viruses [18–20]. Consequently we hypothesized that OvHV-2 encodes miRNAs that target host mRNAs and that these constrain virus pathology in sheep and/or induce MCF pathology in cattle. Identification and characterization of OvHV-2-encoded miRNAs is therefore essential to allow this hypothesis to be addressed.

In a previous study we reported the results of massively parallel sequencing of small RNAs present in the BJ1035 OvHV-2 immortalized bovine LGL cell line and predicted that the virus encodes up to forty-five miRNAs [21]. Eight of these were confirmed by northern hybridization [22]. Here we extend these studies using two PCR protocols to investigate the expression of the other predicted OvHV-2 miRNAs.

Methods

Cell culture

BJ1035 cells, an immortalized bovine T cell line from an animal naturally infected with OvHV-2 [3], was grown in suspension culture in Iscove's Modified Dulbecco's Medium (Invitrogen, Paisley, UK) supplemented with 10% (v/v) foetal calf serum (Sera Laboratories International, Haywards Heath, UK), 1% (v/v) penicillin-streptomycin (Invitrogen), 20 U/ml interleukin 2 (Novartis Pharmaceuticals UK, Camberley, UK) and incubated at 37°C, 5% CO_2. Bovine lymphoid cells were isolated from fresh blood and lymphoblasts generated as described previously [23]. All relevant procedures were approved by the University of Edinburgh Ethical Review Committee and carried out under an Animal (Scientific Procedures) Act 1996 project licence.

Reverse Transcription PCR (RT-PCR)

Bovine lymphoblasts and BJ1035 cells were pelleted by centrifugation and total RNA extracted using Trizol (Invitrogen). cDNA was generated using the miScript II RT Kit (Qiagen, Crawley, UK) that uses oligo-dT to prime reverse transcription. For each predicted miRNA, a specific forward primer spanning the first 15–16 nucleotides of the miRNA was designed (Table S1) allowing subsequent sequence confirmation of the identity of the amplified miRNA RT-PCR was performed using miScript SYBR green PCR kit (Qiagen), with the supplied universal reverse primer and the miRNA specific forward primers using the annealing temperatures shown in Table S1. PCR products were fractionated by electrophoresis using 3% agarose, purified using the Illustra GFX PCR DNA and Gel Band Purification Kits (GE Healthcare, Amersham, UK) and cloned using the TOPO TA Cloning Kit (Invitrogen). Plasmid DNA was isolated using the Qiaprep Spin Miniprep Kit (Qiagen), analysed by restriction enzyme digestion and sequenced (GATC Biotech, London UK).

miRNA specific reverse transcription

Individual miRNA specific primers (Table S2) were used to prime for reverse transcriptase. Each primer also has a 5′ conserved region recognised by a universal reverse primer (5′-GTGCAGGGTCCGAGGT-3′) [24]. An initial reaction to form the hairpin structure of the reverse transcription primer (200 µM) was carried out using the following conditions: 95°C for 30 min, 72°C for 2 min, 37°C for 2 min then 25°C for 2 min. The concentration of the reverse transcription primer after annealing was 50 µM. For the reverse transcription reaction 5 µM reverse transcription primer was used to prime 100 ng of RNA. Conditions for the reverse transcription reaction were as follows: 16°C for 30 min, 42°C for 30 min then 85°C for 5 min. PCR was thenperformed using miRNA specific forward primers (Table S2) and the following conditions: 5 min at 95°C, 40 cycles of: 30 s at

```
                      A    GGC   ACUGUG
miR-216a       5' UAAUCUC GCU    A          A 3'
ovhv2-miR-73-1 5' UAAUCUC GCU    A          A 3'
                      U    CCA   UUGUAA   U
```

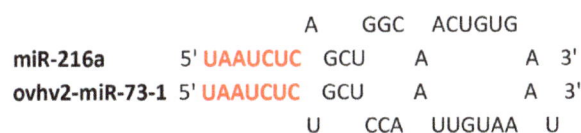

Figure 1. Comparison of the sequences of ovhv2-miR-73-1 and miR-216a. Seed sequences (nt 1-7) are shown in red.

95°C, 30 s at 60°C, 60 s at 72°C; then finally 7 min at 72°C. PCR products were fractionated by electrophoresis using 3% agarose. Reactions were performed in triplicate. The presence of a product in the BJ1035 cells but not in the uninfected bovine lymphoblast cells was taken as proof of OvHV-2 miRNA expression.

Results

Using northern hybridization we have previously demonstrated the expression of the eight of the 45 predicted miRNAs that were represented by the highest number of reads in our parallel sequencing data [22]. RT-PCR using miRNA specific forward primers and a universal reverse primer for the remaining 37 predicted miRNAs initially identified 22 virus-encoded miRNAs (Table S1, Table 1).

To investigate if the remaining 15 miRNAs are expressed, an alternative miRNA specific reverse transcription PCR strategy was adopted. The expression of a predicted miRNA (ovhv2-miR-73-1) that was shown to have seed sequence homology but no 3′ sequence homology with mammalian miR-216a (Figure 1) was also analysed by this method. The presence of a product in the BJ1035 cells but not in the uninfected bovine lymphoblast cells was taken as proof of OvHV-2 miRNA expression. As the forward primer ends at the nucleotide adjacent to that from which cDNA is primed, sequencing of the product would generate only primer sequence. To confirm that amplification was from miRNA and not genomic DNA a no RT control was performed and no amplification was observed with any primer set. Expression of a further 5 miRNAs, including ovhv2-miR-73-1, was confirmed, (Figure 2). Figure 3 shows the location and direction of transcription of the thirty-five validated OvHV-2-encoded miR-NAs.

Discussion

The number of miRNAs expressed by individual herpesviruses ranges from 8 to 50 [25] and here we demonstrate that OvHV-2 encodes 35 miRNAs. Using a predictive algorithm Walz *et al.* [26] predicted 61 hairpin sites in OvHV-2 that might encode miRNAs; 32 of which we have now confirmed to be expressed (Figure 3, Table 1), three of our validated miRNAs were not predicted by Walz *et al.*. All of the validated miRNAs expressed by OvHV-2 are transcribed in the same orientation, right to left. By convention virus-encoded miRNAs are named in relation to the nearest open reading frame (ORF) transcribed in the same direction as the miRNA; we have followed this convention in naming the OvHV-2-encoded miRNAs. Those identified in Levy *et al.* and discussed in Riaz *et al.*[22,27] have been renamed to adhere to this nomenclature (Table 1). Two miRNAs are encoded at the left hand end of the genome in the region between the terminal repeat and the 3′ end of ORF Ov2, these have been named ovhv2-miR-Ov2-1 and ovhv2-miR-Ov2-2 (ovhv2-miR-1 in Levy *et al.* 2012[22]). The OvHV-2 genome, like that of AlHV-1 and equine herpesvirus 2 (EHV-2) contains two large regions of the genome with no predicted open reading frames [28]. The majority (30) of the identified miRNAs are encoded as two clusters at either end of the larger of these two regions. One cluster, spanning 4377 bp at the left end of this region, contains 27 miRNAs; a smaller cluster of three miRNAs is encoded in a 320 bp region at the right hand end of this region (Figure 3). These miRNAs have been named ovhv2-miR-17-1 to -30. Ovhv2-mir-17- 29, -20, -17, -10, -6, -3 and -1 were previously designated ovhv2-miR-2 to -8. One miRNA is encoded in the non-coding region situated toward the right end of the genome and is designated ovhv2-miR-73-1. The remaining miRNAs are encoded within ORFs 24 and 61 and are designated ovhv2-miR-24-1 and ovhv2-miR-61-1.

ovhv2-miR-73-1 was the only OvHV-2-encoded miRNA to show seed sequence homology to any other reported miRNA, miR-216a (Figure 1). This miRNA is broadly conserved in vertebrates and targets *PTEN* and *YBX1* [29,30] down regulation of which can lead to increased cell survival, hypertrophy, sclerosis, and a decreased cellular response to stress [31], all symptoms observed in MCF. We are currently investigating the cellular genes targeted by ovhv2-miR-73-1.

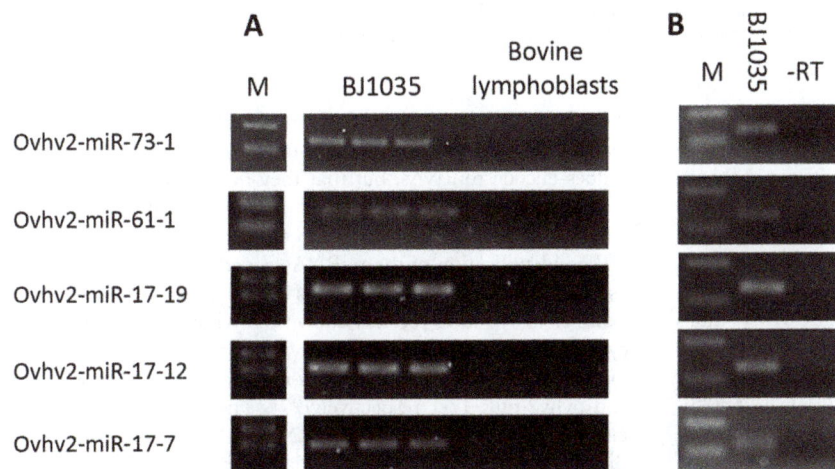

Figure 2. Analysis of OvHV-2-encoded miRNA expression using miRNA specific RT-PCR. A) Expression of five predicted OvHV-2-encoded miRNAs in BJ1035 cells but not uninfected bovine lymphoblasts was confirmed by miRNA specific RT-PCR. Each assay was carried out in triplicate. M: 50 bp and 100 bp markers B) miRNA specific RT-PCR was carried out along with an no RT (-RT) control.

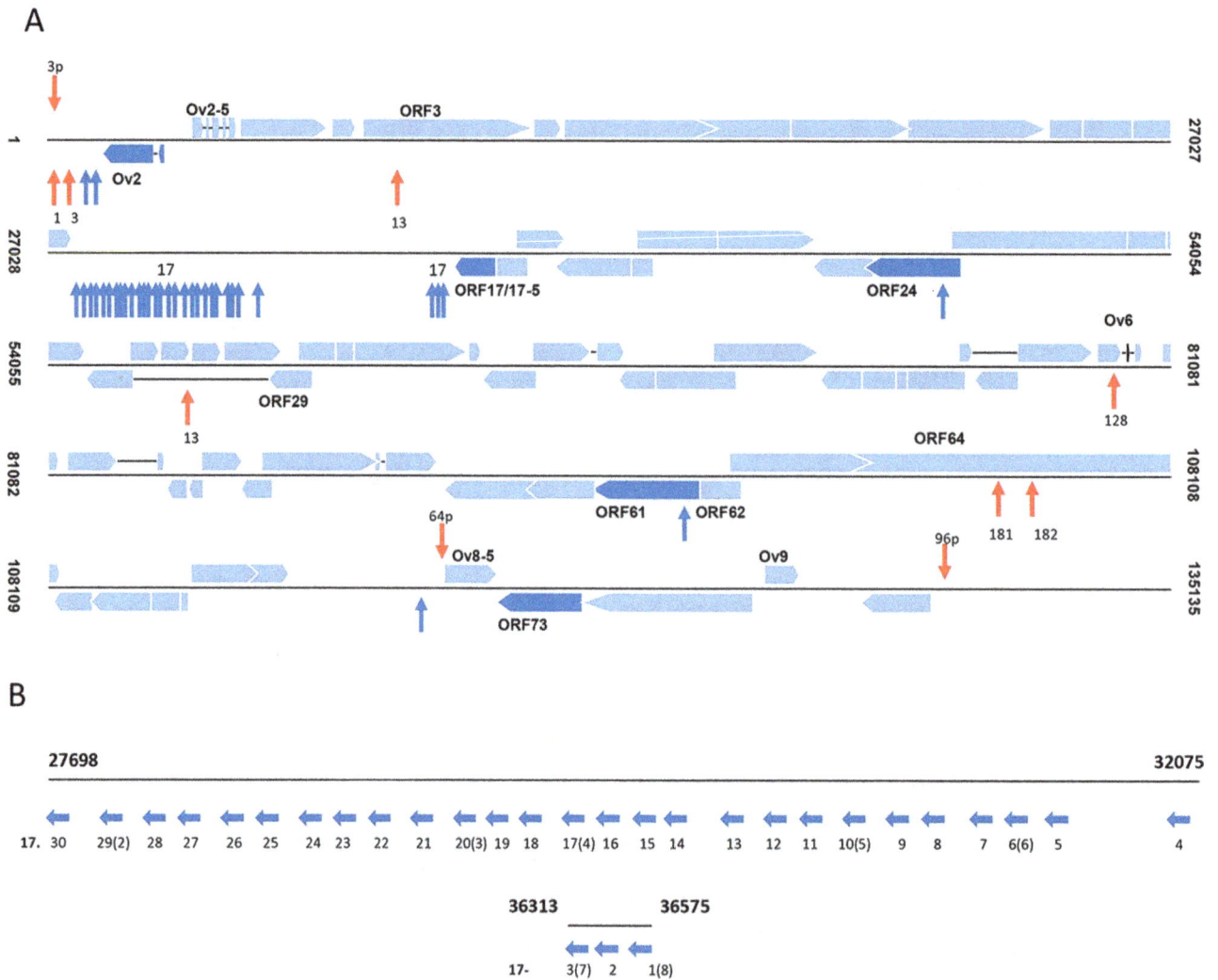

Figure 3. Location of miRNAs in the OvHV-2 genome. A) The relative positions of the predicted miRNAs in the OvHV-2 genome are shown. Numbering is from Hart *et al.*[28]. The genome is represented by a thin line and open reading frames (ORFs) are indicated by blue boxes. Boxes above the line represent ORFs transcribed left to right; those below the line represent ORFs which are transcribed right to left. Only those ORFs adjacent to predicted miRNAs are named. Arrows indicate the position of the predicted miRNAs; arrows above the line represent miRNAs transcribed left to right, those below the line represent miRNAs which are transcribed right to left. Dark blue vertical arrows indicate validated miRNAs. Red arrows indicate non-validated miRNAs named according to the groups listed in Table 1. Those OvHV-2 ORFs closest to validated miRNAs and after which those miRNAs are named are shown in darkblue. B) The locations of ovhv2-miR-17-1 to -30 are shown in more detail.

AlHV-1 is the causative agent of wildebeest-associated MCF and the sequence identity between the individual ORFs of OvHV-2 and AlHV-1 varies from 22–83% ([28]). No significant sequence similarity was found between the non-coding regions of the two viruses and Blastn analysis failed to identify miRNAs in the AlHV-1 genome with sequence homology to any OvHV-2 miRNA. A lack of conservation of miRNAs between closely-related viruses has also been observed in different Marek's disease virus strains [32].

Herpesviruses are generally host species specific and are considered to have co-evolved with their natural host [33]. Herpesvirus-encoded miRNAs have been shown to regulate both virus and host gene expression [12–17] and it is likely that these miRNAs have also co-evolved with their host targets. The different disease outcomes seen in sheep (natural, co-evolved host) and cattle ("foreign" host may be the result of different virus:host interactions. Our hypothesis is that OvHV-2-miRNAs interact differently with sheep and cattle genes and that these differences play a role in the differing disease outcomes. It is likely that AlHV-1 does encode miRNAs, but that they have co-evolved to target wildebeest (natural host) genes in a similar manner to which OvHV-2 miRNAs have evolved to target sheep genes.

The identification of the miRNAs encoded by OvHV-2 allows us to study how these miRNAs affect host and virus gene expression. We have recently shown that viral genes ORF20 (cell cycle inhibition), ORF 50 (reactivation) and ORF 73 (latency maintenance) are targeted by ovhv-miR-17-29; ovhv2-miR-17-10 and ovhv2-miR-17-1 respectively[27]. The identification of host targets of the 35 OvHV2-miRNAs is not straightforward. Bioinformatic analysis of potential targets for the OvHV2-miRNAs in the sheep and cattle genome resulted in the identification of more than 100,000 possible targets in each genome, an unrealistic number to investigate. We are current using experimental approaches to investigate cellular targets of the OvHV-2-miRNAs.

Supporting Information

Table S1 Sequences of specific forward PCR primers and related annealing temperatures. The sequence of the forward primers and annealing temperatures used to analyse expression of the predicted ovhv2-miRNAs are shown. Those miRNAs which were successfully validated using approach are shown in bold. "Group 1" etc. represent predicted miRNAs which were not shown to be expressed.

Table S2 Sequence of miRNA specific Reverse transcription primers and specific 5′ forward primers. For each of the miRNAs which were not validated using the miScript

assay, the sequence of the primers used to prime cDNA synthesis, the specific 5′ forward primers and the sequence of the universal reverse PCR primer are shown. "Group 1" etc. represent predicted miRNAs which were not shown to be expressed.

Acknowledgments

We thank Dr G Russell, Moredun Research Institute, for the kind gift of BJ1035 cells.

Author Contributions

Conceived and designed the experiments: KN RGD JH FG. Performed the experiments: KN CSL SE. Analyzed the data: KN JH FG RGD. Wrote the paper: RGD.

References

1. Russell GC, Stewart JP, Haig DM (2009) Malignant catarrhal fever: A review. Veterinary Journal 179: 324–335.
2. Meier-Trummer CS, Ryf B, Ackermann M (2010) Identification of peripheral blood mononuclear cells targeted by Ovine herpesvirus-2 in sheep. Veterinary Microbiology 141: 199–207.
3. Schock A, Collins RA, Reid HW (1998) Phenotype, growth regulation and cytokine transcription in Ovine Herpesvirus-2 (OHV-2)-infected bovine T-cell lines. Veterinary Immunology and Immunopathology 66: 67–68.
4. Sun JC, Lanier LL (2011) NK cell development, homeostasis and function: parallels with CD8(+) T cells. Nature Reviews Immunology 11: 645–657.
5. Reid HW, Buxton D, Pow I, Finlayson J (1989) Isolation and characterisation of lymphoblastoid cells from cattle and deer affected with 'sheep-associated' malignant catarrhal fever. Res Vet Sci 47: 90–96.
6. Bartel DP (2009) MicroRNAs: Target Recognition and Regulatory Functions. Cell 136: 215–233.
7. Carthew RW, Sontheimer EJ (2009) Origins and Mechanisms of miRNAs and siRNAs. Cell 136: 642–655.
8. Kim VN, Han J, Siomi MC (2009) Biogenesis of small RNAs in animals. Nature Reviews Molecular Cell Biology 10: 126–139.
9. Cullen BR (2009) Viral and cellular messenger RNA targets of viral microRNAs. Nature 457: 421–425.
10. Glazov EA, Horwood PF, Assavalapsakul W, Kongsuwan K, Mitchell RW, et al. (2010) Characterization of microRNAs encoded by the bovine herpesvirus 1 genome. Journal of General Virology 91: 32–41.
11. Grey F, Hook L, Nelson J (2008) The functions of herpesvirus-encoded microRNAs. Medical Microbiology and Immunology 197: 261–267.
12. Dolken L, Krmpotic A, Kothe S, Tuddenham L, Tanguy M, et al. (2010) Cytomegalovirus microRNAs facilitate persistent virus infection in salivary glands. PLoS Pathog 6: e1001150.
13. Gottwein E, Cullen BR (2010) A Human Herpesvirus MicroRNA Inhibits p21 Expression and Attenuates p21-Mediated Cell Cycle Arrest. Journal of Virology 84: 5229–5237.
14. Lu F, Stedman W, Yousef M, Renne R, Lieberman PM (2010) Epigenetic Regulation of Kaposi's Sarcoma-Associated Herpesvirus Latency by Virus-Encoded MicroRNAs That Target Rta and the Cellular Rbl2-DNMT Pathway. Journal of Virology 84: 2697–2706.
15. Qin Z, Kearney P, Plaisance K, Parsons CH (2010) Kaposi's sarcoma-associated herpesvirus (KSHV)-encoded microRNA specifically induce IL-6 and IL-10 secretion by macrophages and monocytes. Journal of Leukocyte Biology 87: 25–34.
16. Seto E, Moosmann A, Groemminger S, Walz N, Grundhoff A, et al. (2010) Micro RNAs of Epstein-Barr Virus Promote Cell Cycle Progression and Prevent Apoptosis of Primary Human B Cells. PLoS Pathogens 6.
17. Zhao YG, Yao YX, Xu HT, Lambeth L, Smith LP, et al. (2009) A Functional MicroRNA-155 Ortholog Encoded by the Oncogenic Marek's Disease Virus. Journal of Virology 83: 489–492.
18. Feederle R, Haar J, Bernhardt K, Linnstaedt SD, Bannert H, et al. (2011) The Members of an Epstein-Barr Virus MicroRNA Cluster Cooperate To Transform B Lymphocytes. Journal of Virology 85: 9801–9810.
19. Feederle R, Linnstaedt SD, Bannert H, Lips H, Bencun M, et al. (2011) A Viral microRNA Cluster Strongly Potentiates the Transforming Properties of a Human Herpesvirus. Plos Pathogens 7.
20. Zhao Y, Xu H, Yao Y, Smith LP, Kgosana L, et al. (2011) Critical Role of the Virus-Encoded MicroRNA-155 Ortholog in the Induction of Marek's Disease Lymphomas. Plos Pathogens 7.
21. Levy CS (2011) Identification and Characterisation of Ovine Herpesvirus 2 microRNAs. PhD Thesis University of Edinburgh.
22. Levy CS, Hopkins J, Russell G, Dalziel RG (2012) Novel virus-encoded microRNA molecules expressed by ovine herpesvirus 2 immortalized bovine T cells. Journal of General Virology 93: 150–154.
23. Bujdoso R, Young P, Hopkins J, McConnell I (1990) IL-2 like activity in lymph fluid following in vivo antigen challenge. Immunology 69: 45–51.
24. Varkonyi-Gasic E, Wu R, Wood M, Walton EF, Hellens RP (2007) Protocol: a highly sensitive RT-PCR method for detection and quantification of microRNAs. Plant Methods 3.
25. Grundhoff A, Sullivan CS (2011) Virus-encoded microRNAs. Virology 411: 325–343.
26. Walz N, Christalla T, Tessmer U, Grundhoff A (2010) A Global Analysis of Evolutionary Conservation among Known and Predicted Gammaherpesvirus MicroRNAs. Journal of Virology 84: 716–728.
27. Riaz A, Dry I, Levy CS, Hopkins J, Grey F, et al. (2014) Ovine herpesvirus-2-encoded microRNAs target virus genes involved in virus latency. Journal of General Virology 95: 472–480.
28. Hart J, Ackermann M, Jayawardane G, Russe G, Haig DM, et al. (2007) Complete sequence and analysis of the ovine herpesvirus 2 genome. Journal of General Virology 88: 28–39.
29. Kato M, Putta S, Wang M, Yuan H, Lanting L, et al. (2009) TGF-beta activates Akt kinase through a microRNA-dependent amplifying circuit targeting PTEN. Nature Cell Biology 11: 881–U263.
30. Kato M, Wang L, Putta S, Wang M, Yuan H, et al. (2010) Post-transcriptional Up-regulation of Tsc-22 by Ybx1, a Target of miR-216a, Mediates TGF-beta-induced Collagen Expression in Kidney Cells. Journal of Biological Chemistry 285: 34004–34015.
31. Evdokimova V, Ruzanov P, Anglesio MS, Sorokin AV, Ovchinnikov LP, et al. (2006) Akt-mediated YB-1 phosphorylation activates translation of silent mRNA species. Molecular and Cellular Biology 26: 277–292.
32. Yao Y, Zhao Y, Xu H, Smith LP, Lawries CH, et al. (2007) Marek's disease virus type 2 (MDV-2)-encoded microRNAs show no sequence conservation with those encoded by MDV-1. Journal of Virology 81: 7164–7170.
33. McGeoch DJ, Rixon FJ, Davison AJ (2006) Topics in herpesvirus genomics and evolution. Virus Research 117: 90–104.

12

Overall Decrease in the Susceptibility of *Mycoplasma bovis* to Antimicrobials over the Past 30 Years in France

Anne V. Gautier-Bouchardon[1,2], **Séverine Ferré**[1,2], **Dominique Le Grand**[3,4], **Agnès Paoli**[3,4], **Emilie Gay**[5], **François Poumarat**[3,4]*

1 ANSES, Laboratoire de Ploufragan/Plouzané, Unité Mycoplasmologie-Bactériologie, Ploufragan, France, 2 Université Européenne de Bretagne, Rennes, France, 3 ANSES, Laboratoire de Lyon, UMR Mycoplasmoses des Ruminants, Lyon, France, 4 Université de Lyon, VetAgro Sup, UMR Mycoplasmoses des Ruminants, Marcy L'Etoile, France, 5 ANSES, Laboratoire de Lyon, Unité Epidémiologie, Lyon, France

Abstract

Mycoplasma (M.) bovis is frequently implicated in respiratory diseases of young cattle worldwide. Today, to combat *M. bovis* in Europe, only antimicrobial therapy is available, but often fails, leading to important economical losses. The antimicrobial susceptibility of *M. bovis* is not covered by antimicrobial resistance surveillance networks. The objectives of this study were to identify resistances that were acquired over the last 30 years in France and to determine their prevalence within comtemporary strains. The minimum inhibition concentration (MIC) values of 12 antimicrobials, considered active on *M. bovis*, were compared, using an agar dilution method, between 27 and 46 *M. bovis* isolates respectively obtained in 1978–1979 and in 2010–2012 from 73 distinct respiratory disease outbreaks in young cattle all over France. For eight antimicrobials, resistances were proven to be acquired over the period and expressed by all contemporary strains. The increase of the MIC value that inhibited 50% of the isolates (MIC_{50}) was: i) substantial for tylosin, tilmicosin, tulathromycin and spectinomycin, from 2 to >64, 2 to >128, 16 to 128 and 4 to >64 μg/mL, respectively, ii) moderate for enrofloxacin, danofloxacin, marbofloxacin and oxytetracycline, from 0.25 to 0.5, 0.25 to 0.5, 0.5 to 1, 32 to >32 μg/mL, respectively. No differences were observed for gamithromycin, tildipirosin, florfenicol and valnemulin with MIC_{50} of 128, 128, 8, <0.03 μg/mL, respectively. If referring to breakpoint MIC values published for respiratory bovine pathogens, all contemporary isolates would be intermediate *in vivo* for fluoroquinolones and resistant to macrolides, oxytetracycline, spectinomycin and florfenicol.

Editor: Mitchell F. Balish, Miami University, United States of America

Funding: Research was supported by ANSES. The funders had no role in the study design, data collection and analysis, decision to publish, or preparation of the manuscript.

Competing Interests: The authors have declared that no competing interest exist.

* E-mail: francois.poumarat@anses.fr

Introduction

Formerly the name "mycoplasma" has commonly denoted bacteria of the class Mollicutes, nowadays it refers exclusively to members of the genus *Mycoplasma*. This genus comprises the simplest life forms that can self-replicate and includes major human and animal pathogens that cause diseases whose occurrence has long been underestimated [1]. All Mycoplasmas are cell-wall less bacteria and therefore are naturally resistant to all antimicrobial families that block cell wall synthesis (e.g. β-lactams and glycopeptides).

In cattle, *Mycoplasma (M.) bovis* causes respiratory disease, mastitis, arthritis and otitis [2]. It is now known that this mycoplasma species is frequently implicated in cases of bovine respiratory disease (BRD) in calves raised in feedlots worldwide [3]: it has been isolated in 40% of BRD outbreaks in the UK [3]; 25 to 80% in Italy [4,5]; 25 to 54% in Israel [6]; and 25% to 90% in France [7,8]. In these cases of BRD, *M. bovis* mostly occurs in coinfection with viruses and/or other bacteria but is often the only etiological agent in the chronic forms of BRD, which respond poorly to antimicrobials [2,9,10]. Today, only antimicrobials and sanitary controls are available to combat *M. bovis* infections.

Commercial vaccines are only available in a few countries and their efficacy is subject to debate [11–13].

Assessing the susceptibility of mycoplasmas to antimicrobials is difficult. Some characteristics of these organisms, such as their slow growth, small size and complex growth media requirements are incompatible with the standard procedures used to test the susceptibility of classic bacteria to antimicrobials such as the disk diffusion method. The Clinical and Laboratory Standards Institute (CLSI) has only recently established standardised antimicrobial susceptibility tests to determine the minimal inhibitory concentrations (MIC) for human mycoplasma pathogens [14]. However, these procedures cannot be used for all mycoplasmas because nutritional requirements, metabolic capacities and fitness vary among species [14]. For veterinary mycoplasma species, recommendations to control the main sources of experimental bias were proposed in 2000 by the International Research Programme on Comparative Mycoplasmology (IRPCM) [15]. Today there is no veterinary reference strain well characterized for MICs to be shared for quality control purposes, which is a major hurdle to compare results from different studies. Moreover, the absence of established antimicrobial breakpoint concentrations for mycoplasmas makes it difficult to evaluate the likely *in vivo* therapeutic efficacy from MIC data established *in vitro*.

Several studies on the susceptibility of *M. bovis* to antimicrobials have been published [6,16–25] but recent ones are scarce [23,24] or have not been published so far [Gosney and Ayling, unpublished results; Cai *et al.*, unpublished results]. The experimental procedures used vary considerably: MIC tests were carried out using either the liquid broth microdilution method [16,19,20,22,23,25], the solid agar dilution method [24] or the E test® [6,21]. Measuring mycoplasma growth is difficult in liquid and solid media because broth turbidity is difficult to measure in a standardised way and colony size on agar can be microscopic. In broth, growth is measured indirectly by a color change of a pH indicator with the inclusion of a substrate, typically glucose, arginine or urea, according to the species. Because *M. bovis* does not use any of these substrates, alternative indirect assay methods have been specifically developed based on either tetrazolium reduction [16]; alamarBlue®, a color redox indicator [22,23]; or phosphatase [6]. Growth has also been directly measured either by observing colonies on agar plates under a stereomicroscope [6,21,24] or by observing pellets after centrifuging the cultures [19]. The reference *M. bovis* type strain ATCC 25523 has often been used as a control [6,15,16,21,22,24]; the large disparities in observed MIC values, from 5 to 8 two-fold dilutions for some antimicrobials, illustrates the difficulty in comparing studies carried out using different methods.

Reports, for most antimicrobials except fluoroquinolones, give MICs that are distributed over a large range of dilutions and suggest that strains greatly vary in their susceptibility, but without any clear separation of sub-populations. Comparative studies using a unique technique reduce the technical bias and prove to be more instructive. Cai *et al.* [unpublished results] showed that over a 20 year period in Canada, *M. bovis* acquired high and frequent resistance to oxytetracycline and macrolides. In Israel, isolates from indigenous cattle proved to be less susceptible to macrolides than those from imported bovines [6]. Strains isolated from mastitis are less susceptible than those isolated from BRD [23; Gosney and Ayling, unpublished results]. Thus the susceptibility pattern of *M. bovis* to antibiotics seems to have changed over the last few decades but in a heterogeneous way, varying according to the date of isolation, the geographical origin, the type of livestock production system and disease. Thereby, changes of susceptibility must be assessed, first and foremost at a local scale as well as by type of livestock production system [6].

The increase in antimicrobial resistance has become a real public health problem and in many countries there is growing pressure to control this resistance in both humans and animals. Curbing the progression of antimicrobial resistance includes setting up integrated treatments based on antimicrobial susceptibility tests and statistics from antimicrobial resistance surveillance networks for animal bacterial pathogens. However, mycoplasmas are generally not covered by these European networks [26]. Respiratory disease accounts for 20% of overall antibiotic consumption in cattle in France [27]. Given the high frequency of occurrence of *M. bovis* in BRD cases and its direct involvement in the chronic forms that are difficult to cure, mycoplasmas cannot be overlooked in the treatment of BRD and the antimicrobial susceptibility patterns of *M. bovis* must be updated and assessed at a regional level.

The objectives of the present study were to identify any evolution in antimicrobial susceptibility of *M. bovis* for the main classes of antimicrobials used to treat BRD in France by comparing strains isolated 30 years apart and then to assess the prevalence of the acquired resistances on a national level today.

Materials and Methods

Selection and Characteristics of M. bovis Isolates

The *M. bovis* isolates selected for this study came from the collection of the French national surveillance network of ruminants mycoplasmoses (VIGIMYC) [28]. Isolation was performed in Anses or in VIGIMYC-partner laboratories and identification was performed in Anses as previously decribed [29,30]. Isolates were preserved lyophilised or −80°C frozen.

Only *M. bovis* isolated from BRD in young cattle were selected. Then two distinct groups were chosen according to the isolation date and the geographical origin: 27 "old" isolates collected in the 1978–1979 period from 27 distinct outbreaks in 20 French *départements* and 46 "contemporary" isolates collected between 2010 and 2012 from 46 distinct outbreaks in 29 French *départements*. In each of the two groups, half of the calves had been weaned and half had not. Likewise, for half of the isolates, only *M. bovis* had been isolated and for the other half, *M. bovis* had been isolated along with other bacteria, mainly *Mannheimia (M.) haemolytica*, *Pasteurella (P.) multocida* and *Trueperella (formerly Arcanobacterium) pyogenes*. In addition, 97 other *M. bovis* isolates collected between 2010 and 2012 across 33 French *départements* were tested for resistance to enrofloxacin. These isolates came from 90 BRD, three arthritis, three otitis and one mastitis outbreaks.

Preparation of Inoculum for MIC Assays

Mycoplasma cultures were prepared in appropriate media from several colonies picked on agar plates after isolation. Cultures were frozen in multiple aliquots at −80°C in 15% (v/v) glycerol. To confirm species identity and to detect any mixtures of mycoplasma species, one aliquot was checked by membrane filtration dot-immunobinding tests [30] against ruminants' mycoplasma species. For each isolate, three aliquots were used to determine the number of colony forming units (CFU) per mL by performing serial 10-fold dilutions in broth, plating each dilution on agar, incubating the plates and then counting colonies with a stereomicroscope. Final CFU/mL concentrations were expressed as the mean.

Antimicrobial Agents Tested

Two groups of antimicrobials were successively tested.

First, six widely used antimicrobials (group n°1), from five antimicrobial classes that are likely to be active on mycoplasmas, were tested on 27 old and 46 contemporary isolates: enrofloxacin (fluoroquinolone), oxytetracycline (tetracycline), spectinomycin (aminocyclitol), florfenicol (amphenicol), tylosin and tilmicosin (macrolides). The enrofloxacin susceptibility was further tested on 97 additional comtemporary *M. bovis* isolates.

Then six other antimicrobials (group n°2) were tested simultaneously on 27 old and 30 of the 46 contemporary isolates used with group n°1: two fluoroquinolones (marbofloxacin and danofloxacin), three macrolides (tulathromycin, gamithromycin and tildipirosin) that are indicated for BRD and one pleuromutilin (valnemulin) indicated for porcine and poultry mycoplasmas.

Most antimicrobials were purchased from Sigma. Tulathromycin, gamithromycin and tildipirosin were provided by Zoetis (formerly Pfizer), Merial and MSD (formerly SP Intervet), respectively. For each antimicrobial agent, the same batch was used for all the assays.

Preparation of Antimicrobial Dilutions

Antimicrobials in powdered form were weighed and dissolved according to the manufacturer's instructions and drug purity. The stock solutions were prepared on the day of the MIC assay and the dilutions for use in individual MIC assays were made up in accordance with published CLSI procedures [31].

Method of MIC Evaluation

MIC assays were performed using the agar dilution method according to recommendations by Waites et al. [14].

Commercial mycoplasma agar medium similar to modified Hayflick medium [15] and provided by Indicia Biotechnology was chosen since Indicia medium is recommended for growing ruminant and avian mycoplasmas and has given satisfactory performance with M. bovis. A single batch of medium without any inhibitor (antimicrobial or thallium acetate) was used for all MIC assays.

Doubling dilutions of the antimicrobial agents were incorporated into molten agar plates and 12 to 14 dilutions of each drug were tested. Then 1 μL of each strain diluted to yield 3×10^5 to 3×10^6 CFU/mL was spotted on the agar plates using a multipoint inoculator: 60 strains were simultaneously tested on the same plate for each antimicrobial dilution. Plates were incubated in ambient air with 5% CO_2 at 37°C for 4 days. The MIC was read as the lowest antimicrobial concentration that prevented colony formation when the antimicrobial-free control plate demonstrated growth of approximately 30 to 300 CFU per spot of inoculum. MIC assays were repeated three times from three distinct aliquots of each strain and for each antimicrobial drug and final results were expressed as the median of the three MIC values.

Antimicrobials from each group were tested simultaneously on 27 old and 30 contemporary isolates in the same assay. Two other assays were conducted on 16 additional contemporary strains for group n°1 antimicrobials and on 97 contemporary strains for enrofloxacin.

Quality Control Strains

Three mycoplasma strains were included as quality control strains for each assay: the M. bovis type strain PG45 isolated in 1962 (ATCC 25523), the M. bovis 1067 French field strain isolated in 1983 and proven to be pathogenic [32], and the Mycoplasma gallisepticum type strain ATCC 15302 that has been used as quality control strain several times before [33]. The Staphylococcus aureus type strain ATCC 29213, a standard for quality control for antimicrobial disk and dilution susceptibility tests for bacteria isolated from animals [31] was also tested in the same conditions (agar medium, drug dilutions and incubation) in order to validate the results obtained.

Stastistical Analysis

To compare MIC distribution, a log2 transformation of the MIC data was first applied so that the variable became continuous. The Mann-Whitney test was then used to compare log2 (MIC) of old and contemporary strains of M. bovis for each antimicrobial, to test if one population had higher values than the other. The Mann-Whitney test is a non-parametric test and can be used with small samples [34]. The significance level was set to 0.05.

Results

The procedure used in this study proved to be reproducible and accurate. The MICs of the M. gallisepticum ATCC 15302 strain and that of the two M. bovis strains (ATCC 25523 and 1067) were tested nine and six times, respectively, for each of the six antimicrobials of the group n°1. The variability of MIC values was always within one dilution of the median value. The 780 measurements of MICs were each repeated three times; in 99.5% of the cases, the observed values were within two successive

dilutions and in the remaining 0.5% of the cases, within three. The MIC values obtained for M. gallisepticum were identical to those reported in other studies [33]. Those of Staphyloccocus aureus ATCC 29213 were consistent with the standard reference values established by the CLSI for antimicrobial susceptibility tests using a dilution method for bacteria isolated from animals [31]. Therefore, the Indicia agar medium used in the assays did not modify the availability of antimicrobials compared to Mueller Hilton medium used in standardised MIC tests for classic bacteria. Thus the scale of MIC values obtained in this study is comparable to that of standardised tests for classic bacteria.

All MIC results are shown in Figures 1 and 2. For nine of the twelve antimicrobials tested, strain susceptibility changed significantly over time ($p < 0.05$), with contemporary strains showing decreased susceptibility except for florfenicol for which susceptibility increased slightly. No significant change in isolates' susceptibility was observed for gamithromycin, tildipirosin or valnemulin. The drop in susceptibility was substantial for tylosin, tilmicosin, spectinomycin and tulathromycin, with shifts in the MIC_{50} (the MIC value that inhibited 50% of the isolates) from 2 to >64, 2 to >128, 4 to >64 and 16 to 128 μg/mL, respectively. The three fluoroquinolones and oxytetracycline MIC only increased by one two-fold dilution, with shifts in the MIC_{50} from 0.25 to 0.5 μg/mL for enrofloxacin and danofloxacin, from 0.5 to 1 μg/mL for marbofloxacin and from 32 to >32 μg/mL for oxytetracycline. The screening of 97 additional contemporary M. bovis isolates for enrofloxacin susceptibility did not reveal any burgeoning of high level resistance in France.

The antimicrobial susceptibility pattern of contemporary M. bovis isolates was very homogeneous. Regardless of the antimicrobial tested, more than 77% of the strains were centred on the same MIC value or 100% showed very high MICs (spectinomycin, tylosin, tilmicosin) or very low MICs (valnemulin). Furthermore the eight resistances that have been selected over the three last decades are now observed simultaneously in 100% of M. bovis isolates.

The effectiveness of antimicrobials in the treatment of BRD can be estimated by comparing in vitro MIC values to MIC breakpoints established by the CLSI. As breakpoints were not available for veterinary mycoplasmas, MIC values were compared to breakpoints given for respiratory bovine pathogens (Pasteurellaceae) [31]. The mean MIC values of tylosin, tilmicosin, oxytetracycline, spectinomycin and tulathromycin for contemporary M. bovis strains are clearly greater than the CLSI thresholds. It is therefore very likely that these antimicrobials are not active in vivo. For florfenicol, 94% of strains are right at the threshold of resistance. For fluoroquinolones, all strains are classified as intermediate. Breakpoints are not available for gamithromycin and tildipirosin, but the MIC_{50} (128 μg/mL) is much greater than the maximum concentrations used for respiratory infections at therapeutic doses, 18 and 15 μg/g of lung homogenate, respectively [35,36].

Discussion

As with all Mollicutes, M. bovis is naturally resistant to β-lactams and glycopeptides, but also to polymyxins, sulfonamides, trimethoprim, nalidixic acid, rifampicin and lincomycin [37]. This study shows that M. bovis strains recently isolated in France (2010–2012) have become less susceptible to other antimicrobials that, until now, have been recommended or likely to be of interest for treating mycoplasmoses.

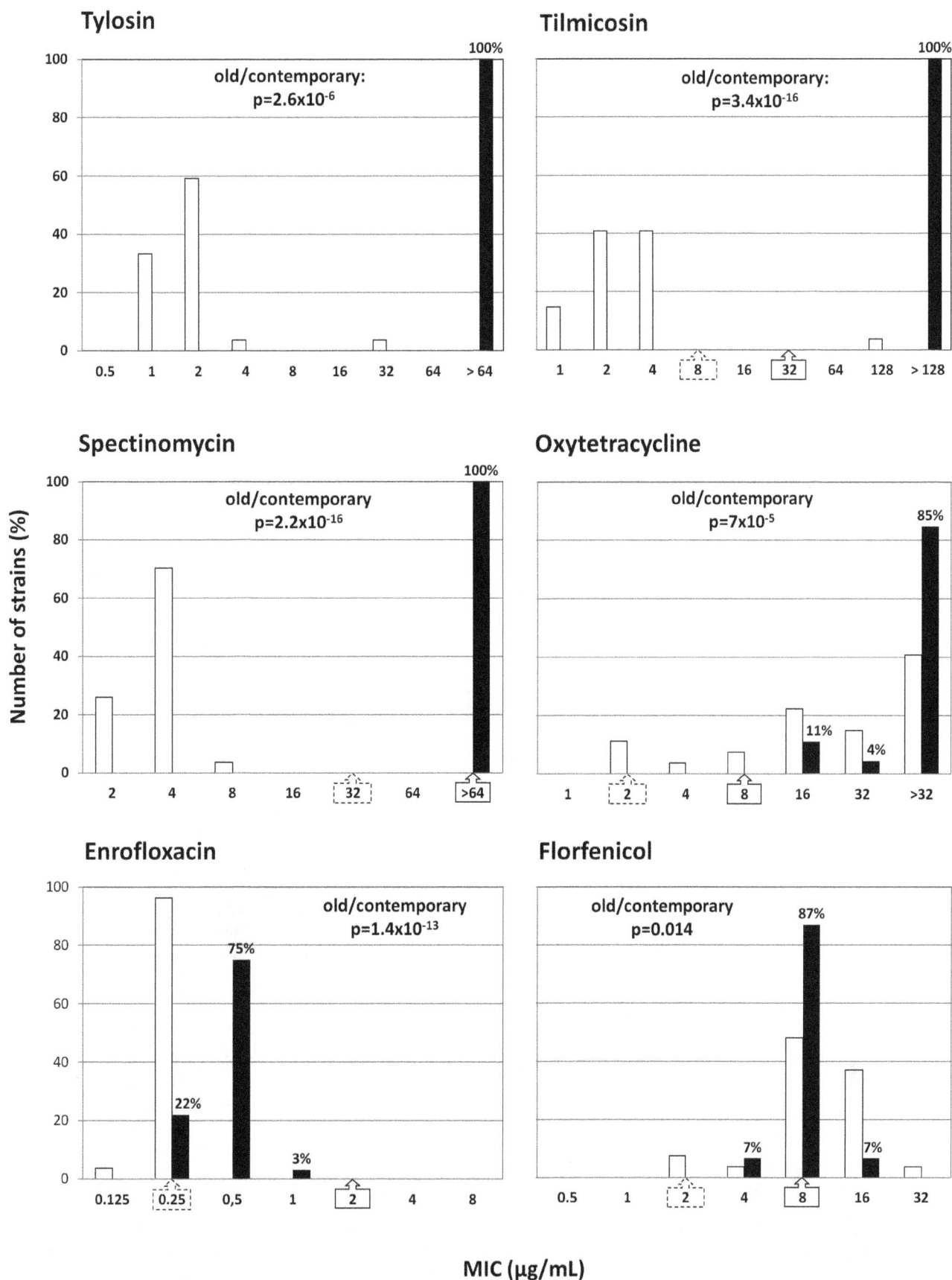

Figure 1. Distribution (%) of MIC values (in μg/mL) of group n°1 antimicrobials. MICs of tylosin, tilmicosin, spectinomycin, oxytetracycline and florfenicol for 27 *M. bovis* strains isolated in 1978–1979 (white bars) and 46 isolated in 2010–2012 (black bars). MICs of enrofloxacin, for 27 *M.*

bovis strains isolated in 1978- 1979 (white bars) and 143 *M. bovis* strains isolated in 2010–2012 (black bars). When available, CLSI breakpoints for bovine *Pasteurellaceae* are given under the X axis: - strains with MIC values less than or equal to the dilution indicated in the dotted-line arrow are susceptible, - strains with MIC values greater than the dilution indicated in the full-line arrow are resistant, - all other strains are intermediate.

Procedure was Repeatable and Accurate, and Sampling Adequately Chosen to Address the Objectives

The agar dilution method was used in this study because it has been recommended for *M. bovis* by the IRPCM [15]. This method has been infrequently used in previous studies because it is very labour-intensive, but it ensures a better standardisation than liquid microdilution methods. The indirect assessment of growth by the use of a substrate in broth microdilution tests is imprecise. The change in colour (of the broth) occurs gradually and requires a high titre of mycoplasmas. Measurement of *M. bovis* growth in liquid media is less standardised than for most other mycoplasma species because *M. bovis* does not utilise commonly used substrates (glucose or arginine). Furthermore, substrate oxidation kinetics for *M. bovis* can vary with strain [38], therefore generally requiring readings at several intervals. By contrast, agar dilution method can be used to test a large number of strains simultaneously on the same batch of agar with the same antimicrobial dilution (via the use of a multipoint inoculator) and growth can be directly and unambiguously assayed by direct observation of colonies under a stereomicroscope.

The unimodal or bimodal distribution of MIC values within the *M. bovis* sample obtained in the present study for all the tested antimicrobials contrasted sharply with the distributions reported in most previous studies [6,19–24]. The MIC values reported for most antimicrobials in these studies, with the exception of fluoroquinolones, were scattered over a large range of dilutions. This scatter, to some extent, may be due to bias of the methods employed or to the choice of samples. Indeed the margin of error of a measurement of MIC in Mollicutes can be high, even in strictly standardised conditions, particularly for certain antimicrobials such as macrolides [14]. The procedure used in the present study was based on the agar dilution method recommended by CLSI for human mycoplasmas [14] and proved to be highly repeatable and accurate. Sampling heterogeneity can also cause scattered MIC values because the susceptibility pattern of *M. bovis* strains varies considerably with region, isolation date, disease and production practices [6, 23, Gosney and Ayling, unpublished results]. To limit sampling bias as much as possible, we chose to compare strains that were clearly different with respect to their date of isolation, but comparable in terms of country origin, disease, animal age class and organ.

The Susceptibility of *M. bovis* to Antimicrobials Dramatically Decreased over the Last Decades

Over the 30-year interval between isolate samplings, the susceptibility of *M. bovis* decreased significantly for eight antimicrobials of tetracycline, fluoroquinolone, aminocyclitol, and macrolide families that are considered to be active on mycoplasmas.

All MIC values of spectinomycin and oxytetracycline towards contemporary French strains became very high. The wide distribution of MIC values for oxytetracycline in the old strains population suggests that less susceptible strains had arisen by 1978–79 for this antimicrobial, which was placed on the market in the 1950s. Such steep susceptibility decreases for these antimicrobials were not observed in other studies. Several recent studies show that the MIC_{90} values for spectinomycin in Britain, the USA, Canada and Japan are still less than 32 µg/mL [22, 24; Gosney

and Ayling, unpublished results; Cai *et al.*, unpublished results] and less than 16 µg/mL for oxytetracycline in Britain, Israel, and the USA [6, 22, Gosney and Ayling, unpublished results].

For first-generation macrolides (tylosin, tilmicosin), the same steep decrease in susceptibility as in France was described worldwide, first in the UK in the 1990s [19] and then in USA, Israel, Canada and Japan [6, 22, 24, Cai *et al.*, unpublished results]. For the new-generation macrolides, gamithromycin and tildipirosin, MICs were high for both old and contemporary strains, pointing to a putative natural resistance as observed for erythromycin. In fact, these high values cannot be attributed to a lack of availability of the antimicrobials in the agar medium as MIC values obtained against the *M. gallisepticum* ATCC 15302 strain were very low (<0.03 and 0.25 for gamithromycin and tildipirosin, respectively). For tulathromycin, old strains were significantly more susceptible, but several old strains with intermediate MIC level were observed before tulathromycin was placed on the market (European agreement obtained in 2004). As resistance for tylosin and tilmicosin in the period before 1980 was observed for only one isolate, the occurrence of these less susceptible old strains could be better explained by naturally resistant variants than a putative cross-resistance with first generation macrolides. Interestingly, two distinct populations were also observed in a study on the action of tulathromycin based on 53 European *M. bovis* strains isolated between 1980–2002, with MIC_{50} of 0.25 and >64 µg/mL, respectively [39].

The decrease in susceptibility with respect to fluoroquinolones is significant but low (only one dilution). Although there has been a recent report of *M. bovis* mastitis strains with very high MICs for enrofloxacin [Gosney and Ayling, unpublished results], further screening of 97 additional contemporary isolates did not reveal any burgeoning resistance of high level in France.

For florfenicol, only a little but significant increase of susceptibility was observed between old and contemporary strains. The MIC_{50} remained constant at 8 µg/mL. However, seven old strains were more susceptible with MICs of 2 µg/mL. MIC_{90} values of less than 2 µg/mL have also been reported in a recent study [40]. This suggests that the susceptibility of French old strains may have already changed in 1978–79 with respect to the natural level of susceptibility. This early change in susceptibility may be a consequence of the massive use of chloramphenicol – which has a common cross-resistance mechanism with florfenicol [41] – between 1950 and 1967 (the year it was taken off the market).

The Prevalence of Multi-resistant *M. bovis* Strains is Very High now in France

In this study, resistances proved to be acquired over the last 30 years for eight antimicrobials, simultaneously affected all the contemporary strains. This 100% prevalence of multi-resistant strains was obtained on a large and diversified sample of strains and may be close to the current national prevalence. That is exceptional in terms of bacterial resistance. Similar findings have been recently reported in UK [Gosney and Ayling, unpublished results] and Canada [Cai *et al.*, unpublished results] but to a lesser extent with respect to number of antimicrobial agents associated with resistance and level of prevalence. This phenomenon cannot be attributed to a simple sampling bias, because the 46 tested strains were isolated from 46 different outbreaks that occurred in

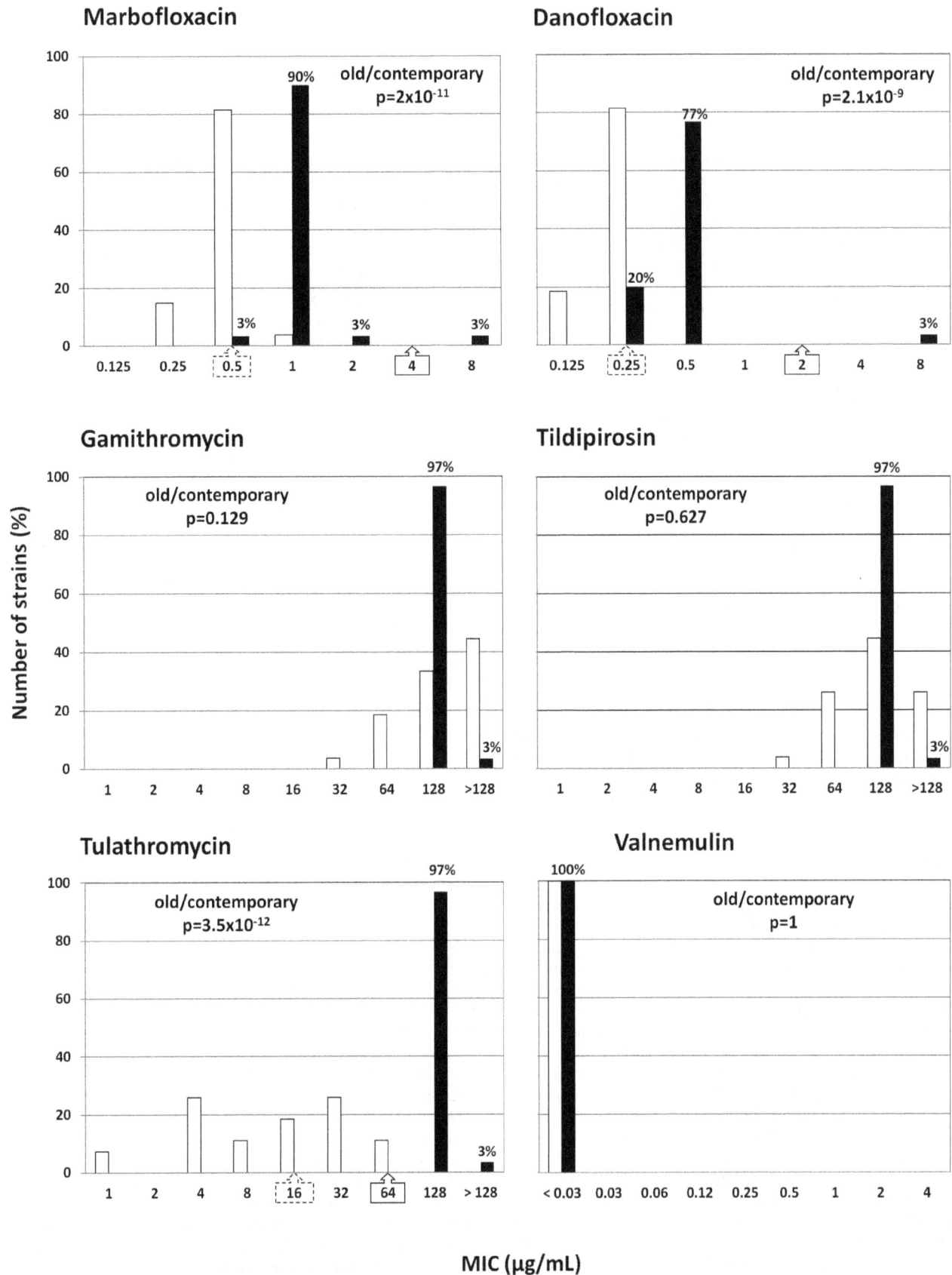

Figure 2. Distribution (%) of MIC values (in μg/mL) of group n°2 antimicrobials. MICs of marbofloxacin, danofloxacin, gamithromycin, tildipirosin, tulathromycin, valnemulin for 27 *M. bovis* strains isolated in 1978–1979 (white bars) and 30 *M. bovis* strains isolated in 2010–2012 (black bars). When available, CLSI breakpoints for bovine *Pasteurellaceae* are given under the X axis: - strains with MIC values less than or equal to the

dilution indicated in the dotted-line arrow are susceptible, - strains with MIC values greater than the dilution indicated in the full-line arrow are resistant, all other strains are intermediate.

25 *départements* across France over a period of two years. The probability of a direct link between all these outbreaks is therefore very low. However the spread of a unique clone of *M. bovis* across all of France could explain a unique resistance pattern for all isolates. The spread of enrofloxacin-resistant strains documented in Israel was not clonal in nature [42]. Sub-typing studies on *M. bovis* conducted locally in feedlots in France [43] and at the national level in other countries [44–47], have concluded that the genetic diversity in contemporary mycoplasma outbreaks is usually high, but with a clonal origin in Austria [48]. This hypothesis is currently being explored by our laboratory as far as French isolates are concerned.

The Pressure and Strategy of Antimicrobial Therapy could be Major Selective Factors of Resistance

The pressure of antimicrobial therapy could be a major selective factor in *M. bovis*, as is the case for other mycoplasma species. Experimental data based on *in vitro* cultures in the presence of antimicrobials confirms that mycoplasmas can very rapidly acquire resistance to antimicrobials. High levels of resistance to macrolides and enrofloxacin in *M. gallisepticum*, *M. synoviae* and *M. iowae* have been obtained in only a few passages [33]. During experimental infections in swine and chicken, infected by *M. hyopneumoniae* and *M. synoviae*, respectively, clones resistant to enrofloxacin have been isolated after only two treatments at therapeutic doses and were directly linked to a point mutation in the "quinolone-resistance determining region" of a topoisomerase gene [49,50]. The rapidity with which resistance is selected may be related to the high mutation rate in mycoplasmas, likely due to a deficit in genetic information dedicated to DNA repair in mycoplasma genomes [51]. Horizontal gene transfer is also an essential factor in the spread of resistance in other bacteria. In mycoplasmas, the possibility of frequent and large transfers that had been predicted earlier from *in silico* data [52] was very recently demonstrated *in vitro* [53]. However to date the only resistance genes known in mycoplasmas to be carried on a mobile genetic element (conjugative transposon) are the *tet*M gene that encode a tetracycline resistance [37].

The strategy of antibiotherapy could also be a predominant factor in the spread of resistant strains. In *M. pneumoniae*, macrolide-resistant strains, unknown before 2000, now represent 10%, 40% and 80% of strains isolated in Europe, Japan, and China, respectively, after outbreaks of worldwide epidemics in 2010–2011 [54]. The pronounced differences in incidence among countries may be explained by more extensive macrolide use in Asia for pneumonia treatment [54]. It may be the same for *M. bovis*. BRD is a multifactorial disease in which several agents occur simultaneously or sequentially, including viruses, mycoplasmas and classic bacteria, mainly *Pasteurellaceae*. The susceptibility of *Pasteurellaceae* to antimicrobials is closely monitored in France (RESAPATH network) [55]. Based on statistics from the network, first-line treatments recommended for BRD today in France target only these *Pasteurellaceae* and do not take into account mycoplasmas. Thus, antimicrobial drugs that are often inappropriate for mycoplasmas, such as β-lactams, that are very active on *Pasteurellaceae*, are frequently used. It is likely that the administered antimicrobial treatments, by eliminating other competing bacteria, actually promote mycoplasmosis and lead to the more chronic forms described for *M. bovis* [2] and therefore to additional antimicrobial treatments. Furthermore, the absence of any

systematic diagnosis for *M. bovis* and the lack of recent statistical data on its recent susceptibility pattern may result in unsuitable treatment leading to persistence and selection of even more resistant strains. In support of this hypothesis, high levels of resistance have also been found in *M. bovirhinis*, a frequent but non-pathogenic resident of the respiratory tract [24].

Most Currently Used Antimicrobials would now be Inactive or Weakly Active on *M. bovis* Diseases but Further Investigations are Needed to Confirm

Choosing first-line active drugs to fight respiratory infections *in vivo* is the key for this type of epidemiological situation. Since there is no standard breakpoint for *M. bovis*, several authors [6,21–23,42] used breakpoints based on epidemiological and pharmacokinetic criteria established by the CLSI for bovine *Pasteurellaceae* [31]. These bacteria occur in the same disease (i.e. BRD) and at the same level (extra-cellular and in deep lung) as *M. bovis*. The conditions for reaching therapeutic concentrations *in situ* are therefore theoretically equivalent. Moreover, the scale of MIC values obtained in this study has proven comparable to that of standardised tests for classic bacteria.

Refering to CLSI breakpoints when available, 100% of contemporary *M. bovis* strains would not be inhibited *in vivo* by any antimicrobial tested in the study, except fluoroquinolones when a high dosage can be used. Very low MIC values (<0.03 μg/mL) obtained for valnemulin are therapeutically interesting, but this antimicrobial is currently used only in swine and poultry and is somewhat toxic in various animal species. This antimicrobial, administered by the oral route, has experimentally proven to be effective in calves infected with *M. bovis* strains with a MIC of 0.0625 μg/mL [56].

Conclusions on the likely therapeutic effectiveness of these antimicrobials must be taken with caution: results on *in vivo* and *in vitro* susceptibility are not always concordant. Some treatments seem to be effective in experimental infection models despite the use of strains with high MIC values [3]. Accordingly, tulathromycin has proven effective despite a MIC of >64 μg/mL on the assayed *M. bovis* strain [39]. The efficacy of gamithromycin on a *M. bovis* strain has also been proven experimentally in an infection model [57]. In contrast, therapeutic failures have been observed experimentally with *M. bovis*, *M. hyopneumoniae* and *M. synoviae* [49,50,58] despite the high susceptibility of inoculated strains. Other factors could indirectly affect the efficacy of a treatment, such as the production of biofilms by mycoplasmas [59] or systematic reinfection after treatment [47].

Finally the frequency of resistant strains in this study may be overestimated compared to that of currently circulating strains. The strains tested in this study came from diagnostic laboratories that were usually called after treatment failures. Antibio-surveillance networks are based on the same type of reporting and the possible overestimation does not lead to erroneous public/animal health measures. However, the rapidity of adaptation in mycoplasmas may exacerbate this bias in estimation. For instance, *M. agalactiae* isolates obtained from goats herds with clinical symptoms of *M. agalactiae* mastitis featured higher MIC values for many antimicrobials compared with isolates from asymptomatic animals [60].

Conclusion

It is now generally accepted that *M. bovis* is frequently involved in bovine diseases such as mastitis, arthritis, otitis media, and particularly respiratory disease worldwide. The rapid decrease in susceptibility of this pathogen to antimicrobials is of high concern, particularly because it causes over-consumption of antimicrobials including those that are critical for human health. It is now important to set up systematic screening of *M. bovis*, adapt BRD treatment strategies accordingly, monitor the overall susceptibility of mycoplasmas to potentially active antimicrobials and determine their actual therapeutic activity *in vivo*. However, given the current situation and the speed at which resistance appears to be selected in mycoplasmas, alternative control measures must be rapidly set up, such as preventive health measures and the development of vaccines.

Acknowledgments

We express our gratitude to the VIGIMYC staff, V. Lefriand and P. Cuchet for technical assistance and to F. Tardy and I. Kempf for critical reading of the manuscript.

Author Contributions

Conceived and designed the experiments: AGB FP DLG SF. Performed the experiments: AGB SF AP FP. Analyzed the data: AGB FP EG. Wrote the paper: AGB FP. Critically reviewed and approved the manuscript: DLG EG.

References

1. Citti C, Blanchard A (2013) Mycoplasmas and their host: emerging and re-emerging minimal pathogens. Trends Microbiol 21: 196–203.
2. Maunsell FP, Woolums AR, Francoz D, Rosenbusch RF, Step DL, et al. (2011) *Mycoplasma bovis* infections in cattle. J Vet Intern Med 25: 772–783.
3. Nicholas RA (2011) Bovine mycoplasmosis: silent and deadly. Vet Rec 168: 459–462.
4. Radaelli E, Luini M, Loria GR, Nicholas RA, Scanziani E (2008) Bacteriological, serological, pathological and immunohistochemical studies of *Mycoplasma bovis* respiratory infection in veal calves and adult cattle at slaughter. Res Vet Sci 85: 282–290.
5. Giovannini S, Zanoni MG, Salogni C, Cinotti S, Alborali GL (2013) *Mycoplasma bovis* infection in respiratory disease of dairy calves less than one month old. Res Vet Sci 95: 576–579.
6. Gerchman I, Levisohn S, Mikula I, Lysnyansky I (2009) In vitro antimicrobial susceptibility of *Mycoplasma bovis* isolated in Israel from local and imported cattle. Vet Microbiol 137: 268–275.
7. Arcangioli MA, Duet A, Meyer G, Dernburg A, Bezille P, et al. (2008) The role of *Mycoplasma bovis* in bovine respiratory disease outbreaks in veal calf feedlots. Vet J 177: 89–93.
8. Poumarat F, Perrin M, Gauthier N, Lepage D, Martel J-L (1988) Pathologie respiratoire des veaux de nurserie et des taurillons. Prévalence de *Mycoplasma bovis* parmi les différentes étiologies infectieuses au travers d'enquêtes réalisées en région Rhône-Alpes. Rec Med Vet 164: 625–632.
9. Gagea MI, Bateman KG, Shanahan RA, van Dreumel T, McEwen BJ, et al. (2006) Naturaly occurring *Mycoplasma bovis*-associated pneumonia and polyar-thritis in feedlot beef calves. J Vet Diagn Invest 18: 29–40.
10. Caswell JL, Bateman KG, Cai HY, Castillo-Alcala F (2010) *Mycoplasma bovis* in respiratory disease of feedlot cattle. Vet Clin North Am Food Anim Pract 26: 365–379.
11. Maunsell FP, Donovan GA, Risco C, Brown MB (2009) Field evaluation of a *Mycoplasma bovis* bacterin in young dairy calves. Vaccine 27: 2781–2788.
12. Mulongo M, Prysliak T, Perez-Casal J (2013) Vaccination of feedlot cattle with extracts and membrane fractions from two *Mycoplasma bovis* isolates results in strong humoral immune responses but does not protect against an experimental challenge. Vaccine 31: 1406–1412.
13. Soehnlen MK, Aydin A, Lengerich EJ, Houser BA, Fenton GD, et al. (2011) Blinded, controlled field trial of two commercially available *Mycoplasma bovis* bacterin vaccines in veal calves. Vaccine 29: 5347–5354.
14. Waites KB, Duffy LB, Bébéar CM, Matlow A, Talkington DF, et al. (2012) Standardized methods and quality control limits for agar and broth microdilu-tion susceptibility testing of *Mycoplasma pneumoniae*, *Mycoplasma hominis*, and *Ureaplasma urealyticum*. J Clin Microbiol 50: 3542–3547.
15. Hannan PC (2000) Guidelines and recommendations for antimicrobial minimum inhibitory concentration (MIC) testing against veterinary mycoplasma species. International Research Programme on Comparative Mycoplasmology. Vet Res 31: 373–395.
16. ter Laak EA, Noordergraaf JH, Verschure MH (1993) Susceptibilities of *Mycoplasma bovis*, *Mycoplasma dispar*, and *Ureaplasma diversum* strains to antimicro-bial agents in vitro. Antimicrob Agents Chemother 37: 317–321.
17. Ball HJ, Reilly GAC, Bryson DG (1995) Antibiotic susceptibility of *Mycoplasma bovis* strains isolated in Northern Ireland. Irish Vet J 48: 316–318.
18. Mazzolini E, Agnoletti F, Friso S (1997) Farmaco sensibilita dei micoplasmi respiratori del bovino. Obiettivi Doc Vet 1: 61–66.
19. Ayling RD, Baker SE, Peek ML, Simon AJ, Nicholas RA (2000) Comparison of in vitro activity of danofloxacin, florfenicol, oxytetracycline, spectinomycin and tilmicosin against recent field isolates of *Mycoplasma bovis*. Vet Rec 146: 745–747.
20. Thomas A, Nicolas C, Dizier I, Mainil J, Linden A (2003) Antibiotic susceptibilities of recent isolates of *Mycoplasma bovis* in Belgium. Vet Rec 153: 428–431.
21. Francoz D, Fortin M, Fecteau G, Messier S (2005) Determination of *Mycoplasma bovis* susceptibilities against six antimicrobial agents using the E test method. Vet Microbiol 105: 57–64.

22. Rosenbusch RF, Kinyon JM, Apley M, Funk ND, Smith S, et al. (2005) In vitro antimicrobial inhibition profiles of *Mycoplasma bovis* isolates recovered from various regions of the United States from 2002 to 2003. J Vet Diagn Invest 17: 436–441.
23. Soehnlen MK, Kunze ME, Karunathilake KE, Henwood BM, Kariyawasam S, et al. (2011) In vitro antimicrobial inhibition of *Mycoplasma bovis* isolates submitted to the Pennsylvania Animal Diagnostic Laboratory using flow cytometry and a broth microdilution method. J Vet Diagn Invest 23: 547–51.
24. Uemura R, Sueyoshi M, Nagatomo H (2010) Antimicrobial susceptibilities of four species of mycoplasma isolated in 2008 and 2009 from cattle in Japan. J Vet Med Sci 72: 1661–1663.
25. Hannan PC, Windsor GD, de Jong A, Schmeer N, Stegemann M (1997) Comparative susceptibilities of various animal-pathogenic mycoplasmas to fluoroquinolones. Antimicrob Agents Chemother 41: 2037–2040.
26. de Jong A, Thomas V, Klein U, Marion H, Moyaert H, et al. (2013) Pan-European resistance monitoring programmes encompassing food-borne bacteria and target pathogens of food-producing and companion animals. Int J Antimicrob Agents 41: 403–409.
27. Gay E, Cazeau G, Jarrige N, Calavas D (2012) Utilisation des antibiotiques chez les ruminants domestiques en France: résultats d'enquêtes de pratiques auprès d'éleveurs et de vétérinaires. Bull Epid Santé Anim Alim 53: 8–10.
28. Chazel M, Tardy F, Le Grand D, Calavas D, Poumarat F (2010) Mycoplasmoses of ruminants in France: recent data from the national surveillance network. BMC Vet Res 6: 32.
29. Tardy F, Gaurivaud P, Tricot A, Maigre L, Poumarat F (2009) Epidemiological surveillance of mycoplasmas belonging to the "*Mycoplasma mycoides*" cluster: is DGGE fingerprinting of 16S rRNA genes suitable? Lett Appl Microbiol 48: 210–217.
30. Poumarat F, Perrin B, Longchambon D (1991) Identification of ruminant mycoplasma by dot-immunobinding on membrane filtration (MF dot). Vet Microbiol 29: 329–338.
31. CLSI (2008) Performance standards for antimicrobial disk and dilution susceptibility tests for bacteria isolated from animals; Approved Standard-Third Edition. CLSI document M31-A3. Wayne, PA: Clinical and Laboratory Standards Institute.
32. Hermeyer K, Buchenau I, Thomasmeyer A, Baum B, Spergser J, et al. (2012) Chronic pneumonia in calves after experimental infection with *Mycoplasma bovis* strain 1067: characterization of lung pathology, persistence of variable surface protein antigens and local immune response. Acta Vet Scand 54: 9.
33. Gautier-Bouchardon AV, Reinhardt AK, Kobisch M, Kempf I (2002) In vitro development of resistance to enrofloxacin, erythromycin, tylosin, tiamulin and oxytetracycline in *Mycoplasma gallisepticum*, *Mycoplasma iowae* and *Mycoplasma synoviae*. Vet Microbiol 88: 47–58.
34. Hollander M, Wolfe DA (1999) Nonparametric Statistical Methods. 2nd edition. New York: John Wiley & Sons. 787 p.
35. Menge M, Rose M, Bohland C, Zschiesche E, Kilp S, et al. (2012) Pharmacokinetics of tildipirosin in bovine plasma, lung tissue, and bronchial fluid (from live, nonanesthetized cattle). J Vet Pharmacol Ther 35: 550–559.
36. Huang RA, Letendre LT, Banav N, Fischer J, Somerville B (2010) Pharmacokinetics of gamithromycin in cattle with comparison of plasma and lung tissue concentrations and plasma antibacterial activity. J Vet Pharmacol Ther 33: 227–237.
37. Bébéar CM, Kempf I (2005) Antimicrobial therapy and antimicrobial resistance. In: Blanchard A, Browning G, editors. Mycoplasmas: Molecular Biology Pathogenicity and Strategies for Control. Poole, UK: Horizon Bioscience. 535–568.
38. Khan LA, Loria GR, Ramirez AS, Nicholas RA, Miles RJ, et al. (2005) Biochemical characterisation of some non fermenting, non arginine hydrolysing mycoplasmas of ruminants. Vet Microbiol 109: 129–134.
39. Godinho KS, Rae A, Windsor GD, Tilt N, Rowan TG, et al. (2005) Efficacy of tulathromycin in the treatment of bovine respiratory disease associated with induced *Mycoplasma bovis* infections in young dairy calves. Vet Ther 6: 96–112.

40. Thiry J, Rubion S, Sarasola P, Bonnier M, Hartmann M, et al. (2011) Efficacy and safety of a new 450 mg/ml florfenicol formulation administered intramuscularly in the treatment of bacterial bovine respiratory disease. Vet Rec 169: 526.

41. Arcangioli MA, Leroy-Setrin S, Martel JL, Chaslus-Dancla E (2000) Evolution of chloramphenicol resistance, with emergence of cross-resistance to florfenicol, in bovine *Salmonella Typhimurium* strains implicates definitive phage type (DT) 104. J Med Microbiol 49: 103–110.

42. Lysnyansky I, Mikula I, Gerchman I, Levisohn S (2009) Rapid detection of a point mutation in the *parC* gene associated with decreased susceptibility to fluoroquinolones in *Mycoplasma bovis*. Antimicrob Agents Chemother 53: 104–108.

43. Arcangioli MA, Aslan H, Tardy F, Poumarat F, Le Grand D (2011) The use of pulsed-field gel electrophoresis to investigate the epidemiology of *Mycoplasma bovis* in French calf feedlots. Vet J 192: 96–100.

44. McAuliffe L, Kokotovic B, Ayling RD, Nicholas RA (2004) Molecular epidemiological analysis of *Mycoplasma bovis* isolates from the United Kingdom shows two genetically distinct clusters. J Clin Microbiol 42: 4556–4565.

45. Pinho L, Thompson G, Rosenbusch R, Carvalheira J (2012) Genotyping of *Mycoplasma bovis* isolates using multiple-locus variable-number tandem-repeat analysis. J Microbiol Methods 88: 377–385.

46. Aebi M, Bodmer M, Frey J, Pilo P (2012) Herd-specific strains of *Mycoplasma bovis* in outbreaks of mycoplasmal mastitis and pneumonia. Vet Microbiol 157: 363–368.

47. Castillo-Alcala F, Bateman KG, Cai HY, Schott CR, Parker L, et al. (2012) Prevalence and genotype of *Mycoplasma bovis* in beef cattle after arrival at a feedlot. Am J Vet Res 73: 1932–1943.

48. Spergser J, Macher K, Kargl M, Lysnyansky I, Rosengarten R (2013) Emergence, re-emergence, spread and host species crossing of *Mycoplasma bovis* in the Austrian Alps caused by a single endemic strain. Vet Microbiol 164: 299–306.

49. Le Carrou J, Laurentie M, Kobisch M, Gautier-Bouchardon AV (2006) Persistence of *Mycoplasma hyopneumoniae* in experimentally infected pigs after marbofloxacin treatment and detection of mutations in the *parC* gene. Antimicrob Agents Chemother 50: 1959–1966.

50. Le Carrou J, Reinhardt AK, Kempf I, Gautier-Bouchardon AV (2006) Persistence of *Mycoplasma synoviae* in hens after two enrofloxacin treatments and detection of mutations in the *parC* gene. Vet Res 37: 145–154.

51. Rocha E, Sirand-Pugnet P, Blanchard A (2005) Genome analysis: recombination, repair. In: Blanchard A, Browning G, editors. Mycoplasmas: Molecular Biology Pathogenicity and Strategies for Control. Poole, UK: Horizon Bioscience. 31–73.

52. Sirand-Pugnet P, Lartigue C, Marenda M, Jacob D, Barre A, et al. (2007) Being pathogenic, plastic, and sexual while living with a nearly minimal bacterial genome. PLoS Genet 3: e75.

53. Dordet Frisoni E, Marenda MS, Sagne E, Nouvel LX, Blanchard A, et al. (2013) ICEA of *Mycoplasma agalactiae*: a new family of self-transmissible integrative elements that confers conjugative properties to the recipient strain. Mol Microbiol 89: 1226–1239.

54. Bébéar C (2012) Infections due to macrolide-resistant *Mycoplasma pneumoniae*: now what? Clin Infect Dis 55: 1650–1651.

55. Madec J-Y, Jouy E, Haenni M, Gay E (2012) Le réseau Résapath de surveillance de l'antibiorésistance des bactéries pathogènes chez les animaux: évolution du réseau et des résistances depuis dix ans. Bull Epid Santé Anim Alim 53: 16–19.

56. Stipkovits L, Ripley PH, Tenk M, Glavits R, Molnar T, et al. (2005) The efficacy of valnemulin (Econor) in the control of disease caused by experimental infection of calves with *Mycoplasma bovis*. Res Vet Sci 78: 207–215.

57. Lechtenberg KF, Tessman RK, Chester ST (2011) Efficacy of gamithromycin injectable solution for the treatment of *Mycoplasma bovis* induced pneumonia in cattle. Intern J Appl Res Vet Med 9: 233–240.

58. Poumarat F, Le Grand D, Philippe S, Calavas D, Schelcher F, et al. (2001) Efficacy of spectinomycin against *Mycoplasma bovis* induced pneumonia in conventionally reared calves. Vet Microbiol 80: 23–35.

59. McAuliffe L, Ellis RJ, Miles K, Ayling RD, Nicholas RA (2006) Biofilm formation by mycoplasma species and its role in environmental persistence and survival. Microbiology 152: 913–922.

60. Paterna A, Sanchez A, Gomez-Martin A, Corrales JC, De la Fe C, et al. (2013) In vitro antimicrobial susceptibility of *Mycoplasma agalactiae* strains isolated from dairy goats. J Dairy Sci 96: 1–4.

13

A Blueberry-Enriched Diet Attenuates Nephropathy in a Rat Model of Hypertension via Reduction in Oxidative Stress

Carrie M. Elks[1,4], Scott D. Reed[2], Nithya Mariappan[1], Barbara Shukitt-Hale[3], James A. Joseph[3], Donald K. Ingram[4]*, Joseph Francis[1]*

1 Comparative Biomedical Sciences, Louisiana State University School of Veterinary Medicine, Baton Rouge, Louisiana, United States of America, 2 Neurosignaling Laboratory, Pennington Biomedical Research Center, Louisiana State University System, Baton Rouge, Louisiana, United States of America, 3 United States Department of Agriculture-Agriculture Research Services, Human Nutrition Research Center on Aging, Tufts University, Boston, Massachusetts, United States of America, 4 Nutritional Neuroscience and Aging Laboratory, Pennington Biomedical Research Center, Louisiana State University System, Baton Rouge, Louisiana, United States of America

Abstract

Objective and Background: To assess renoprotective effects of a blueberry-enriched diet in a rat model of hypertension. Oxidative stress (OS) appears to be involved in the development of hypertension and related renal injury. Pharmacological antioxidants can attenuate hypertension and hypertension-induced renal injury; however, attention has shifted recently to the therapeutic potential of natural products as antioxidants. Blueberries (BB) have among the highest antioxidant capacities of fruits and vegetables.

Methods and Results: Male spontaneously hypertensive rats received a BB-enriched diet (2% w/w) or an isocaloric control diet for 6 or 12 weeks or 2 days. Compared to controls, rats fed BB-enriched diet for 6 or 12 weeks exhibited lower blood pressure, improved glomerular filtration rate, and decreased renovascular resistance. As measured by electron paramagnetic resonance spectroscopy, significant decreases in total reactive oxygen species (ROS), peroxynitrite, and superoxide production rates were observed in kidney tissues in rats on long-term dietary treatment, consistent with reduced pathology and improved function. Additionally, measures of antioxidant status improved; specifically, renal glutathione and catalase activities increased markedly. Contrasted to these observations indicating reduced OS in the BB group after long-term feeding, similar measurements made in rats fed the same diet for only 2 days yielded evidence of increased OS; specifically, significant increases in total ROS, peroxynitrite, and superoxide production rates in all tissues (kidney, brain, and liver) assayed in BB-fed rats. These results were evidence of "hormesis" during brief exposure, which dissipated with time as indicated by enhanced levels of catalase in heart and liver of BB group.

Conclusion: Long-term feeding of BB-enriched diet lowered blood pressure, preserved renal hemodynamics, and improved redox status in kidneys of hypertensive rats and concomitantly demonstrated the potential to delay or attenuate development of hypertension-induced renal injury, and these effects appear to be mediated by a short-term hormetic response.

Editor: Carmine Zoccali, L' Istituto di Biomedicina ed Immunologia Molecolare-Consiglio Nazionale delle Ricerche, Italy

Funding: This work is funded by the National Institutes of Health Grant 2 P50AT002776 from the National Center for Complementary and Alternative Medicine (NCCAM) and by the Office of Dietary Supplements (ODS) pilot grant and National Heart, Lung, and Blood Institute grant HL-80544-05 to Dr. Joseph Francis. The funders had no role in study design, data collection and analysis, decision to publish, or preparation of the manuscript.

Competing Interests: The authors have declared that no competing interests exist.

* E-mail: jfrancis@lsu.edu (JF); donald.ingram@pbrc.edu (DKI)

Introduction

Oxidative stress produced by overproduction of reactive oxygen species/reactive nitrogen species (RONS) or inefficient antioxidant defenses appears to be involved in the development and progression of hypertension and hypertension-induced renal injury [1,2]. The detrimental role of RONS in hypertension-induced renal injury has fostered an increased interest in the therapeutic potential of antioxidants; however, the majority of studies thus far have employed synthetic antioxidants to prevent or attenuate the detrimental effects of ROS both *in vivo* and *in vitro*. Recently, attention has been directed to natural products as sources of antioxidants [3]. Most plant cells contain antioxidant mechanisms to detoxify free radicals, which are produced during normal cellular metabolic processes [4]. In particular, small berry fruits have been demonstrated to have high contents of several antioxidant compounds, including anthocyanins and phenolics. These metabolites function to protect plants against photodynamic reactions by quenching ROS, and have been suggested to have protective effects against several human diseases [5,6].

Blueberries (BB; *Vaccinium spp.*) have among the highest antioxidant capacities of fruits and vegetables tested to date, and contain polyphenols such as anthocyanins, proanthocyanidins, and phenolic acids, and flavanols [7]. BB-enriched diets and BB extracts have been shown to attenuate and even improve age-related behavioral and neuronal deficits in rodents [8–11]. BB supplementation can also attenuate proinflammatory cytokine production in rat glial cells [12] and protect the rat heart from ischemia [13]. Additionally, hypertensive rats on BB-supplemented diets exhibit significantly lower systolic and mean arterial pressures and renal nitrite content [14]. Therefore, it is plausible to suggest that dietary BB supplementation may have a tissue-protective effect in various pathologic conditions. In this light, the general objective of the current study was to assess the chronic effects of a BB-enriched diet on blood pressure (BP) and renal hemodynamics in a rat model of hypertension-induced renal injury. The hypothesis was that the dietary BB supplementation would reduce oxidative stress and thus attenuate renal damage. As an extension of this hypothesis, rats were also subjected to a short-term (2-day) exposure of the BB-supplemented diet to determine whether a hormetic effect would be observed. Hormesis has been proposed as the mechanism mediating the protective effects of many plant products [15,16]. Specifically, the hypothesis was that during short-term exposure, increased RONS production would be observed which would lead to up-regulation of antioxidant defense mechanisms to enhance long-term protection.

Materials and Methods

Ethics Statement

All experimental procedures were in compliance with all applicable principles set forth in the National Institutes of Health Guide for the Care and Use of Laboratory Animals (Publication No.. 85-23, revised 1996). This study was approved by the Institutional Animal Care and Use Committee of the Louisiana State University School of Veterinary Medicine (protocol approval number 09-008).

Experimental Design

Experiment 1: Chronic feeding studies. Forty-eight male stroke-prone spontaneously hypertensive rats (SHRSP) and thirty-two male normotensive Wistar-Kyoto (WKY) rats were used for chronic feeding studies. Rats were 7 weeks old with baseline body weights between 130 and 150 grams. Rats were randomly divided into four diet groups for each chronic study: WKY control (WC), WKY blueberry (WBB), SHRSP control (SC), or SHRSP BB (SBB). Animals were fed control or BB-enriched diets for 6 weeks or 12 weeks. All animals in all groups were provided 1% sodium chloride in tap water for the duration of both chronic studies. All animals were subjected to acute determination of glomerular filtration rate and renal plasma flow, as previously described [17], at the end of the 6-week or 12-week feeding periods. Rats were euthanized, kidneys were excised, and cortex and medulla separated for analyses. Kidneys were formalin-fixed, paraffin-embedded, and then sectioned (3 um); sections were placed on slides and stained with Masson's Trichrome for evaluation by a veterinary pathologist who was blinded to experimental conditions.

Experiment 2: Short-term feeding studies in SHRSP rats. For short-term feeding studies to evaluate hormetic effects, 24 additional 7-week-old male SHRSP were used. Rats (n = 12 in each group) were fed control or BB-enriched diets for 2 days. Rats were euthanized after which heart, brain, kidney, and liver tissues were collected. In both 2-day and chronic studies, fresh tissues were used for electron paramagnetic resonance (EPR) spectroscopy studies, and frozen tissues were used for antioxidant studies.

Diets

Diets were prepared by Harlan Teklad (Madison, WI) using a reformulated NIH-31 diet by adding 20 g/kg lyophilized BB or 20 g/kg dried corn. To prepare the 2% BB diet, the berries were homogenized in water, centrifuged, lyophilized and added to the NIH-31 rodent chow. The amount of corn in the control diet was adjusted to compensate for the added volume of BB, in order to make the two diets isocaloric [18]. Food consumption was measured weekly for the chronic feeding studies by weighing feed before placing it in each cage, and subtracting the weight of remaining feed at the end of each week. Rats maintained on BB diets for 6 weeks consumed an average of 371 mg/day (WBB) or 374 mg/day (SBB) of lyophilized blueberries, roughly equivalent to 4.1 g/day or 4.2 g/day, respectively, of fresh blueberries. Rats maintained on BB diets for 12 weeks consumed an average of 397 mg/day (WBB) or 399 mg/day (SBB) of lyophilized blueberries, roughly equivalent to 4.4 g/day or 4.5 g/day, respectively, of fresh blueberries.

Blood pressure measurements

In rats from all chronic feeding groups, tail blood pressures (BP) were measured noninvasively using a Coda 6 Volume-Pressure Recording System (Kent Scientific, Torrington, CT), as previously described [1,19]. Briefly, eight unanesthetized rats from each group were warmed to an ambient temperature of 30°C by placing them in a holding device mounted on a thermostatically controlled warming plate. Tail cuffs were placed on animals, and animals were allowed to acclimate to cuffs for 10 minutes prior to each pressure recording session. All animals were habituated to the blood pressure system and to the holders daily for one week prior to the initiation of experimental measurements. All measurements were taken within the same 2-hour time window each day. Each session consisted of 30 cycles. BP was measured on five consecutive days each week, and values were averaged from at least six consecutive cycles. BP was measured at baseline (7 weeks of age) and then weekly until the end of either chronic study period.

Acute renal clearance experiments

Nine rats from each 6-week feeding group and nine rats from each 12-week feeding group were subjected to renal clearance experiments at the end of their respective feeding periods as previously described [1]. Briefly, each rat was anesthetized with Inactin (thiobutabarbital; 100 mg/kg), the right inguinal area was shaved, a small (<2 cm) incision made, and femoral vessels isolated. The right femoral artery was cannulated with heparin-primed (100 U/ml) PE-50 polyethylene tubing connected to a pressure transducer (PowerLab data acquisition system; ADInstruments, Colorado Springs, CO) for continuous measurement of arterial pressure. The right femoral vein was catheterized with heparin-primed PE-50 tubing for infusion of solutions at 20 μl/min. An isotonic saline solution containing 6% albumin was infused during surgery. After surgery, the infusion fluid was changed to isotonic saline containing 2% bovine serum albumin (BSA), 7.5% inulin (Inutest), and 1.5% PAH, and a 300 ul bolus of this solution was administered at the start of each clearance experiment. The bladder was exposed via a suprapubic incision and catheterized with a PE-200 tube (with one end flanged) for gravimetric urine collection. After a 15- to 20-minute stabilization period, a 30-minute clearance period was conducted to assess values of renal hemodynamic parameters. An arterial blood sample was collected at the end of the 30-minute clearance collection period for measurement of plasma inulin and PAH concentrations. Plasma inulin and PAH concentrations were measured colorimetrically to determine glomerular filtration rate (GFR) and renal plasma flow (RPF), respectively.

Electron paramagnetic resonance (EPR) spectroscopy

Total ROS, superoxide, and peroxynitrite production rates were measured in pieces of kidney cortex or medulla (chronic and 2-day feeding studies) and in liver and cerebral cortex (2-day feeding study) via EPR spectroscopy as previously described [1,19–24]. In this EPR protocol, 'total ROS' represents all reactive oxygen species; however, the major sources trapped by the spin trap used are superoxide, hydrogen peroxide, and hydroxyl radical, with other species as minimal contributors. Briefly, tissue pieces were incubated at 37°C with 6.6 µl of CMH (200 µM) for 30 minutes for ROS measurement; 1.5 µl of PEG-SOD (50 U/µl) for 30 minutes, then CMH for an additional 30 minutes for superoxide measurement; or 30 µl of CPH (500 µM) for 30 minutes for peroxynitrite measurement. Aliquots of incubated probe media were then taken in 50 µl disposable glass capillary tubes (Noxygen Science Transfer and Diagnostics, Elzach, Germany) for determination of total ROS, superoxide, or peroxynitrite production, under previously established EPR settings.

Measurement of renal catalase and glutathione levels

Catalase activity and total glutathione (GSH) levels were measured in kidney cortex and medulla (chronic and 2-day feeding studies) and also in liver and left ventricle (2-day feeding study) using commercially available kits (Cayman Chemical, Ann Arbor, MI) according to manufacturer's instructions, as previously described [1,25].

Measurement of urine creatinine levels

Creatinine was quantified in urine with a QuantiChrom Creatinine kit (BioAssay Systems, Hayward, CA) according to manufacturer's instructions, as previously described [17].

Measurement of urine and tissue nitrate/nitrite levels

Total nitrate/nitrite levels in kidney cortex and medullary tissues and in urine were quantified with a Nitrate/Nitrite Colorimetric Assay kit (Cayman Chemical, Ann Arbor, MI), according to manufacturer's instructions.

Statistical analyses

A two-way ANOVA (strain x diet) was used to analyze blood pressure, food consumption, body weight, physiological, biochemical, and EPR data at each time-point. Where significant main effects or interactions were found, individual planned comparisons were made using Student's t-tests for all other chronic feeding study data specifically to compare WC and WBB animals; WC and SC animals; and SC and SBB animals. T-tests were also used to compare results from SHR C and SHR BB groups for the 2-day feeding study. In all cases, p≤0.05 was accepted as the level of statistical significance.

Results

A. Chronic feeding studies

Body weight and food intake. Consistent with past studies using similar dietary formulations [8,13,14,26], weekly food consumption and body weight gain did not differ among any of the diet groups in the chronic feeding studies. Mean starting body weights in the WKY and SHR animals at baseline before assignment to groups were 138±3 g and 142±2 g, respectively; at the end of the 6 week study, the mean body weights were as

follows: WC = 252±9 g; WBB = 246±3 g; SC = 250±3 g; and SBB = 252±3 g. At the end of the 12 week study, mean body weights were as follows: WC = 346±4 g; WBB = 342±5 g; SC = 334±6 g; and SBB = 333±8 g.

Effect of chronic BB feeding on blood pressures and renal hemodynamic parameters. Figure 1 presents the BP trends for each group of rats in both the 6-week and 12-week studies. Compared to SC rats, the mean arterial and systolic pressures of the SBB rats were significantly lower by the second week of the 6-week and 12-week studies, and remained significantly lower for the remainders of both chronic studies.

Table 1 presents the renoprotective effects of BB diet in SHRSP rats fed for 6 weeks or 12 weeks. Glomerular filtration rate and renal blood flow were higher, and renal vascular resistance was lower, in 6-week and 12-week SBB rats when compared to SC rats. There were no significant differences in renal hemodynamic or BP measures between WC or WBB animals.

Effect of chronic BB feeding on cortical and medullary free radical production rates. The decreases in total ROS, superoxide, and peroxynitrite seen with chronic BB feeding for 6 or 12 weeks appear in Table 2. For both 6- and 12-week studies, SBB rats exhibited significantly lower free radical production rates than SC rats.

Effect of chronic BB feeding on catalase and glutathione activities. The increases in cortical and medullary catalase and glutathione activities noted with chronic BB-enriched diet feedings appear in Figures 2 and 3, respectively. For both chronic feeding studies, SBB rats exhibited significantly higher catalase and glutathione activities than SC rats. There were no differences in antioxidant activities between WC and WBB rats at the conclusion of the 6- or 12-week studies.

Effect of chronic BB feeding on renal pathology. Representative photomicrographs of kidneys from each 6-week and 12-week rat group appear in Figures 4 and 5, respectively. The kidneys of WC and WBB rats fed for 6 weeks exhibited similar appearances histologically. Kidneys of WC and WBB rats exhibited mild to moderate periarterial fibrosis, occasional tubular degeneration and dilation, mild glomerular parietal metaplasia, and minimal arterial hyperplasia. The kidneys of SBB rats fed for 6 weeks had relatively little renal pathologic change, with mild glomerular parietal metaplasia, occasional tubular degeneration and dilation and minimal periarterial fibrosis. The kidneys of SC rats, however, fed for 6 weeks had greater incidences of glomerular parietal metaplasia, tubular degeneration and dilation, and periarterial, interstitial, and periglomerular fibrosis, along with moderate to marked arterial myointimal hyperplasia.

In the kidneys of rats fed for 12 weeks, the amount of interstitial, periarterial, and periglomerular fibrosis was greater in all four groups than at six weeks. The SC rat kidneys had severe arterial changes which often were attended by evidence of renal hypoxia (tubular degeneration and necrosis). Arteries were frequently thrombosed and often had evidence of recanalization. The 12 week SC rat kidneys also had the most severe fibrosis, arterial myointimal hyperplasia, tubular degeneration and necrosis, and evidence of hemoglobin and proteinaceous casts. Though much less severe, the SBB rat kidneys did exhibit arterial myointimal hyperplasia with occasional mononuclear inflammatory cells present in the interstitium surrounding arteries. Kidneys of WC and WBB rats fed for 12 weeks exhibited much less severe changes, but showed the same trends.

B. Short-term feeding studies in SHRSP rats

Body weights. No significant differences were found in body weights between control- or BB-diet fed SHRSP rats in the 2-day

A. 6 week feeding

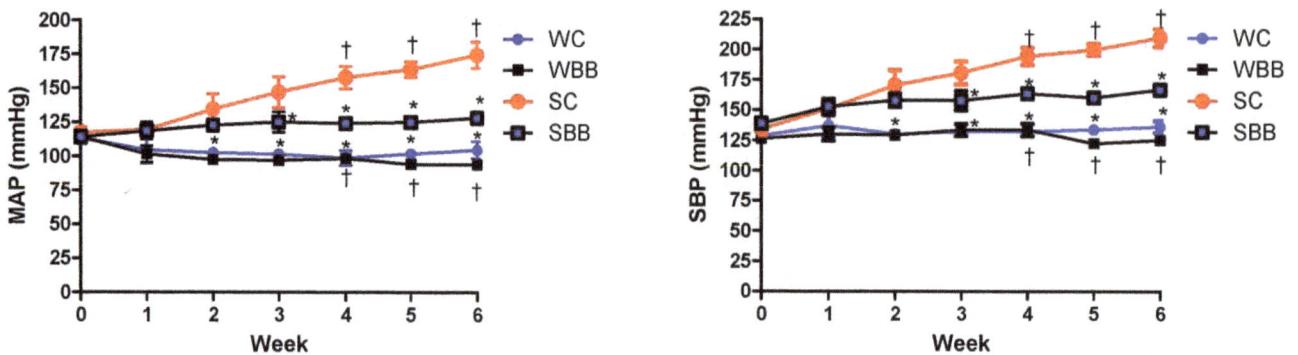

B. 12 week feeding

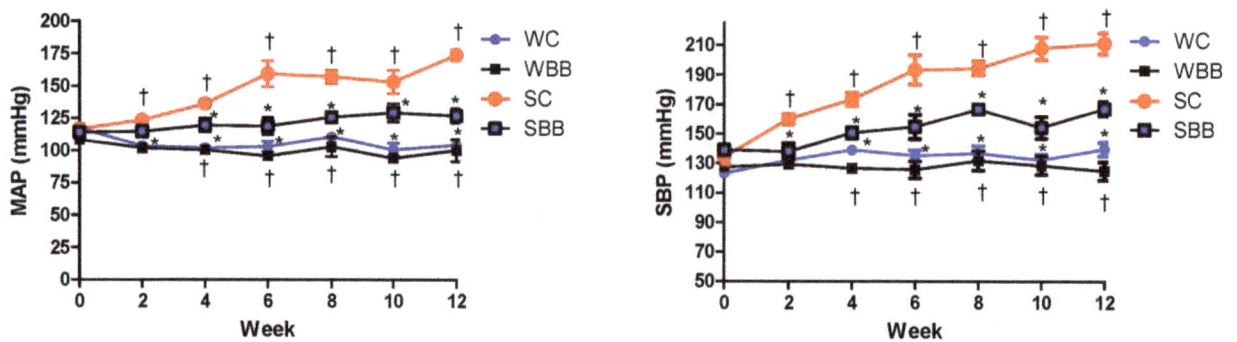

Figure 1. Blueberry-enriched diet delays the progression of hypertension. Mean arterial and systolic blood pressures were assessed in rats fed a control diet or a blueberry-enriched diet for 6 weeks (A) or 12 weeks (B). * p<0.05 vs. SC; † p<0.05 vs. SBB.

Table 1. Renal hemodynamic indices in control- or blueberry-fed rats after 6 weeks or 12 weeks of feeding.

		WC (n = 9)	WBB (n = 9)	SC (n = 9)	SBB (n = 9)
6 WEEKS	**GFR** (ml/min/g KW)	0.95±0.05$^#$	0.92±0.05	0.59±0.04$^{*\$}$	0.97±0.07$^#$
	RBF (ml/min/g KW)	7.98±0.25$^#$	8.42±0.32	5.96±0.35$^{*\$}$	7.71±0.17$^#$
	RVR (mmHg/ml/min/g KW)	13.33±0.70$^#$	14.28±1.24	28.04±1.39$^{*\$}$	13.34±0.63$^#$
	Urine Cr (mg/dl)	161.2±7.7$^#$	142.3±12.9	70.1±4.8$^{*\$}$	121.5±8.2$^#$
	FE$_{Na}$ (%)	0.28±0.02$^#$	0.32±0.03	0.59±0.04$^{*\$}$	0.38±0.04$^#$
	KW/BW (mg/g)	3.68±0.04$^#$	3.70±0.04	4.73±0.05*	4.72±0.06
12 WEEKS	**GFR**	0.90±0.06$^#$	1.11±0.09	0.53±0.04$^{*\$}$	1.02±0.07$^#$
	RBF	7.03±0.25$^#$	8.42±0.75	3.62±0.22$^{*\$}$	6.80±0.59$^#$
	RVR	15.98±1.14$^#$	14.05±1.41	36.71±2.10$^{*\$}$	15.49±1.22$^#$
	Urine Cr	119.0±9.0$^#$	119.8±12.3	66.6±4.2$^{*\$}$	129.1±12.2$^#$
	FE$_{Na}$	0.36±0.02$^#$	0.34±0.03	0.67±0.03$^{*\$}$	0.46±0.04$^#$
	KW/BW	3.13±0.05$^#$	3.14±0.06	4.98±0.15$^{*\$}$	4.48±0.05$^#$

Abbreviations used: WC = WKY corn-fed, WBB = WKY blueberry-fed, SC = SHRSP corn fed, SBB = SHRSP blueberry-fed, GFR = glomerular filtration rate, RBF = renal blood flow, RVR = renal vascular resistance, KW = kidney weight, Cr = creatinine, FE$_{Na}$ = fractional excretion of sodium.
*p≤0.05 vs. WC;
$^#$p≤0.05 vs. SC;
$^\$$p≤0.05 vs. SBB.

Table 2. Total ROS, superoxide, and peroxynitrite production rates as measured by EPR in tissues of control- or blueberry-fed rats after 6 or 12 weeks of feeding.

	WC (n = 8-10)	WBB (n = 8-10)	SC (n = 8-10)	SBB (n = 8-10)
	KIDNEY CORTEX			
Total ROS (uM/mg protein/minute)				
6 weeks	0.067±0.012[#]	0.099±0.005[$]	0.199±0.027[*$]	0.069±0.011[#]
12 weeks	0.115±0.013[#]	0.112±0.009[$]	0.429±0.038[*$]	0.195±0.026[#]
Superoxide (uM/mg protein/minute)				
6 weeks	0.040±0.014[#]	0.028±0.006	0.136±0.026[*$]	0.030±0.007[#]
12 weeks	0.067±0.018[#]	0.063±0.013	0.165±0.013[*$]	0.063±0.006[#]
Peroxynitrite (uM/mg protein/minute)				
6 weeks	0.017±0.002[#]	0.022±0.003[$]	0.053±0.011[*$]	0.011±0.003[#]
12 weeks	0.020±0.006[#]	0.028±0.004	0.111±0.021[*$]	0.028±0.020[#]
	KIDNEY MEDULLA			
Total ROS				
6 weeks	0.057±0.011[#]	0.087±0.007[$]	0.188±0.025[*$]	0.118±0.010[#]
12 weeks	0.157±0.014[#]	0.151±0.018	0.314±0.017[*$]	0.170±0.017[#]
Superoxide				
6 weeks	0.056±0.011[#]	0.051±0.013	0.122±0.009[*$]	0.048±0.011[#]
12 weeks	0.079±0.012[#]	0.085±0.008	0.194±0.017[*$]	0.089±0.019[#]
Peroxynitrite				
6 weeks	0.027±0.006[#]	0.021±0.005	0.050±0.005[*$]	0.025±0.005[#]
12 weeks	0.052±0.017[#]	0.065±0.005[$]	0.128±0.009[*$]	0.089±0.019[#]

Abbreviations used: WC = WKY corn-fed, WBB = WKY blueberry-fed, SC = SHRSP corn fed, SBB = SHRSP blueberry-fed, ROS = reactive oxygen species.
*$p \leq 0.05$ vs. WC;
[#]$p \leq 0.05$ vs. SC;
[$]$p \leq 0.05$ vs. SBB.

feeding study. Ending body weights were 161 ± 5 g for rats fed the control diet and 163 ± 5 g for rats fed the BB diet.

Effect of short-term BB feeding on cortical and medullary free radical production rates. As noted in Table 3, significant increases in production rates of total ROS, superoxide, and peroxynitrite were observed in cerebral cortex, liver, kidney cortex, and kidney medulla of SHRSP rats fed a BB diet for 2 days compared to those on control diet.

Effect of short-term BB feeding on catalase and glutathione levels. Table 4 depicts the catalase and glutathione levels recorded in heart, liver, and kidney tissues of 2-day BB-fed SHRSP when compared to control diet-fed SHRSP. In the left ventricle and kidney cortex of SHRSP fed BB-diet for 2 days, catalase levels were increased when compared to those of SHRSP fed a control diet for 2 days. However, total GSH levels were lower in the left ventricle of 2 day BB-fed rats when compared to 2-day control diet-fed rats, with no significant changes in GSH levels noted in other tissues assayed.

Discussion

Primary (essential) hypertension remains a major cause of morbidity and mortality in Western society, and continues to be a leading cause of heart and kidney diseases [27]. The cause(s) of primary hypertension remain elusive; however, oxidative stress and proinflammatory cytokine production are known contributors [28,29]. Nephropathy resulting from hypertension is the second leading cause of end-stage renal disease in the United States [27]; therefore, the most effective way to avoid the development of

hypertensive nephropathy is to prevent hypertension or to delay its progression. In many cases, hypertension can be attenuated with pharmacological treatments including, but not limited to: diuretics, beta receptor antagonists, angiotensin converting enzyme antagonists, and angiotensin II receptor antagonists; however, these commonly used anti-hypertensives can also have undesirable side effects. Therefore, it is valuable to consider natural products, such as foods, as potentially therapeutic sources of antioxidants for a variety of conditions.

Thus far, a variety of pharmacotherapies have proven successful in decreasing renal damage in hypertensive animals; however, the possible benefits of dietary interventions have only recently come into focus. BB-enriched diets have been shown to decrease renal nitrite content, protect the myocardium from ischemia, and correct neurological deficits in rats [8,10-14]. In the present study, we show for the first time that regular dietary supplementation with blueberries in SHRSP rats preserves renal hemodynamics and prevents oxidative stress in the kidney. We also demonstrate that BB may act via a hormetic mechanism in preventing long-term oxidative stress in the SHRSP rat.

After 6 weeks and 12 weeks of BB feeding, GFR and RBF measures were higher, estimated RVR was lower, renal free radical production was attenuated, and renal catalase and glutathione levels were preserved in BB-fed SHRSP when compared to those of SHRSP maintained on a control diet. The results of our chronic feeding experiments also demonstrate that total ROS, superoxide, and peroxynitrite production rates were significantly lower and antioxidant activities were significantly higher in BB-fed SHRSP than in corn-fed SHRSP. These results

A. 6 week feeding

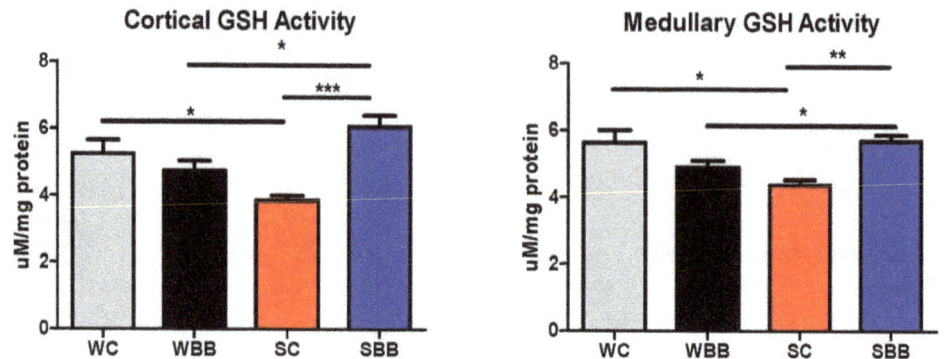

B. 12 week feeding

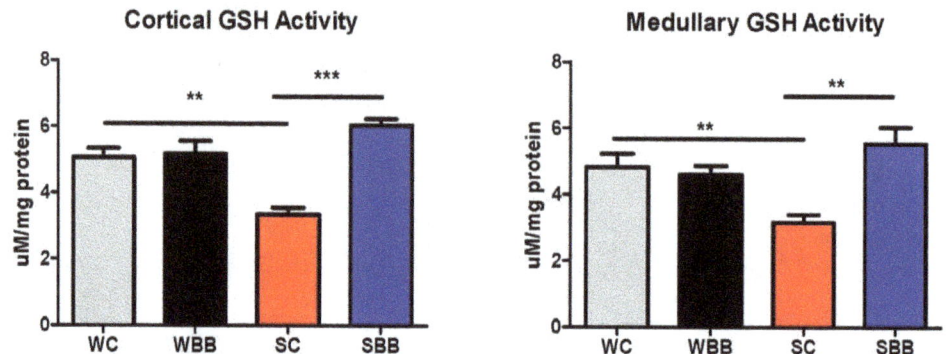

Figure 2. Blueberry-enriched diet improves glutathione activity in hypertensive rats. Glutathione activities were assessed in renal cortical and medullary tissues of rats fed a control diet or a blueberry-enriched diet for 6 weeks (A) or 12 weeks (B). $^*p<0.05$; $^{**}p<0.01$; $^{***}p<0.001$.

clearly demonstrate a protective antioxidant effect of BB feeding. The imbalance between superoxide production and NO production in the kidney is a primary contributor to renal oxidative stress and salt-sensitive hypertension [30,31]. Oxidative stress is further enhanced in the kidneys of SHRSP that are salt-loaded (as were the SHRSP in this study) [31,32]. We demonstrate here that the BB diet protected against oxidative renal damage by attenuating free radical production and preserving catalase and glutathione levels, and thereby improving BP and renal hemodynamics.

A possible mechanism for this renoprotection may be the scavenging of superoxide in kidney tissues, which has been shown to lower BP in various models of hypertension [31,33]. BB are known scavengers of RONS, including superoxide, *in vitro* [34]. In further support of a renal superoxide scavenging mechanism, we found that the cortical and medullary production rates of peroxynitrite in BB-fed rats from both 6- and 12-week time-points were significantly lower compared to rats fed the control diet, as were urinary nitrate/nitrite and tissue nitrate/nitrite levels (Table 5). Further study is needed to determine conclusively whether this effect is responsible for the renoprotection afforded by chronic BB feeding. These chronic feeding studies were not intended to analyze specific signaling pathways responsible for preservation of renal hemodynamics and/or reduction of oxidative stress in the kidneys of hypertensive animals on a BB-enriched diet, but rather as a proof of concept. One assertion that can be made on the basis of these findings is that alterations in signaling were likely associated with decreases in RONS production and improvements in RONS scavenging.

Our results from the 2-day feeding study indicate that a hormetic effect of BB may indeed exist in the prevention of hypertension-induced renal hemodynamic alterations. The 'xeno-hormesis' hypothesis proposes that animal species have evolved the ability to use chemical cues from plant species to mount a preemptive defense response that increases its chances of survival [16,35]. Polyphenols, among other phytochemicals, are thought to exert many of their beneficial effects via hormetic mechanisms [35]. In contrast to the clear evidence of reduced RONS production in the long-term studies, results from the 2-day feeding study indicated significant increases in total ROS, superoxide, and peroxynitrite production in kidney, brain, and liver tissues of BB-fed rats when compared to corn-fed rats. As a response to this situation, increased catalase activities were found with 2-day BB feeding, but only in kidney cortex and left ventricular tissues. Overall, the EPR and antioxidant assay results suggest that, in the case of BB feeding, an initial oxidative stimulus is produced, which is presumably required for the antioxidant defense to be activated, thereby supporting the assertion that a hormetic effect is involved in the protection afforded by BB *in vivo*. Since we evaluated hormetic responses only at the 2-day time-point of BB exposure, further analysis is required to document in detail the kinetics of ROS production and antioxidant responses.

In summary, our experiments examining rats chronically maintained on a BB-enriched diet for 6 or 12 weeks found preservation of renal hemodynamics and decreased blood pressure. Further, the BB diet decreased RONS production and preserved the status of some endogenous antioxidant systems in

A. 6 week feeding

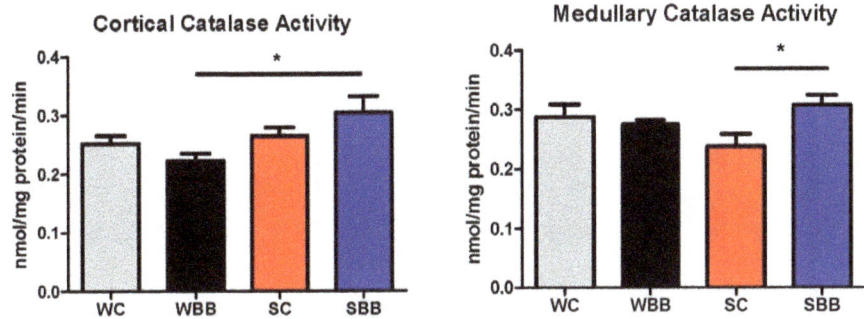

Cortical Catalase Activity

*

WC   WBB   SC   SBB

Medullary Catalase Activity

*

WC   WBB   SC   SBB

B. 12 week feeding

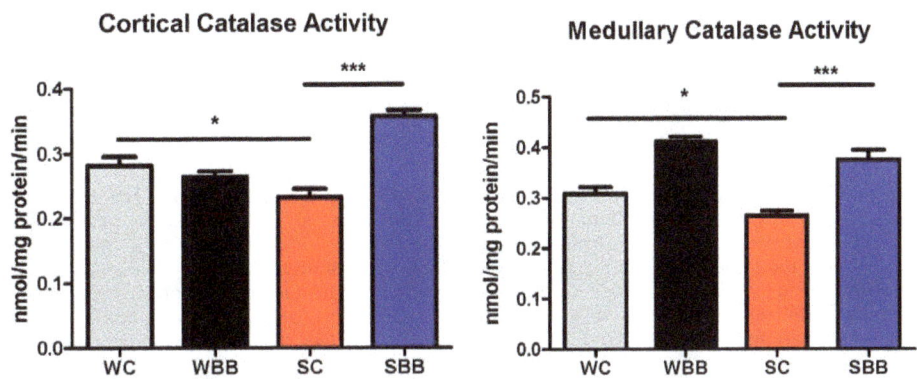

Cortical Catalase Activity

*   ***

WC   WBB   SC   SBB

Medullary Catalase Activity

*   ***

WC   WBB   SC   SBB

Figure 3. Blueberry-enriched diet improves catalase activity in hypertensive rats. Catalase activities were assessed in renal cortical and medullary tissues of rats fed a control diet or a blueberry-enriched diet for 6 weeks (A) or 12 weeks (B). $^{*}p<0.05$; $^{**}p<0.01$; $^{***}p<0.001$.

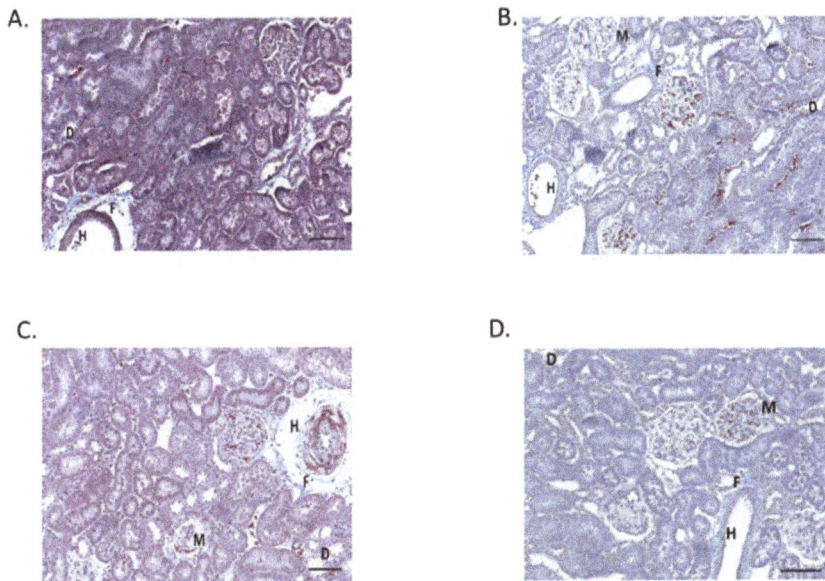

Figure 4. Blueberry-enriched diet improves renal pathology in hypertensive rats fed for 6 weeks. Trichrome-stained kidney sections were evaluated by a veterinary pathologist who was blinded to experimental conditions. Kidneys from (A) WC and (B) WBB rats exhibited similar histological appearance, with mild pathologic changes. Kidneys from (C) SC rats exhibited greater incidence and severity of pathologic change, while kidneys from (D) SBB rats exhibited very little pathologic change. Scale bar = 200 um. F = fibrosis, H = vascular smooth muscle hypertrophy, D = tubular degeneration and ectasia, and M = glomerular parietal metaplasia.

A.

B.

C.

D.

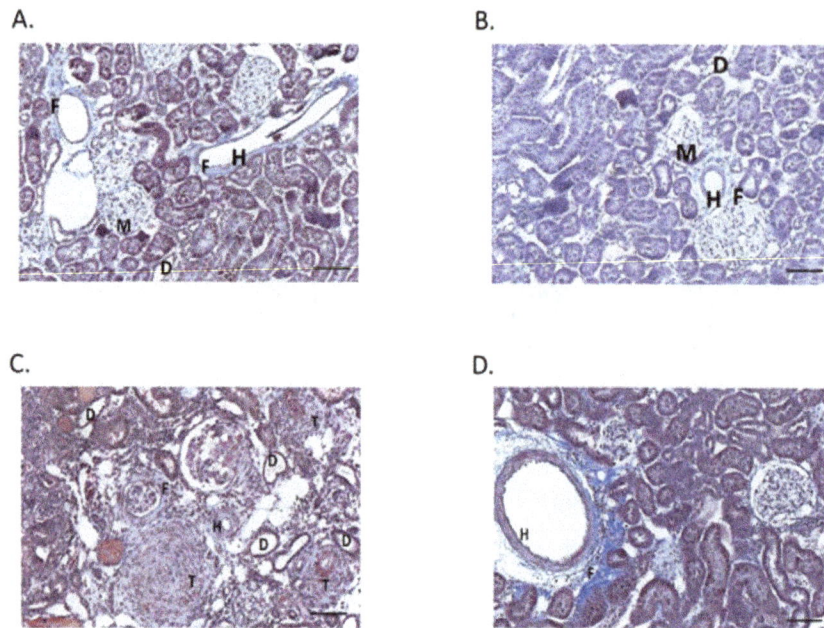

Figure 5. Blueberry-enriched diet improves renal pathology in hypertensive rats fed for 12 weeks. Trichrome-stained kidney sections were evaluated by a veterinary pathologist who was blinded to experimental conditions. In all four 12-week groups, the amount of interstitial, periarterial, and periglomerular fibrosis was greater than at six weeks. The SC rat kidneys (C) had severe arterial changes, with evidence of hypoxia. Kidneys from the SC rats also had the most severe fibrosis, arterial myointimal hyperplasia, tubular degeneration and necrosis, and evidence of hemoglobin and proteinaceous casts. The SBB rat kidneys (D) did exhibit arterial myointimal hyperplasia, though it was much less severe. Kidneys of WC (A) and WBB (B) rats fed for 12 weeks exhibited much less severe changes, but showed the same trends. Scale bar = 200 um. F = fibrosis, H = vascular smooth muscle hypertrophy, T = organizing thrombus, D = tubular degeneration and ectasia, and M = glomerular parietal metaplasia.

the kidney cortex and medulla of chronically fed hypertensive rats. The beneficial effects of the BB diet may be due to a hormetic effect, as evidenced by our results from the 2-day feeding

experiment, where RONS production was increased in all tissues of BB-fed animals, while responses of the catalase and glutathione systems were in a state of flux, with some systems elevated at that time-point and others unresponsive. While the current results indicate major therapeutic benefits of the BB diet on renal function and pathology, it should be acknowledged that the effects reported pertain to prevention of the pathogenesis rather than treatment of

Table 3. Total ROS, superoxide, and peroxynitrite production rates as measured by EPR in tissues of control- or blueberry-fed rats after 2 days of feeding.

	Corn (n = 7)	Blueberry (n = 7)	P
CEREBRAL CORTEX			
Total ROS	0.126±0.008	0.156±0.015	0.0417
Superoxide	0.024±0.003	0.039±0.005	0.0087
Peroxynitrite	0.005±0.001	0.022±0.003	0.0004
LIVER			
Total ROS	0.371±0.026	0.530±0.057	0.0129
Superoxide	0.150±0.007	0.246±0.023	0.0046
Peroxynitrite	0.014±0.002	0.042±0.007	0.0069
KIDNEY CORTEX			
Total ROS	0.140±0.013	0.210±0.022	0.0289
Superoxide	0.041±0.005	0.063±0.004	0.0275
Peroxynitrite	0.015±0.002	0.034±0.004	0.0044
KIDNEY MEDULLA			
Total ROS	0.146±0.011	0.189±0.019	0.0136
Superoxide	0.060±0.011	0.106±0.025	0.0258
Peroxynitrite	0.035±0.006	0.075±0.011	0.0158

Abbreviations used: WC = WKY corn-fed, WBB = WKY blueberry-fed, SC = SHRSP corn fed, SBB = SHRSP blueberry-fed, ROS = reactive oxygen species.

Table 4. Catalase and total glutathione (GSH) levels as measured by colorimetric assays in tissues of control- or blueberry-fed rats after 2 days of feeding.

	Corn (n = 8-10)	Blueberry (n = 8-10)	P
LEFT VENTRICLE			
Catalase	0.293±0.019	0.373±0.022	0.0285
Total GSH	2.68±0.243	1.89±0.213	0.0495
LIVER			
Catalase	0.287±0.011	0.276±0.016	n.s.
Total GSH	1.91±0.159	1.85±0.065	n.s.
KIDNEY CORTEX			
Catalase	0.246±0.012	0.306±0.020	0.0331
Total GSH	2.11±0.187	2.23±0.091	n.s.
KIDNEY MEDULLA			
Catalase	0.325±0.010	0.310±0.028	n.s.
Total GSH	2.23±0.207	2.17±0.065	n.s.

Abbreviations used: WC = WKY corn-fed, WBB = WKY blueberry-fed, SC = SHRSP corn fed, SBB = SHRSP blueberry-fed, GSH = glutathione.

Table 5. Urine and tissue nitrate/nitrite levels as measured by colorimetric assay in control- or blueberry-fed rats after 6 or 12 weeks of feeding.

	WC (n = 6)	WBB (n = 6)	SC (n = 6)	SBB (n = 6)
Urinary NOx (umol/mg creatinine)				
6 weeks	1.16±0.18[#]	0.57±0.10	2.01±0.27[*$]	0.97±0.13[#]
12 weeks	1.08±0.15[#]	0.62±0.12	3.85±0.68[*$]	2.09±0.31[#]
Cortical NOx (umol/mg protein)				
6 weeks	1.18±0.08[#]	1.34±0.14	1.92±0.17[*]	1.80±0.11
12 weeks	1.40±0.09[#]	1.09±0.06	2.29±0.22[*$]	1.33±0.18[#]
Medullary NOx (umol/mg protein)				
6 weeks	1.57±0.21[#]	1.66±0.17	3.08±0.53[*$]	1.41±0.18[#]
12 weeks	1.82±0.28[#]	1.84±0.23	4.78±0.46[*$]	1.97±0.20[#]

Abbreviations used: WC = WKY corn-fed, WBB = WKY blueberry-fed, SC = SHRSP corn fed, SBB = SHRSP blueberry-fed, NOx = nitrate/nitrite.
[*]$p \leq 0.05$ vs. WC;
[#]$p \leq 0.05$ vs. SC;
[$]$p \leq 0.05$ vs. SBB.

the condition. Additional experiments will need to be conducted to assess treatment potential. In support of this possibility, the same BB diet has been shown to both confer protection against myocardial ischemia when started before the occurrence of myocardial infarction [13] as well as protection from further myocardial dysfunction when started two weeks after myocardial infarction [36]. These results in the myocardium indicate the potential for BB to be used as a preventative and as a treatment. We are planning follow-up experiments in this regard. This is the first demonstration, to our knowledge, of the effectiveness of a readily available natural product in an acceptable, consumable quantity to significantly attenuate hypertension-induced renal functional alterations.

References

1. Elks CM, Mariappan N, Haque M, Guggilam A, Majid DS, et al (2009) Chronic NF-κB blockade reduces cytosolic and mitochondrial oxidative stress and attenuates renal injury and hypertension in SHR. Am J Physiol Renal Physiol 296: F298–305.

2. Wilcox CS (2005) Oxidative stress and nitric oxide deficiency in the kidney: a critical link to hypertension? American Journal of Physiology - Regulatory, Integrative and Comparative Physiology 289: R913–R935.

3. Newman DJ, Cragg GM (2007) Natural Products as Sources of New Drugs over the Last 25 Years ⊥. Journal of Natural Products 70: 461–477.

4. Baker CJ, Orlandi EW (1995) Active oxygen in plant pathogenesis. Annual Review of Phytopathology 33: 299–321.

5. Wang SY, Jiao H (2000) Scavenging capacity of berry crops on superoxide radicals, hydrogen peroxide, hydroxyl radicals, and singlet oxygen. J Agric Food Chem 48: 5677–5684.

6. Spormann TM, Albert FW, Rath T, Dietrich H, Will F, et al. (2008) Anthocyanin/polyphenolic–rich fruit juice reduces oxidative cell damage in an intervention study with patients on hemodialysis. Cancer Epidemiology Biomarkers & Prevention 17: 3372–3380.

7. Smith MAL, Marley KA, Seigler D, Singletary KW, Meline B (2000) Bioactive Properties of Wild Blueberry Fruits. Journal of Food Science 65: 352–356.

8. Joseph JA, Shukitt-Hale B, Denisova NA, Bielinski D, Martin A, et al. (1999) Reversals of Age-Related Declines in Neuronal Signal Transduction, Cognitive, and Motor Behavioral Deficits with Blueberry, Spinach, or Strawberry Dietary Supplementation. J Neurosci 19: 8114–8121.

9. Bickford PC, Gould T, Briederick L, Chadman K, Pollock A, et al. (2000) Antioxidant-rich diets improve cerebellar physiology and motor learning in aged rats. Brain Research 866: 211–217.

10. Joseph JA, Shukitt-Hale B, Casadesus G (2005) Reversing the deleterious effects of aging on neuronal communication and behavior: beneficial properties of fruit polyphenolic compounds. The American Journal of Clinical Nutrition 81: 313S–316S.

11. Ramassamy C (2006) Emerging role of polyphenolic compounds in the treatment of neurodegenerative diseases: a review of their intracellular targets. European Journal of Pharmacology 545: 51–64.

12. Lau FC, Bielinski DF, Joseph JA (2007) Inhibitory effects of blueberry extract on the production of inflammatory mediators in lipopolysaccharide-activated BV2 microglia. Journal of Neuroscience Research 85: 1010–1017.

13. Ahmet I, Spangler E, Shukitt-Hale B, Juhaszova M, Sollott SJ, et al. (2009) Blueberry-enriched diet protects rat heart from ischemic damage. PLoS ONE 4: e5954.

14. Shaughnessy KS, Boswall IA, Scanlan AP, Gottschall-Pass KT, Sweeney MI (2009) Diets containing blueberry extract lower blood pressure in spontaneously hypertensive stroke-prone rats. Nutrition Research 29: 130–138.

15. Mattson MP (2008) Dietary factors, hormesis and health. Ageing Research Reviews 7: 43–48.

16. Lamming DW, Wood JG, Sinclair DA (2004) Small molecules that regulate lifespan: evidence for xenohormesis. Mol Microbiol 53: 1003–1009.

17. Elks CM, Mariappan N, Haque M, Guggilam A, Majid DSA, et al. (2009) Chronic NF-κB blockade reduces cytosolic and mitochondrial oxidative stress and attenuates renal injury and hypertension in SHR. Am J Physiol Renal Physiol 296: F298–305.

18. Goyarzu P, Malin DH, Lau FC, Taglialatela G, Moon WD, et al. (2004) Blueberry supplemented diet: effects on object recognition memory and nuclear factor-kappa B levels in aged rats. Nutritional Neuroscience 7: 75–83.

19. Agarwal D, Haque M, Sriramula S, Mariappan N, Pariaut R, et al. (2009) Role of proinflammatory cytokines and redox homeostasis in exercise-induced delayed progression of hypertension in spontaneously hypertensive rats. Hypertension 54: 1393–1400.

20. Cardinale JP, Sriramula S, Pariaut R, Guggilam A, Mariappan N, et al. (2010) HDAC inhibition attenuates inflammatory, hypertrophic, and hypertensive responses in spontaneously hypertensive rats. Hypertension 56: 437–444.

21. Ebenezer PJ, Mariappan N, Elks CM, Haque M, Francis J (2009) Diet-induced renal changes in Zucker rats are ameliorated by the superoxide dismutase mimetic TEMPOL. Obesity (Silver Spring) 17: 1994–2002.

22. Ebenezer PJ, Mariappan N, Elks CM, Haque M, Soltani Z, et al. (2009) Effects of pyrrolidine dithiocarbamate on high-fat diet-induced metabolic and renal alterations in rats. Life Sci 85: 357–364.

Acknowledgments

We express our deepest regret for the loss of our colleague, Dr. James A. Joseph, who passed away on June 1, 2010. Dr. Joseph conducted pioneering work in the health benefits of berry fruits. The authors gratefully acknowledge Sherry Ring and Alexander Castillo for their technical assistance.

Author Contributions

Conceived and designed the experiments: CME BSH JAJ DKI JF. Performed the experiments: CME SDR NM. Analyzed the data: CME DKI. Contributed reagents/materials/analysis tools: CME SDR BSH JAJ DKI JF. Wrote the paper: CME SDR DKI.

23. Mariappan N, Elks CM, Fink B, Francis J (2009) TNF-induced mitochondrial damage: a link between mitochondrial complex I activity and left ventricular dysfunction. Free Radic Biol Med 46: 462–470.

24. Mariappan N, Elks CM, Sriramula S, Guggilam A, Liu Z, et al. (2010) NF-κB-induced oxidative stress contributes to mitochondrial and cardiac dysfunction in type II diabetes. Cardiovascular Research 85: 473–483.

25. Mariappan N, Soorappan RN, Haque M, Sriramula S, Francis J (2007) TNF-alpha-induced mitochondrial oxidative stress and cardiac dysfunction: restoration by superoxide dismutase mimetic Tempol. Am J Physiol Heart Circ Physiol 293: H2726–2737.

26. Malin DH, Lee DR, Goyarzu P, Chang Y-H, Ennis LJ, et al. (2011) Short-term blueberry-enriched diet prevents and reverses object recognition memory loss in aging rats. Nutrition 27: 338–342.

27. Rosamond W, Flegal K, Furie K, Go A, Greenlund K, et al. (2008) Heart disease and stroke statistics--2008 Update: a report from the American Heart Association Statistics Committee and Stroke Statistics Subcommittee. Circulation 117: e25–146.

28. Guijarro C, Egido J (2001) Transcription factor-κB (NF-κB) and renal disease. Kidney Int 59: 415–424.

29. Wilcox CS, Welch WJ (2001) Oxidative stress: cause or consequence of hypertension? Experimental Biology and Medicine 226: 619–620.

30. Ma XL, Gao F, Nelson AH, Lopez BL, Christopher TA, et al. (2001) Oxidative inactivation of nitric oxide and endothelial dysfunction in stroke-prone spontaneous hypertensive rats. J Pharmacol Exp Ther 298: 879–885.

31. Majid DS, Kopkan L (2007) Nitric oxide and superoxide interactions in the kidney and their implication in the development of salt-sensitive hypertension. Clin Exp Pharmacol Physiol 34: 946–952.

32. Manning RD Jr., Meng S, Tian N (2003) Renal and vascular oxidative stress and salt-sensitivity of arterial pressure. Acta Physiol Scand 179: 243–250.

33. Tian N, Thrasher KD, Gundy PD, Hughson MD, Manning RD, Jr. (2005) Antioxidant treatment prevents renal damage and dysfunction and reduces arterial pressure in salt-sensitive hypertension. Hypertension 45: 934–939.

34. Neto CC (2007) Cranberry and blueberry: evidence for protective effects against cancer and vascular diseases. Mol Nutr Food Res 51: 652–664.

35. Howitz KT, Sinclair DA (2008) Xenohormesis: sensing the chemical cues of other species. Cell 133: 387–391.

36. Ahmet I, Spangler E, Shukitt-Hale B, Joseph JA, Ingram DK, et al. (2009) Survival and Cardioprotective Benefits of Long-Term Blueberry Enriched Diet in Dilated Cardiomyopathy Following Myocardial Infarction in Rats. PLoS ONE 4: e7975.

14

Daily Treatment with SMTC1100, a Novel Small Molecule Utrophin Upregulator, Dramatically Reduces the Dystrophic Symptoms in the *mdx* Mouse

Jonathon M. Tinsley[1]*, Rebecca J. Fairclough[2], Richard Storer[1], Fraser J. Wilkes[1], Allyson C. Potter[2], Sarah E. Squire[2], Dave S. Powell[2], Anna Cozzoli[3], Roberta F. Capogrosso[3], Adam Lambert[1], Francis X. Wilson[1], Stephen P. Wren[1], Annamaria De Luca[3], Kay E. Davies[2]*

1 Summit plc, Abingdon, United Kingdom, 2 MRC Functional Genomics Unit, Department of Physiology Anatomy and Genetics, University of Oxford, Oxford, United Kingdom, 3 Unit of Pharmacology, Department of Pharmaco-biology, University of Bari "A. Moro", Bari, Italy

Abstract

Background: Duchenne muscular dystrophy (DMD) is a lethal, progressive muscle wasting disease caused by a loss of sarcolemmal bound dystrophin, which results in the death of the muscle fibers leading to the gradual depletion of skeletal muscle. There is significant evidence demonstrating that increasing levels of the dystrophin-related protein, utrophin, in mouse models results in sarcolemmal bound utrophin and prevents the muscular dystrophy pathology. The aim of this work was to develop a small molecule which increases the levels of utrophin in muscle and thus has therapeutic potential.

Methodology and Principal Findings: We describe the *in vivo* activity of SMT C1100; the first orally bioavailable small molecule utrophin upregulator. Once-a-day daily-dosing with SMT C1100 reduces a number of the pathological effects of dystrophin deficiency. Treatment results in reduced pathology, better muscle physiology leading to an increase in overall strength, and an ability to resist fatigue after forced exercise; a surrogate for the six minute walk test currently recommended as the pivotal outcome measure in human trials for DMD.

Conclusions and Significance: This study demonstrates proof-of-principle for the use of *in vitro* screening methods in allowing identification of pharmacological agents for utrophin transcriptional upregulation. The best compound identified, SMT C1100, demonstrated significant disease modifying effects in DMD models. Our data warrant the full evaluation of this compound in clinical trials in DMD patients.

Editor: Paul Dent, Virginia Commonwealth University, United States of America

Funding: This work was supported by the Medical Research Council, Muscular Dystrophy Campaign, Muscular Dystrophy Association USA, Association Francaise contre les Myopathies, and Telethon Italy. The funders had no role in study design, data collection and analysis, decision to publish, or preparation of the manuscript.

Competing Interests: JMT, RS, FJW, AL, FXW, SPW are employed by Summit plc. KED is a shareholder of Summit plc.

* E-mail: Jon.Tinsley@summitplc.com (JMT); kay.davies@dpag.ox.ac.uk (KED)

Introduction

Duchenne muscular dystrophy (DMD) is a lethal X-linked recessive muscle wasting disease caused by mutations in the dystrophin gene (for review see [1]). Affected boys are ambulatory until about 12 years of age but often live into their twenties with recent improvements in respiratory support. Many boys show an abnormal ECG in the late stages of the diseases and cardiomyopathy is also a general feature. The milder form of the disease known as Becker muscular dystrophy (BMD) is also characterized by cardiac defects despite BMD patients often being ambulant in their 50s and 60s. Thus, any therapy for the disease would need not only to target skeletal, but also cardiac muscle.

Currently there is no effective treatment for DMD. Various strategies developed to alleviate the symptoms include steroid treatment, anti-inflammatory agents, and growth hormone and myostatin inhibitors (for review see [2]). More recently, genetic approaches have been tested in DMD patient trials. In particular, readthrough of stop codons has been attempted in the 10–15% of patients that have mutations resulting in premature stop codons resulting in dystrophin deficiency. An orally delivered small molecule, Ataluren, recently entered a phase IIb trial. The six minute walk distance test [3] (6MWD) was used as the primary efficacy endpoint as the ability to walk further after treatment is considered by the regulatory authorities as a major improvement in the quality of life for these patients. Unfortunately, after conclusion of the trial, no statistically significant increase in the distance travelled using the 6MWD was reported. Skipping of exon 51, which targets up to 13% of patients, represents the monoskipping therapy which would be applicable to the largest proportion of DMD patients. Antisense molecules, delivered either intravenously or sub-cutaneously, have shown some restoration of dystrophin to a variable degree in patients [4,5]. Next generation trials are planned with constructs which increase the efficiency of delivery of the antisense oligonucleotides. The efficacy of this approach was demonstrated using the dystrophin/utrophin knock-out mouse, where restoration of muscle function was demonstrated [6]. To treat more patients, different antisense sequences will need to be developed to target other exons and the regulatory authorities may treat each of these new constructs as a new drug. The ideal scenario would be to develop multi-exon skipping [7] but this may only be achieved using AAV delivery which faces immunological problems.

We have taken an alternative pharmacological approach to DMD by developing an orally bioavailable small molecule which should be appropriate to treat all patients irrespective of their mutation and target both skeletal and cardiac muscle. Building on our work in the *mdx* mouse, which demonstrated that the loss of dystrophin could be compensated for by increasing the levels of the dystrophin-related protein, utrophin, we have developed novel small molecules which can transcriptionally upregulate the utrophin gene. The demonstration that increased utrophin can reduce the muscular dystrophy in the *mdx* mouse has been confirmed by others [8–11]. Our early data from the *mdx* mouse suggested that increasing the levels of utrophin over two-fold would be of great benefit [12].

SMT C1100 was the final product of an exhaustive chemical screening and optimisation campaign. In this paper we present evidence confirming an overall two-fold increase in both utrophin RNA and protein resulting in a significant reduction in dystrophic symptoms and increased muscle function in dystrophin-deficient *mdx* mice. This was a comprehensive study looking at the beneficial effects of daily dosing of SMT C1100 in both sedentary *mdx* and the more severely affected forced exercise model. If the results obtained here using SMT C1100 translated across to DMD patients then undoubtedly this would be a disease modifying therapy for DMD.

Methods

Ethics Statement

All animal procedures were performed in accordance with UK Home Office regulations or in accordance with the Italian Guidelines for the use of laboratory animals, which conform with the European Community Directive published in 1986 (86/609/ EEC). The work performed in Oxford was performed under certificate of designation number 30/2306 and project license number 30/2652 following approval by the University of Oxford Departments of Physiology, Anatomy & Genetics and Experimental Psychology Joint Departmental Ethics Review Committee. The work performed by Covance Laboratories Ltd. was performed under certificate of designation number 50/8504 and project license number 60/3774 following approval by the Covance Ethical Review Process. The work in Bari was approved by the central review board under the Italian Minister of Health which authorizes that all animal studies conform to the ethical requirement and current law.

Generation of a utrophin promoter screening cell line

Murine H2K cells [13] were transfected with 8.4 kb of the human utrophin promoter including the first untranslated exon linked to a luciferase reporter gene and stable lines generated for screening (H2K-*mdx* utrnA-luc).

Cell culture

The H2K-*mdx* utrnA-luc cells were maintained in DMEM (Invitrogen) supplemented with 20% Fetal Bovine Serum Gold (PAA), 5% CEE (SLI), 2 mM L-Glutamine (Invitrogen), 1%

Penicillin Streptomycin (Invitrogen) and 2 µg/500 ml Mouse Interferon-γ (Roche). Cells were maintained at 10% CO_2 at 33°C. Normal human skeletal muscle cells (SkMc) were sourced from TCS cell works. Passaging was undertaken according to the supplier's instructions including the use of specialist culture media. Cells were maintained at 5% CO_2 at 37°C.

In vitro assays

For luciferase assays plates were seeded with H2K-*mdx* utrnA-luc at 5000 cells per well. These were incubated in 10% CO_2 and 33°C for 24 h prior to dosing.

All compounds were supplied as a 10 mM solution in dimethyl sulfoxide (DMSO). Cells were treated compounds dissolved in a final concentration of 0.3% DMSO. Assays were performed in triplicate and the compounds were dosed for 48 h. Luciferase levels were measured using the Steady-Glo Luciferase kit (Promega) and the plates were then read using a FLUOstar Optima plate reader (BMG Labtech). The means from the biological triplicates were used in a 4 Parameter Logistic Model to generate an EC_{50} and Hill slope. The software used to calculate this was XLfit version 4.2.2.

Sedentary mice and drug treatment

Three week-old male *mdx* (C57BL/10ScSn-Dmd^{mdx}/J; Charles River Laboratories, MA, USA) littermates were randomly split between 2 groups and treated with SMT C1100 (50 mg/kg) or vehicle only (phosphate buffered saline (PBS), 0.1% Tween-20, 5% DMSO) *via* daily i.p. injection for four weeks. At the end of the drug treatment period mice were sacrificed by CO_2 asphyxiation in accordance with Schedule I of the UK Animals (Scientific Procedures) Act 1986. C57BL/6 contractile properties were measured in EDL muscle dissected from eight week old untreated mice obtained at 4 week of age from Harlan (n = 5). All animal procedures were performed in accordance with UK Home Office regulations. In all other experiments described using the sedentary *mdx* mice dosing was by the oral gavage using a canula to deliver SMTC1100 or vehicle only on a daily basis for 28 days. At the end of this period the mice were sacrificed and muscle and blood samples were taken. Quantification of muscle and plasma levels of SMT C1100 was performed using CD1 mice.

Exercised mice, treadmill running and drug treatment

Most of the experimental procedures conform to the standard operating procedures for pre-clinical tests using *mdx* mice available at http://www.treat-nmd.eu/research/preclinical/SOPs/.

A total of 24 *mdx* male mice of 4–5 weeks of age (Charles River-Italy), and homogeneous for body weight, underwent a 30 min running regime on an horizontal treadmill (Columbus Instruments) at 12 m/min, twice a week (keeping a constant interval of 2–3 days between each trial), for 4–6 weeks, according to a standard protocol [13,14]. Experimental groups were treated as follows: vehicle only (n = 7), SMT C1100 (50 mg/kg; n = 6), α-methyl prednisolone (PDN; 1 mg/kg; n = 5) and combination of SMT C1100 (50 mg/kg) and PDN (1 mg/kg) (n = 6). Age and gender-matched wild type C57/BL10ScSn) or non-exercised *mdx* mice were also used for specific experimental purposes, as indicated in the text. The dose of PDN has been chosen based on our previous studies [14]. The treatment started one day before the beginning of the exercise protocol, and continued until the day of sacrifice. SMT C1100 and the combination of PDN+SMT C1100 were dissolved in 5% DMSO, 0.1% Tween-20 in PBS, whilst PDN was dissolved in sterile water. Drugs were formulated for i.p. injection so that the correct dose was administered in 0.1 ml/10 g. Body weight was assessed weekly, as was fore-limb force by means of a grip strength meter (Columbus Instruments, USA) [14,15]. An exercise resistance test, consisting of horizontal running for 5 min at 5 m/min, then increasing the speed of 1 m/min each minute, was performed on week 0 and after four and five weeks of treatment. The total distance run by each mouse until exhaustion was measured [15]. At the end of the 5th week of exercise/treatment the *ex vivo* experiments were also started. To this aim mice were deeply anesthetized and sacrificed using 1.2 g/kg urethane (i.p.) in accordance with the Italian Guidelines for the use of laboratory animals, which conform with the European Community Directive published in 1986 (86/609/EEC).

Muscle mechanics/electrophysiology

Muscle mechanics were conducted on the extensor digitorum longus (EDL) muscle as previously described [6]. EDL muscles were removed and rapidly placed in the recording chamber for the electrophysiological or isometric recordings. In the recording chambers EDL muscles were bathed at $30 \pm 1°C$ in the following normal physiological solution: NaCl 148 mM, KCl 4.5 mM, $CaCl_2$ 2.0 mM, $MgCl_2$ 1.0 mM, $NaHCO_3$ 12.0 mM, NaH_2PO_4 0.44 mM, glucose 5.55 mM, and continuously gassed with 95% O_2 and 5% CO_2 (pH 7.2–7.4). The mechanical threshold (MT) was determined in EDL muscle fibres by the two microelectrode "point" voltage clamp method, described previously [13,14]. In brief, depolarizing command pulses of variable duration (from 500 to 5 ms at 0.3 Hz) were progressively increased in amplitude from the holding potential (H) of -90 mV until a visible fiber contraction. The mean threshold membrane potential values of individual myofibers (V, in mV) at various pulse durations (t, in ms) allowed the construction of a "strength-duration" curve. The rheobase voltage (R, in mV) was obtained by a non-linear least square algorithm using a previously described equation [14,15].

Protein analyses

A human DMD cell line with a deletion of exons 49 and 50 (generously provided by Vincent Mouly, Paris) was seeded in 6 cm dishes in DMEM (Invitrogen), Medium 199 (20%; Sigma-Aldrich), Fetal Calf Serum (20%; Invitrogen), glutamine and penicillin/streptomycin (Invitrogen) 24 h prior to drug treatment. After three days of drug treatment cells were lysed for 20 min at 4°C in Tris pH6.8 (75 mM), SDS (3.8%), Urea (4 M), glycerol (20%) supplemented with protease inhibitors (1:100; Sigma-Aldrich). Soluble protein was purified at $8000 \times g$ for 20 min at 4°C and 30 µl was size fractionated by 5% Tris-HCL SDS-PAGE gel electrophoresis and transferred to a PVDF membrane (GE Healthcare). Soluble protein was prepared from muscle samples snap frozen in liquid nitrogen and stored at $-80°C$ until use for biochemical analysis. For western blotting, protein was crushed with a pestle in a liquid nitrogen-cooled mortar, solubilised in 50 volumes of single-section western blot lysis buffer [16], vortexed, briefly homogenised and sonicated, heated to 94°C for 4 minutes and centrifuged for 3 min at $15\,000 \times g$ to remove insoluble matter. For western blotting, 50 µl soluble protein extract was separated by 5% Tris-HCL SDS-PAGE gel electrophoresis and transferred onto PVDF (GE Healthcare). Utrophin protein was detected using MANCHO 3 antibody (1:100; kind gift from G.E. Morris, Oswestry, UK) and ECL HRP-conjugated anti-mouse antibody (GE Healthcare). Equal protein loading was corrected by detection of α-actinin (1:200, N-19; Santa Cruz Biotechnology, Inc.) and a HRP-conjugated anti-goat antibody (Sigma). Blots were developed using ECL reagent (GE Healthcare), Densitometry was performed using the freely available web version of Image J (rsbweb.nih.gov/ij/). Immunohistochemistry was carried out as previously described [17].

RNA analyses

For quantitative real time RT-PCR SkMC cells were seeded in six well plates at 25000 cells per well in 3 ml of appropriate media and incubated for 24 h prior to dosing. Compounds were dosed in a final concentration of 1% DMSO for 72 h. RNA was extracted from tissue using a QIAGEN RNeasy® Plus kit (Qiagen) and QiaShredder (Qiagen), using the manufacturer's instructions. The High-Capacity cDNA Reverse Transcriptase Kit (Applied Biosystems) was used according to manufacturer's instructions. Real-time PCR was performed according to the $\Delta\Delta CT$ method [18]. The 7300 Real-Time PCR System from Applied Biosystems was used for this assay along with the 7300 System SDS software with the SDS Relative Quantification Study Plug in. Data was analysed using the 7300 System SDS software with the SDS Relative Quantification Study Plug in.

Blood analyses

Measurements of SMT C1100 plasma concentrations were obtained following RO (retro-orbital) blood sampling on day 1, 24 h after oral dosing with SMT C1100 (50 mg/kg) or vehicle only (0.1% PBS-Tween-20/5% DMSO). Further samples were taken at day 15 and day 28 after the start of dosing.

Blood was collected with non-heparinized hematocrit tubes into serum microtainer tubes and centrifuged for 12 min at 12,000 rpm at 4°C. Serum was stored at $-80°C$ prior to analysis using the CK (NAC) reagent kit in conjunction with the AU 400 Clinical Chemistry analyser (Olympus UK Ltd).

Histological analyses

After 28 days of dosing muscle samples were taken for histopathology and processed by Premier Laboratory LLC (Colorado, U.S.A.). Samples were received in 10% neutral buffered formalin, processed into paraffin, and 5 µm sections and stained for Hematoxylin and Eosin (H&E) and Masson's Trichrome (tibialis anterior, extensor digitorum longus, soleus, and diaphragm). Both the H&E and Masson's Trichrome stained slides were submitted blind to a Board Certified Veterinary Pathologist at Premier Laboratory LLC and scored for the presence of inflammation and fibrosis. A total of five sections from each muscle were analysed.

The muscle fibres were scored according to the following criteria:

Inflammation:

0 = none to minimal - No inflammation within the muscle bundles or inter-bundle connective tissue; occasional mononuclear inflammatory cells may be present but no obvious aggregations.

1 = mild - Occasional mononuclear inflammatory cells in the inter-bundle connective tissue with focal aggregations of mononuclear inflammatory cells.

2 = moderate - Multiple foci of mononuclear inflammatory cell infiltration in the inter-bundle connective tissue; occasional mononuclear inflammatory cells between individual muscle fibres.

3 = severe - Multiple large foci of mononuclear inflammatory cell infiltration in the inter-bundle connective tissue extending into the intra-bundle connective tissue with expansion of the inter-bundle and intra-bundle space.

Fibrosis:

0 = none to minimal - No fibrosis in the muscle bundles or inter-bundle connective tissue; mild expansion of the inter-bundle connective tissue may be present focally.

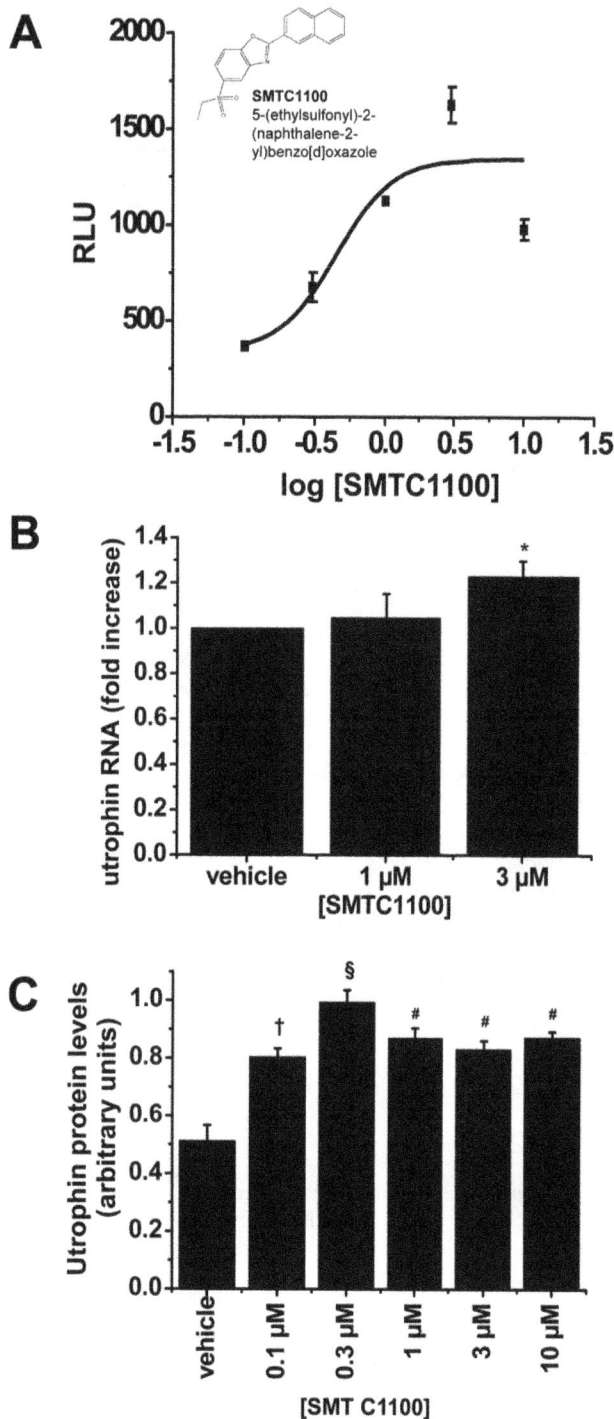

72 hours with six biological replicates. *p = 0.01 relative to vehicle only; (C) Utrophin protein levels in human DMD cell line treated with SMT C1100 (1 μM) or vehicle (0.1% DMSO). Blots were stained with anti-utrophin (MANCHO3; 1:100) and ECL HRP-conjugated anti-mouse antibody (GE Healthcare). Bands were quantified using Image J and arbitrary units represent utrophin levels corrected for equal loading by α-actinin immunostaining. Results represent a mean ± S.E based on n = 3. †p = 0.00683; §p<0.001; #p<0.005 relative to vehicle-treated cells.

1 = mild - Focal expansion of the inter-bundle connective tissue; mild focal expansion of the intra-bundle space may be present.

2 = moderate - Multiple foci of expansion of the connective tissue component in the inter-bundle area; focal intra-bundle increases in connective tissue between individual muscle fibres.

3 = severe - Multiple large foci of connective tissue in the inter-bundle region extending into the intra-bundle connective tissue with expansion of the inter-bundle and intra-bundle space.

In addition two 42-bit color images were captured with a Zeiss AxioCam HR digital camera on a Zeiss Axioskop 2 microscope utilizing AxioVision 4.4 software (Zeiss) of each muscle on the H&E stained slides. Once the images were captured they were white balanced in Adobe Photoshop (Adobe). The proportion of centrally nucleated fibers was determined by analyzing the images and counting the number of centrally located nuclei; a total of two hundred cells per muscle were evaluated. Students' two-tailed t-test was used to compare the groups with significance set at p<0.05.

Statistical Analyses

Significance was calculated using the Student's t test with a two-tailed distribution assuming unequal sample variance. Multiple statistical comparisons between groups, was performed by one-way ANOVA, with Bonferroni's t test post-hoc correction for allowing a better evaluation of intra- and inter-group variability and avoiding false positive.

Results

In vitro upregulation of utrophin

SMT C1100 was identified from an iterative analoging approach from initial hits identified using a human muscle specific utrophin A promoter cell-based assay. Myoblasts (mdx) were cloned from H-2K-tsA58×mdx with an IFN/tsSV40 T-Ag transgene in order to control proliferation and fusion [13]. The screening line named H2K-mdx utrnA-luc contains a stably integrated reporter consisting of 8.4 kb of the human utrophin promoter linked to a luciferase reporter gene. The region of the utrophin promoter contained all the motifs known to control utrophin expression [19,20]. This high throughput screening assay identified a number of luciferase-inducing compounds that also have the ability to increase the transcription of the endogenous mouse UTRN, thus identifying compounds with both human and mouse activity eventually leading to the final optimized compound, SMT C1100 whose chemical structure is shown in Fig. 1A.

SMT C1100 shows a maximal increase of four to five-fold compared to vehicle with an EC$_{50}$ of 0.4 μM (Fig. 1A). In vitro dosing of human myoblasts with SMT C1100 leads to a 25% increase in utrophin mRNA (Fig. 1B) when compared to vehicle-only dosing after three days of treatment. Treatment of human

Figure 1. In vitro activity of SMT C1100. (A) SMT C1100 dose response in murine H2k-mdx utrnA-luc cells expressing the human utrophin promoter linked to a luciferase reporter gene. Cells were treated with compound for 48 h in standard growth medium containing 0.3% DMSO. The chart shows relative luminescence (RLU) in relation to five different doses of SMT C1100. A Four Parameter Logistic Model was used to generate an EC$_{50}$. Points represent a mean ±S.E. of three experiments and are typical of the results for all batches of SMTC1100. The structure for SMTC1100 is shown; (B) SMT C1100 significantly increased mRNA copy number of the utrophin transcript in SkMC cells. In this assay Gene Expression Assay 4326315 was used for β-actin detection and Gene Expression Assay Hu01125984_m1 was used for utrophin transcript detection (both Applied Biosystems). Cells were exposed to SMT C1100 in standard media with 1% DMSO (vehicle) for

DMD cells with SMT C1100 lead to a 2-fold increase in utrophin protein levels at an optimal concentration of 0.3 µM after 3 days of treatment (Fig. 1C).

Plasma levels of SMT C1100

Significant plasma (Fig. 2A) and muscle (Fig. 2B) levels of compound were achieved for several hours following oral administration of SMT C1100 (50 mg/kg). From the EC_{50} data (Fig. 1A), taken together with the levels of utrophin upregulation achieved at various drug concentrations in both DMD and normal myoblasts, we can estimate that the effective concentration required for efficacy would be in the order of 0.5–1 µM. This means that therapeutic levels are achieved in muscle for at least eight hours following dosing.

Toxicological evaluation of SMT C1100

In order to confirm that SMT C1100 had no obvious off target toxicological liabilities mice were dosed with high levels of compound. Overall no toxicologically significant changes in clinical condition, body weight, food consumption, haematology or clinical chemistry parameters were seen during the study. There were no microscopic findings within the comprehensive set of tissues analysed due to effects of SMT C1100. Conclusion from Covance Laboratories Ltd. confirmed that the study did not identify any toxicity that was attributable to dosing with SMTC1100. Based on the conditions of this study, it was considered that no toxicity was determined for SMT C1100 administered by oral gavage to the mouse up to dose levels of 2000 mg/kg/day for 28 days. This information was a key

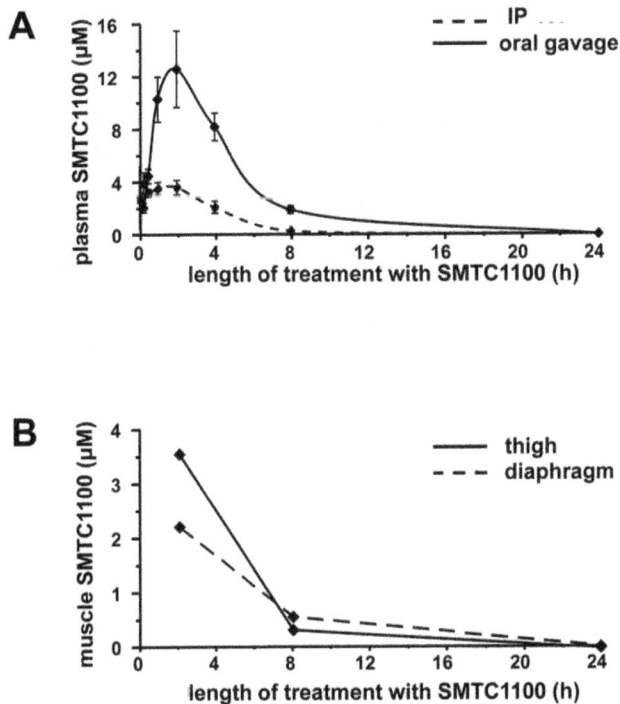

Figure 2. Plasma levels of SMT C1100 in the mouse. (A) SMT C1100 plasma levels were assessed over a 24 h period after oral gavage or i.p. delivery of 50 mg/kg of the compound into wild type CD1 mice. At set time points after administration groups of three animals were taken for blood samples at the times stated in the figure. (B) Thigh and diaphragm samples from CD1 dosed orally with 50 mg/kg were quantified for the presence of SMT C1100.

component of the toxicology assessment which led to a successful clinical trial application and testing in healthy volunteers. This was only one component of a significant package of safety evaluation performed on SMT C1100.

In vivo upregulation of utrophin

To confirm the *in vivo* activity of SMT C1100, the dystrophin-deficient *mdx* mouse was used to monitor any changes in the dystrophic phenotype after chronic dosing for several weeks. To confirm increases in utrophin expression after repeated daily dosing with SMT C1100, muscle samples were taken for RNA and protein analysis. Fig. 3A demonstrates a two-fold increase in utrophin mRNA as determined by quantitative PCR from *mdx* mice dosed daily with SMT C1100 for 28 days compared to vehicle only. Fig. 3B demonstrates significant increases in utrophin protein quantified from western blots of heart; a muscle notoriously difficult to target with systemic administration of putative DMD therapeutics, and diaphragm; the skeletal muscle most affected in sedentary *mdx* mice. Fig. 3C illustrates a qualitative increase in sarcolemmal-bound utrophin in the tibialis anterior (TA) and EDL muscles after repeat dosing with SMT C1100 following muscle sectioning. A similar result has been observed in both diaphragm and hind limb muscles of forced exercise-treated *mdx* mice (data not shown), suggesting no impact of work load on drug action. This data confirms SMT C1100 drives increased utrophin transcriptional expression *in vivo* and, more importantly, demonstrates increased utrophin staining at the required site of action - the sarcolemma - and independently from muscle work load.

Benefits of daily dosing of sedentary *mdx* mice with SMT C1100

In the case of the sedentary *mdx* mouse, there is a significant triggering of muscle degeneration at around 4 weeks which continues for a further 4 weeks where limb muscles then appear to reach stasis and levels of regeneration remain stable. One muscle where continued development of necrosis is seen is the diaphragm muscle. The dosing schedule for SMT C1100-treated mice was a single daily administration from day 21 for a further 28 days. This period of dosing encompassed the necrotic degenerative phase resulting from dystrophin deficiency.

The hypothesis to protect myofibres from damage in the absence of dystrophin is that utrophin, if continually localised to the sarcolemma, will replace dystrophin function. If dystrophin negative fibres are protected from damage for longer by the continued presence of utrophin then the catastrophic secondary effects of regeneration, fibrosis and inflammation should be reduced and muscle should be able to function for longer. All of these endpoints are significantly improved in *mdx* dosed daily with SMT C1100 for several weeks compared to *mdx* dosed with vehicle-only. SMT C1100 addresses the primary cause of fibre loss by protecting the sarcolemma from damage as exemplified by increased resistance to eccentric contractions (Fig. 4A) and a reduction in serum creatine kinase levels (Fig. 4B). At the point where the muscle necrosis is at a maximum, SMT C1100 reduces the release of CK into the plasma by 75% compared to vehicle (Fig. 4B; 15 d after the start of dosing). When degeneration has stabilised there is still significant benefit seen as evidenced by continued lower levels of CK (Fig. 4B, 28 d after start of dosing). This data also demonstrates that beneficial effects of SMT C1100 driven utrophin upregulation must occur within a few days after the start of dosing.

The resultant protection of dystrophin-deficient fibres by continued expression of utrophin resulted in a reduction in the

A

B

C

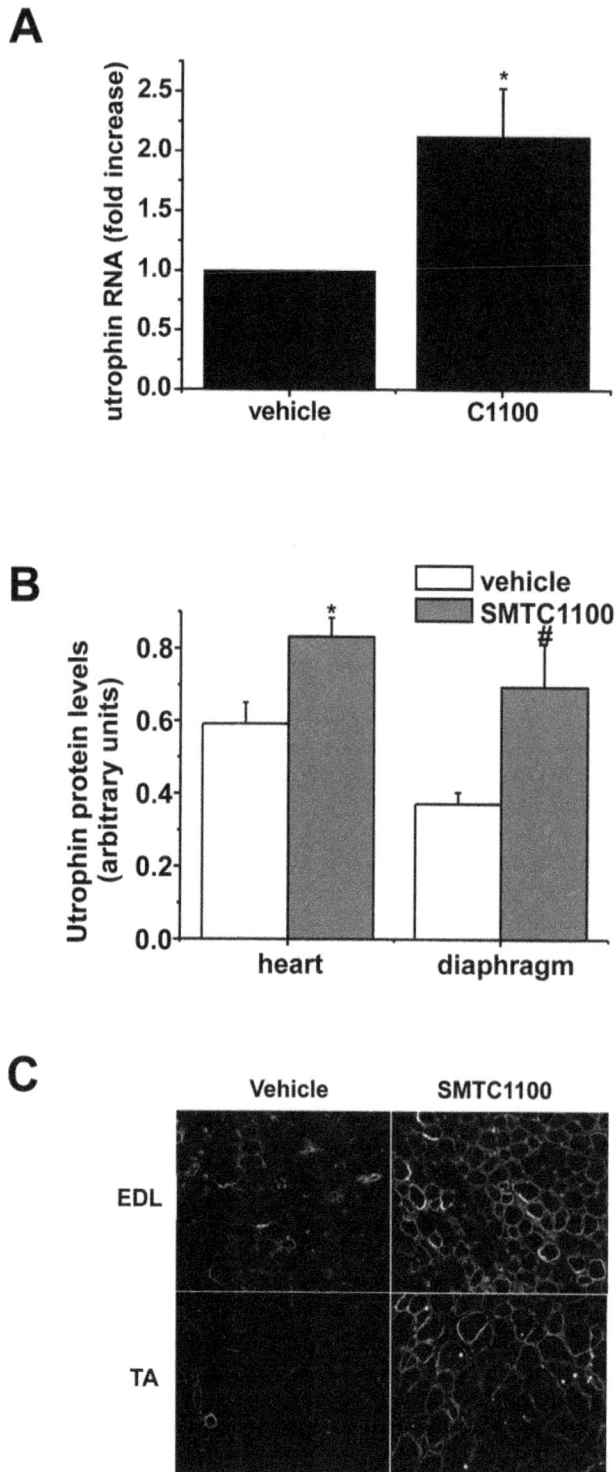

Figure 3. Effect of SMT C1100 on *in vivo* utrophin levels in the *mdx* mouse. (A) Two-fold increase in utrophin mRNA following daily oral administration of *mdx* mice with SMT C1100 (50 mg/kg/day) or vehicle only (PBS-Tween-20 (0.1%)/5% DMSO) from three weeks of age for four weeks. Results represent the mean ± S.E from six mice per treatment group and are corrected for β-actin. *p = 0.019; (B) Utrophin protein levels in heart and diaphragm following treatment of *mdx* mice as described in (A) above. Blots were stained with anti-utrophin (MANCHO3; 1:100) and ECL HRP-conjugated anti-mouse antibody (GE Healthcare). Bands were quantified using Image J and arbitrary units represent utrophin levels corrected for equal loading by α-actinin immunostaining. Results represent a mean ±S.E from eight mice per

treatment group except for heart vehicle only which is based on n = 7. *p<0.01; #p<0.05; (C) Immunohistochemical staining of EDL and TA muscle sections (10 μm; 20× magnification) were prepared from *mdx* mice treated as in (A). Sections were stained with anti-utrophin polyclonal antibody URD40 (1:100) and fluorescein isothiocyanate-conjugated anti-rabbit secondary antibody (1:1000).

level of regeneration taking place in skeletal muscle in *mdx* mice dosed with SMT C1100. This is demonstrated by a significant reduction in the numbers of fibres with centrally localized nuclei, as fibres with peripheral nuclei are thought to be more mature in development and therefore to have been a component of the muscle for longer (Fig. 4C). Significant reduction in centrally nucleated fibres is seen in the skeletal muscles examined including the diaphragm; a more severely affected *mdx* muscle which better mimics the more severe pathology of a DMD patient.

As the cycle of fibre degeneration and regeneration is being slowed by continued utrophin expression in SMT C1100-dosed *mdx* then the cytoplasmic signals to engage in muscle repair responses such as inflammation and fibrosis are reduced. In normal muscle this inflammatory protection response is dampened down as the proliferation of resident satellite cells fuse and reconnects the broken fibres. However, with the constant degeneration, these protection signals are not switched off, resulting in the continued influx of inflammatory cells and fibroblasts, leading to an increasing cascade of further fibre damage and loss of muscle "space" by fibrotic plaques. Treatment with SMT C1100 significantly reduces this damage by virtue of the reduced fibre regeneration. Blinded analysis by a board-certified veterinary pathologist of muscle sections from *mdx* mice dosed with either vehicle or SMTC1100 demonstrated a significant reduction in both inflammation and fibrosis. Whole muscle sections were rated with a pathology score on a scale from normal (0) – mild (1) – moderate (2) – severe (3). Pooled averages of total scoring from the TA, EDL and soleus are shown (Fig. 5A). A qualitative example of the extent of inflammation from a SMT C1100-dosed EDL or vehicle dosed EDL (Fig. 5B) is shown where the SMT C1100 section was scored as mild (occasional mononuclear inflammatory cells in the inter-bundle connective tissue with focal aggregations of mononuclear inflammatory cells) and the *mdx* as moderate (multiple foci of mononuclear inflammatory cell infiltration in the inter-bundle connective tissue; occasional mononuclear inflammatory cells between individual muscle fibres). This data confirms the concept of reduced fibre damage due to utrophin localization leading to reduced inflammation and fibrosis.

Benefits of daily dosing of forced exercise *mdx* mice with SMT C1100

A forced exercise regime of chronic exercise was used as a strategy to worsen the murine pathology [14,21]. Five week old *mdx* mice underwent forced treadmill exercise twice a week and the effects of daily SMT C1100 treatment under this exercise regime were then evaluated.

This exercise protocol significantly worsens *in vivo* parameters readily evaluated by non-invasive approaches, such as fore limb grip and endurance tests. In particular, the exercise protocol induced the typical decrease of fore limb force *in vivo* over time; a reduction which is seldom observed in sedentary *mdx*. SMT C1100-treated *mdx* showed a significant protection against exercise-induced fore limb weakness, as demonstrated by both the maximal strength achieved and the increase in strength after four weeks of dosing (Fig. 6A, B). After four weeks of dosing both

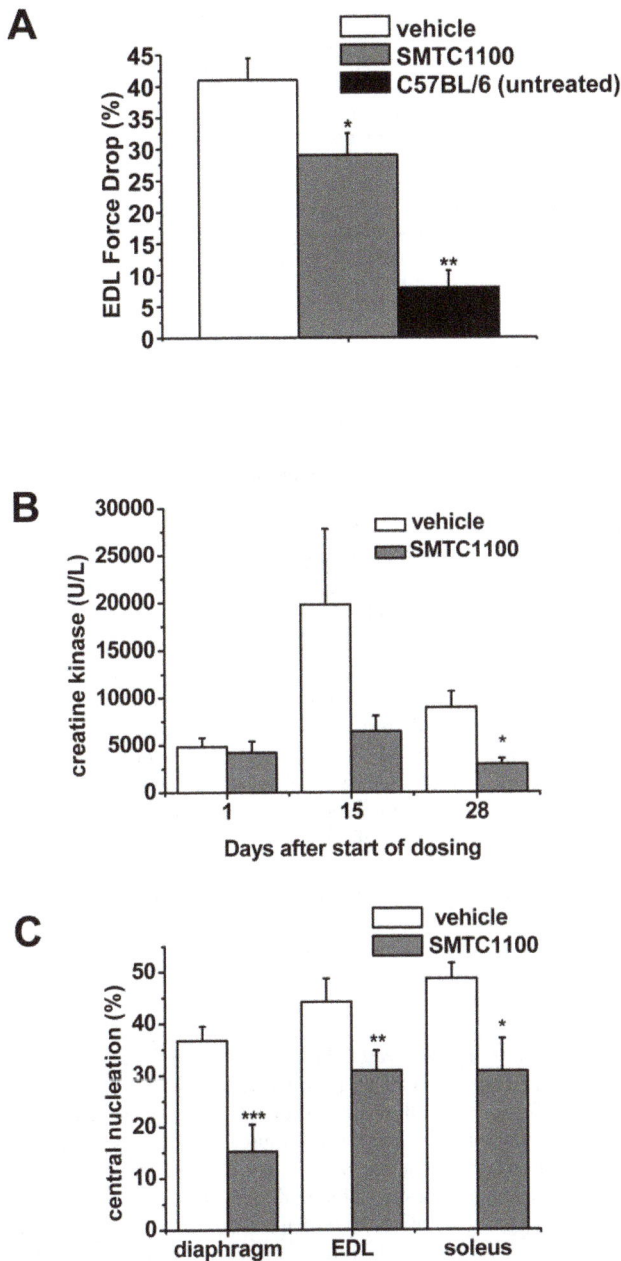

Figure 4. *Ex vivo* analysis of SMT C1100 activity in the *mdx* mouse. (A) *mdx* mice were treated with SMT C1100 (50 mg/kg/day) or vehicle only (0.1% Tween-20/5% DMSO in PBS) via daily i.p. injection from two weeks of age for four weeks. Whilst contracting tetanically, EDL muscles were stretched at 15% of their fibre length. The difference in force produced between the first and fifth stretch is represented as an indicator of the resistance of the muscle to stretch-induced damage. *p<0.05; **p<1.0×10^{-5}; (B) levels of serum creatine kinase following oral gavage of *mdx* mice with 50 mg/kg SMT C1100 or vehicle from three weeks of age for four weeks (C) Muscles from the dosing described in (B) were processed to assess the percentage of centrally nucleated fibres *p<0.01; (C)***p=0.0001; **p=0.005; *p=0.003.

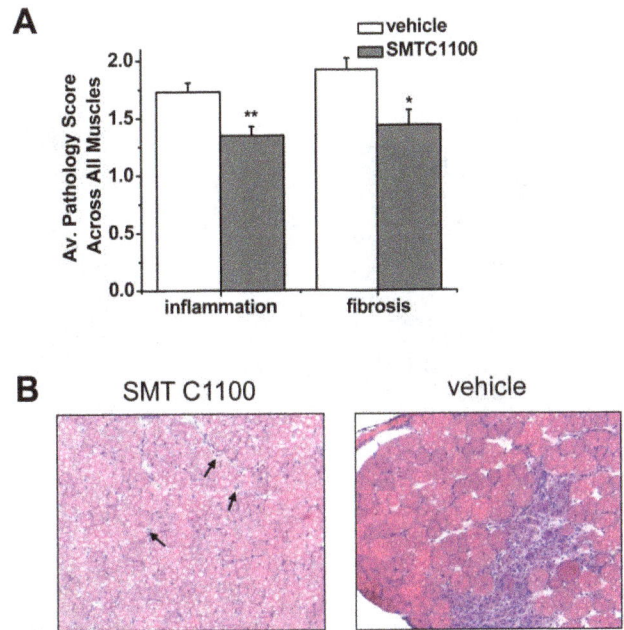

Figure 5. Reduction in secondary pathological features. (A) Data demonstrates the reduction in overall skeletal muscle inflammation and fibrosis from *mdx* treated with SMT C1100 compared to vehicle only. SMT C1100 (50 mg/kg) or vehicle was delivered daily by oral gavage to groups of six *mdx* mice aged around 17 d for a total of 28 days. The TA, EDL, soleus, and diaphragm were removed and five sections from each muscle were stained and analysed blind by a board-certified veterinary pathologist for evidence of inflammation and fibrosis using a standard pathology scoring method described in the methods section. Scoring (0–3) was made for each section from each muscle then averaged for all muscles to give an overall assessment of improvement in the pathological effects of dystrophin deficiency; (B) Qualitative assessment of EDL muscle from SMT C1100-dosed *mdx* scored as 1 = mild - occasional mononuclear inflammatory cells in the inter-bundle connective tissue with focal aggregations of mononuclear inflammatory cells. The arrows mark foci of inflammation. Qualitative assessment of EDL dosed with vehicle and scored as 2 = moderate - multiple foci of mononuclear inflammatory cell infiltration in the inter bundle connective tissue; occasional mononuclear inflammatory cells between individual muscle fibres.

values from the SMT C1100-dosed *mdx* were equivalent to those observed in sedentary *mdx* and wild type mice.

Data with direct relevance to DMD treatment was generated using a fatigue assessment of the mice which underwent forced exercise. Fatigue was assessed in an acute endurance test and estimated as the maximal distance run before exhaustion.

Sedentary *mdx* mice, although run for a shorter distance than wild type [14], maintain the same exercise performance over time, whilst the exercised *mdx* demonstrate a dramatic increase in fatigability between the start and the fourth and fifth week of training (Fig. 6C). A partial restoration of the resistance to fatigue was observed in SMT C1100-dosed mice, with an increase in distance travelled of around 50% compared to vehicle only after 5 weeks of dosing. Interestingly, this effect was similar to that observed in the exercised *mdx* mice treated with PDN; which is currently the gold standard in clinical treatment for Duchenne patients. Significant synergy was observed when SMT C1100 was co-administered with PDN for five weeks. The forced exercise *mdx* were completely resistant to fatigue and were able to continue running as far as the sedentary *mdx* (Fig. 6C). This equated to an increase in distance travelled of around 350% compared to the vehicle-treated forced exercise *mdx*.

Ex vivo analysis on isolated muscles from forced exercise *mdx* mice demonstrated that SMT C1100 exerted a significant amelioration of calcium-dependent functional parameters. These are typically modified in *mdx* muscles due to the altered calcium homeostasis, which in turn is believed to drive the rate of

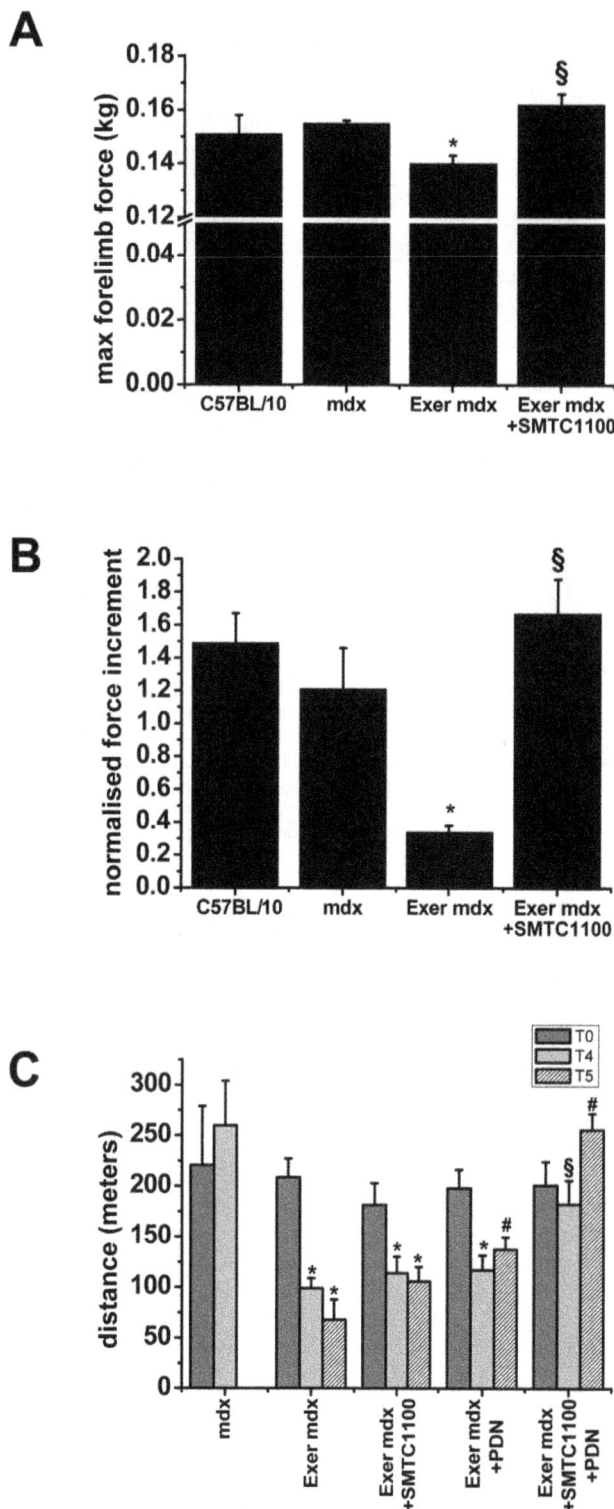

Figure 6. Effect of SMT C1100 on *in vivo* parameters of exercised *mdx* mice. (A) Maximal fore limb strength after 4 weeks of either exercise and/or drug treatment. The values are mean ± SEM from the number of animals shown in each bar (B) Normalized force increment, i.e. difference between the mean values of normalized fore limb strength at time 4 and at time 0. Normalized force values have been calculated for each mouse as the ratio of maximal fore limb strength to mouse body weight. The values are mean ± SE. The SE of ΔNF has been calculated as detailed elsewhere [14,21]. For (A) and (B) statistical significance between groups was evaluated by ANOVA test

for multiple comparison (F-values) and Bonferroni t-test *post hoc* correction. Significantly different versus *sedentary mdx and [§]Exer *mdx*; p<0.05; (C) Resistance to treadmill running, calculated as the maximal distance the mouse can run when undergoing a single bout of treadmill exercise. The values are mean ± SEM from 3–7 mice and show the maximal distance run (in meters) at T0 (start of forced exercise and dosing) and after four (T4) and five weeks (T5). Statistical significance between groups was evaluated by ANOVA test for multiple comparison (F-values) and Bonferroni t-test *post hoc* correction. Highly significant differences were observed between groups and within groups at the different ages (F>10; p<0.005). The symbols show statistical differences *versus sedentary *mdx* at T4 and #versus vehicle-treated exercised *mdx* at either T4 or T5 (p<0.05 and less).

degeneration. In SMT C1100-treated EDL muscle fibres the strength-duration curve describing the mechanical threshold was significantly shifted toward the more positive membrane potential values and almost overlapped with that observed in wildtype myofibres (Fig. 7A). The rheobase value of SMT C1100-treated muscles approached the wild type value (−69.3±0.4 mV), and was approximately 5 mV less negative than that of non-treated exercised group (−70.5±1.2 mV vs. −75±1.5 mV: p<0.05 by Student's t test). Interestingly, this parameter is not ameliorated by a partial increase in dystrophin expression by gentamicin treatment [21]. Similarly, the ratio between twitch and tetanic tension was significantly reduced in SMT C1100-treated exercised *mdx* EDL muscles with respect to untreated counterparts, again demonstrating that SMT C1100 treatment generates similar values to those typically found in wild type EDL muscle (Fig. 7B). The amelioration of calcium-dependent parameters was paralleled by a partial, although significant, 18% decrease in the cytosolic Ca^{2+} level, as determined by fura-2 microspectrofluorimetry [14] (data not shown), thus corroborating that the sarcolemmal bound utrophin stimulated by SMT C1100 treatment can improve calcium-mediate mechanotransduction signalling.

Discussion

This manuscript illustrates the effectiveness of dosing a well-established mouse model of DMD with a novel oral utrophin upregulator for several weeks. SMT C1100 induces increased levels of utrophin RNA in human muscle cells and significantly reduces dystrophin-deficient muscle pathology to such an extent that significant benefit on whole body strength and endurance is observed. Currently PDN and deflazacort are the only drugs approved by the regulatory authorities for the treatment of DMD. We believe that fatigue testing of *mdx* after a regime of forced exercise is a good surrogate for the primary clinical endpoint which will be used in DMD trials, *i.e.* in the 6MWD. Dosing with SMT C1100 alone demonstrated significant benefit in this surrogate model, and the 50% increase in the distance walked would have achieved the required efficacy endpoint if translated over to the 6MWD in DMD trials. Combining doses of SMT C1100 and PDN for several weeks completely prevented fatigue in this model. Thus, the combination of the two drugs with presumed different modes of action protect the muscle from fatiguing with exercise, thereby allowing for significantly increased ambulation. High levels of long term steroid use have unwanted side effects, however a steroid sparing therapy (either reducing dose or frequency to alleviate the unwanted side effects) working synergistically with a utrophin upregulator, has the potential to become the new standard of care for all DMD patients.

These results show proof-of-principle for the development of small molecules able to increase levels of utrophin for the therapy of DMD. The great advantage of this approach is that it will be

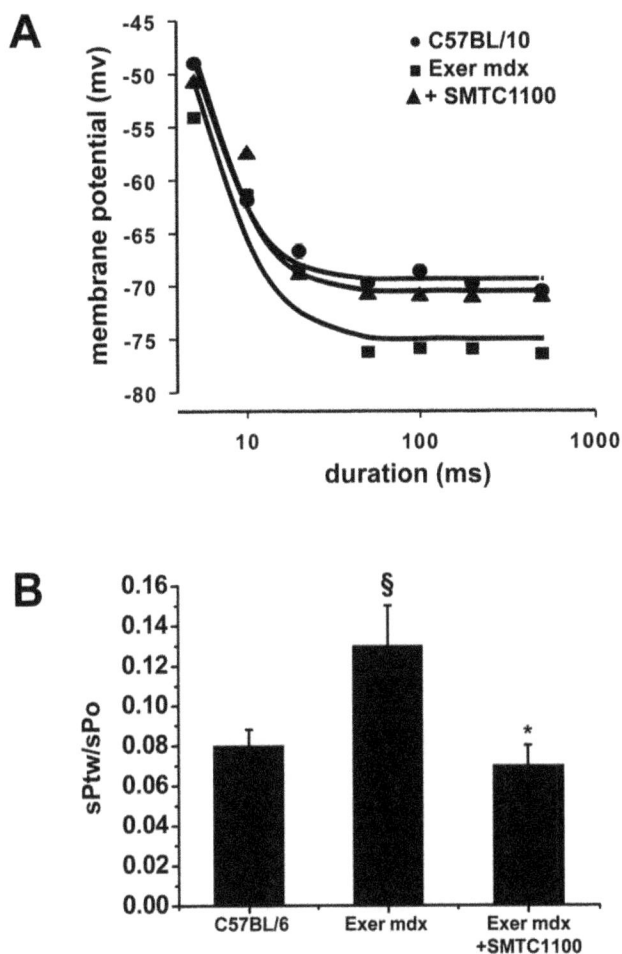

Figure 7. Effect of SMT C1100 treatment on calcium-dependent functional parameters of exercised *mdx* muscles. (A) Strength-duration curves describing the mechanical threshold of treated and/or untreated EDL muscle fibers. The values are means ±S.E.M. (from 10–45 fibers from 3–5 muscles) of the membrane potential at which contraction occurs in response to a depolarizing voltage step of variable duration (5–500 ms) by means of two microelectrode "point" voltage clamp method. The goodness-of-fit has been estimated by χ^2 analysis. Error bars are sometime not detectable if smaller than symbol size. Although not shown for graphical reasons, the threshold values of C1100 treated myofibres are significantly different with respect to those of untreated ones, at each pulse duration ($0.001<p<0.05$ by Student's t test); (B) ratio between twitch (sPtw) and tetanic tension, as mean ±S.E.M. from 5–7 EDL muscles. Significantly different *versus Exer *mdx*; $p<0.05$ and §versus sedentary *mdx*; $p<0.025$.

possible to treat all DMD and Becker patients, irrespective of their dystrophin mutation. In addition, it could also be used in combination with existing/novel strategies in the future, including utrophin stabilisation strategies such as biglycan.

In choosing a dosing route, an orally bioavailable product to be taken at home would be the ideal preference. In short, SMT C1100 has the perfect profile - an oral drug suitable for treating all DMD patients. In the recent clinical trial sponsored by BioMarin, after repeat dosing SMT C1100 (BMN-195) achieved low plasma exposure. This is frequently a problem in Phase I trials and issues of low exposure can often be addressed by developing new formulations of the drug to increase bioavailability. From the data presented here, only modest plasma levels of around 0.5 µM SMT C1100 maintained over several hours are sufficient to generate enough utrophin for substantial benefit. This strongly supports the importance of retesting new formulations of SMT C1100 in new Phase I clinical trials with a view to progressing to DMD patient trials.

Acknowledgments

We thank Covance for designing and conducting the safety evaluation programme for SMT C1100. For the study on exercised *mdx* mice we thank Dr. Karina Litvinova and Dr. Valeriana Sblendorio for assistance with the physiology and in vivo experiments, respectively, Dr. Antonella Liantonio for fura-2 microspectofluometry and Prof. Beatrice Nico for supervision on immunofluorescence and morphological studies. We acknowledge Charles J. Sherr, M.D., Ph.D., a Howard Hughes Medical Institute Investigator at St. Jude Children's Research Hospital, Memphis, USA, who developed the retroviral vector pSRalphaMSV-CDK4-tkneo used to generate the human DMD cell line provided by Vincent Mouly and Gillian Butler-Browne (Institute of Myology, Paris). We further acknowledge Prof. Steve Davies and Dr. Angela Russell (Chemistry Research Laboratories, Oxford University) who performed the initial pilot compound screens. We are grateful to the Medical Research Council, Muscular Dystrophy Campaign, Muscular Dystrophy Association USA and the Association Francaise contre les Myopathies for support of the work in Oxford. The support of Telethon-Italy (project GGP05130) for part of the work conducted in Bari is also gratefully acknowledged.

Author Contributions

Conceived and designed the experiments: JMT RJF KED AC RFC ADL RS FXW. Performed the experiments: RJF ACP SES DSP FJW AL SPW AC RFC. Analyzed the data: JMT RJF ACP SES DSP KED AC RFC ADL RS FJW FXW. Wrote the paper: JMT RJF ADL KED. Obtained permission to use the retroviral vector pSRalphaMSV-CDK4-tkneo used to generate the human DMD cell line: RJF.

References

1. Bogdanovich S, Perkins KJ, Krag TO, Khurana TS (2004) Therapeutics for Duchenne muscular dystrophy: current approaches and future directions. J Mol Med 82: 102–15.
2. Khurana TS, Davies KE (2003) Pharmacological strategies for muscular dystrophy. Nat Rev Drug Discov 2: 379–90.
3. McDonald CM, Henricson EK, Han JJ, Abresch RT, Nicorici A, et al. The 6-minute walk test as a new outcome measure in Duchenne muscular dystrophy. Muscle Nerve 41: 500–10.
4. Goemans NM, Tulinius M, Buyse G, Wilson R, de Kimpe R, et al. (2010) 24 week follow-up data from a phase I/IIa extension study of PRO051/GSK2402968 in subjects with Duchenne muscular dystrophy. Neuromusc Disord 20: 639.
5. Shrewsbury SB, Cirak S, Guglieri M, Bushby K, Muntoni F (2010) Current progress and preliminary results with the systemic administration trial of AVI-4658, a novel phosphorodiamidate morpholino oligomer (PMO) skipping dystrophin exon 51 in Duchenne muscular dystrophy (DMD). Neuromuscular Disorders 20: 639–640.
6. Goyenvalle A, Babbs A, Powell D, Kole R, Fletcher S, et al. (2009) Prevention of Dystrophic Pathology in Severely Affected Dystrophin/Utrophin-deficient Mice by Morpholino-oligomer-mediated Exon-skipping. Mol Ther 18: 198–205.
7. Beroud C, Tuffery-Giraud S, Matsuo M, Hamroun D, Humbertclaude V, et al. (2007) Multiexon skipping leading to an artificial DMD protein lacking amino acids from exons 45 through 55 could rescue up to 63% of patients with Duchenne muscular dystrophy. Hum Mutat 28: 196–202.

8. Amenta AR, Yilmaz A, Bogdanovich S, McKechnie BA, Abedi M, et al. (2011) Biglycan recruits utrophin to the sarcolemma and counters dystrophic pathology in *mdx* mice. Proc Natl Acad Sci U S A 108: 762–7.

9. Krag TO, Bogdanovich S, Jensen CJ, Fischer MD, Hansen-Schwartz J, et al. (2004) Heregulin ameliorates the dystrophic phenotype in *mdx* mice. Proc Natl Acad Sci U S A 101: 13856–60.

10. Peter AK, Marshall JL, Crosbie RH (2008) Sarcospan reduces dystrophic pathology: stabilization of the utrophin-glycoprotein complex. J Cell Biol 183: 419–27.

11. Mattei E, Corbi N, Di Certo MG, Strimpakos G, Severini C, et al. (2007) Utrophin up-regulation by an artificial transcription factor in transgenic mice. PLoS ONE 2: e774.

12. Tinsley J, Deconinck N, Fisher R, Kahn D, Phelps S, et al. (1998) Expression of full-length utrophin prevents muscular dystrophy in *mdx* mice. Nat Med 4: 1441–4.

13. Morgan JE, Beauchamp JR, Pagel CN, Peckham M, Ataliotis P, et al. (1994) Myogenic cell lines derived from transgenic mice carrying a thermolabile T antigen: a model system for the derivation of tissue-specific and mutation-specific cell lines. Dev Biol 162: 486–98.

14. De Luca A, Pierno S, Liantonio A, Cetrone M, Camerino C, et al. (2003) Enhanced dystrophic progression in *mdx* mice by exercise and beneficial effects of taurine and insulin-like growth factor-1. J Pharmacol Exp Ther 304: 453–63.

15. Burdi R, Rolland JF, Fraysse B, Litvinova K, Cozzoli A, et al. (2009) Multiple pathological events in exercised dystrophic mdx mice are targeted by pentoxifylline: outcome of a large array of *in vivo* and *ex vivo* tests. J Appl Physiol 106: 1311–24.

16. Cooper ST, Lo HP, North KN (2003) Single section Western blot: improving the molecular diagnosis of the muscular dystrophies. Neurology 61: 93–7.

17. Squire S, Raymackers JM, Vandebrouck C, Potter A, Tinsley J, et al. (2002) Prevention of pathology in *mdx* mice by expression of utrophin: analysis using an inducible transgenic expression system. Hum Mol Genet 11: 3333–44.

18. Livak KJ, Schmittgen TD (2001) Analysis of relative gene expression data using real-time quantitative PCR and the 2(-Delta Delta C(T)) Method. Methods 25: 402–8.

19. Hirst RC, McCullagh KJ, Davies KE (2005) Utrophin upregulation in Duchenne muscular dystrophy. Acta Myol 24: 209–16.

20. Miura P, Jasmin BJ (2006) Utrophin upregulation for treating Duchenne or Becker muscular dystrophy: how close are we? Trends Mol Med 12: 122–9.

21. De Luca A, Nico B, Rolland JF, Cozzoli A, Burdi R, et al. (2008) Gentamicin treatment in exercised *mdx* mice: Identification of dystrophin-sensitive pathways and evaluation of efficacy in work-loaded dystrophic muscle. Neurobiol Dis 32: 243–53.

15

The Influence of Therapeutic Radiation on the Patterns of Bone Marrow in Ovary-Intact and Ovariectomized Mice

Susanta K. Hui[1,3]*, Leslie Sharkey[2,3], Louis S. Kidder[3], Yan Zhang[3], Greg Fairchild[1], Kayti Coghill[1], Cory J. Xian[5], Douglas Yee[3,4]

1 Department of Therapeutic Radiology, Medical School, University of Minnesota, Minneapolis, Minnesota, United States of America, 2 Department of Veterinary Clinical Sciences, College of Veterinary Medicine, University of Minnesota, St. Paul, Minnesota, United States of America, 3 Masonic Cancer Center, University of Minnesota, Minneapolis, Minnesota, United States of America, 4 Department of Medicine, Medical School, University of Minnesota, Minneapolis, Minnesota, United States of America, 5 Sansom Institute, School of Pharmacy and Medical Sciences, University of South Australia, Adelaide, South Australia, Australia

Abstract

Background: The functional components of bone marrow (i.e., the hematopoietic and stromal populations) and the adjacent bone have traditionally been evaluated incompletely as distinct entities rather than the integrated system. We perturbed this system *in vivo* using a medically relevant radiation model in the presence or absence of ovarian function to understand integrated tissue interaction.

Methodology/Principal Findings: Ovary-intact and ovariectomized mice underwent either no radiation or single fractional 16 Gy radiation to the caudal skeleton (I±R, OVX±R). Marrow fat, hematopoietic cellularity, and cancellous bone volume fraction (BV/TV %) were assessed. Ovariectomy alone did not significantly reduce marrow cellularity in non-irradiated mice (OVX−R vs. I−R, p = 0.8445) after 30 days; however it impaired the hematopoietic recovery of marrow following radiation exposure (OVX+R vs. I+R, p = 0.0092). The combination of radiation and OVX dramatically increases marrow fat compared to either factor alone (p = 0.0062). The synergistic effect was also apparent in the reduction of hematopoietic marrow cellularity (p = 0.0661); however it was absent in BV/TV% changes (p = 0.2520). The expected inverse relationship between marrow adiposity vs. hematopoietic cellularity and bone volume was observed. Interestingly compared with OVX mice, intact mice demonstrated double the reduction in hematopoietic cellularity and a tenfold greater degree of bone loss for a given unit of expansion in marrow fat.

Conclusions/Significance: Ovariectomy prior to delivery of a clinically-relevant focal radiation exposure in mice, exacerbated post-radiation adipose accumulation in the marrow space but blunted bone loss and hematopoietic suppression. In the normally coupled homeostatic relationship between the bone and marrow domains, OVX appears to alter feedback mechanisms. Confirmation of this non-linear phenomenon (presumably due to differential radiosensitivity) and demonstration of the mechanism of action is needed to provide strategies to diminish the effect of radiation on exposed tissues.

Editor: Ganesh Chandra Jagetia, Mizoram University, India

Funding: This work was supported by the National Institutes of Health grants (1R01CA154491-01, 1R03AR055333-01A1 and 1K12-HD055887-01). This work was also supported by PHS Cancer Center Support Grant P30 CA77398 and the Minnesota Medical Foundation (MMF). Susanta K. Hui is a scholar of the BIRCWH (Building Interdisciplinary Careers in Women's Health) program. The funders had no role in study design, data collection and analysis, decision to publish, or preparation of the manuscript.

Competing Interests: The authors have declared that no competing interests exist.

* E-mail: huixx019@umn.edu

Introduction

Radiation is a common treatment modality for almost all cancers. However the impact of irradiation on normal bone and bone marrow and their interactions are not well characterized, despite the importance of understanding the complications of treatment due to the increasing number of long-term cancer survivors. Women in particular may experience accelerated bone loss from anti-cancer therapy (e.g. chemotherapy, endocrine therapy, radiation, chemo-radiation) [1], primarily due to the varying status of the ovarian hormones. Women who undergo

cancer therapy experience a 10–20% increased fracture risk from treatment-induced bone loss compared to healthy patients [2,3]. Furthermore, recovery from skeletal damage induced by radiation in women with differing ovarian function (i.e., pre- and post-menopausal) may have variable responses to anti-resorptive therapy [4]. Thus, we hypothesize that damage and subsequent recovery of the bone and bone marrow after irradiation may depend on ovarian status. This clinical question highlights the importance of fundamental biological investigations into the relationships of bone, marrow components (hemopoietic marrow measured by cellularity, stromal marrow measure by adiposity), and how they are impacted by physiological factors and the treatment of disease.

In the past, bone and hematopoietic tissues have been considered distinct entities, with bone merely providing a physical scaffold for the hematopoietic precursors of the marrow. More recent work emphasizes critical bidirectional biochemical and mechanical communications through which bone metabolism and hematopoiesis are linked [5,6]. This suggests that a more integrated approach to the understanding of radiation-induced injury to these tissues is necessary and emphasizes the interface between basic biology and translational applications in clinical medicine. Mesenchymal stromal cells (MSC) residing in the marrow space give rise to cellular populations of the marrow microenvironment, such as osteoblasts and adipocytes. Because of their pluripotent capability, there has long been an assumption MSC phenotype directly influences bone – related parameters, i.e., increasing marrow adipogenesis is inversely proportional with bone mass [7–10]. MSCs additionally act as key regulators of hematopoiesis. There is evidence that MSC abnormalities contribute to the pathology of hematopoietic diseases, such as myelodysplastic syndrome [11]; that they may play a role in hematopoietic recovery after radiation injury [12]; and that they influence hematopoietic recovery after transplantation [13].

Given advancements in radiation therapy, including radiation-based conditioning regimens for bone marrow transplantation, a comprehensive evaluation of the effects on bone and marrow and their interactions will be crucial for the optimization of therapeutic protocols and the application of rational strategies for patient management. In general, marrow adiposity is shown to be negatively correlated to osteogenic potential [14–17]. These tissue level interactions must be clarified if more in depth investigations of molecular mechanisms are to be undertaken in terms of the relevant biology of the system in disease states. In the current study, we evaluated the effects of clinically relevant doses of radiation on patterns of bone marrow changes in murine models over time, and measured the influence of ovarian function on radiation induced changes in hematopoiesis, adipogenesis and bone mass.

Methods

Four groups of skeletally mature BALB/c female mice (16 weeks old) were used for this study. The schematic representation of the design of this study is described by Figure 1. The first experiment characterized the response of the hematopoietic space to a clinically relevant dose of radiation in intact female mice to establish the kinetics of hematopoietic recovery in the presence of normal ovarian function. The second experiment evaluated the response of bone and hematopoietic marrow space 30 days after radiation exposure in both ovary-intact (I) and ovariectomized (OVX) mice, which were utilized to mimic the clinical management of pre-menopausal and menopausal (spontaneous or induced) cancer patients undergoing radiation therapy (R), with appropriate controls. OVX mice were ovariectomized by the vendor 57 days prior to irradiation (Jackson Laboratory; Bar Harbor, ME). The day of radiation is designated Day 0. Mice were randomly divided into the following groups: 1) "I−R" (intact no radiation, n = 5, 5 and 7 sacrificed at day 3, 8 and 30; 2) "I+R" (intact irradiated, n = 5, 5 and 9 sacrificed at day 3, 8 and 30); 3) "OVX−R" (OVX no radiation, n = 7 sacrificed at day 30); and 4) "OVX+R" (OVX irradiated, n = 8 sacrificed at day 30). This study was approved by the University of Minnesota Institutional Animal Care and Use Committee (IACUC).

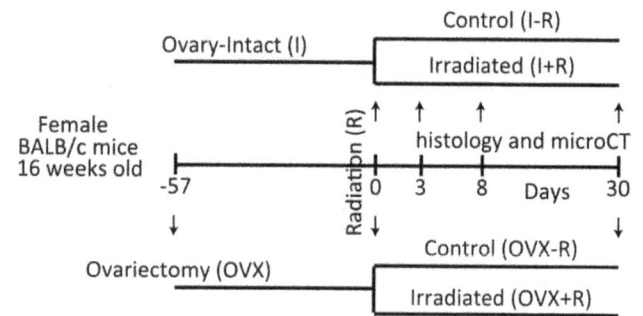

Figure 1. Experimental Plan Schematic. Sixteen week old BALB/c mice were ovariectomized (OVX) and maintained in the vivarium for 57 days in order to attain skeletal hemostasis. Both intact (I) and OVX mice were then irradiated with 16Gy delivered to the caudal skeleton or maintained as controls. Groups of animals were euthanized at 3, 8, and 30 days post irradiation in order to perform histological evaluations of the distal femur; microCT measurements were conducted at the 30 day time point only.

Animal Husbandry

Mice were weighed prior to irradiation and daily following irradiation for 10 days, as well as prior to placement in metabolic collection cages. Mice were housed 3–5 per cage, in a temperature- and humidity-controlled room with free access to a standard rodent chow containing 18.6% protein, 1% calcium, and 1.5 IU/g vitamin D_3 (2018; Harlan Teklad, Madison, WI) and water. Mice were acclimated to a 12-hour light/dark cycle. There was small weight loss (0.5 to 1gm) in radiation group compared to non-irradiated group as expected. This small change in body weight however is not expected to affect the results of our study.

Radiation Delivery

Details of radiation delivery are described by our previous publication [4]. Briefly, all mice in the I+R and OVX+R groups were anesthetized using a 0.05 mL intraperitoneal injection of a cocktail of 2.0 mL ketamine, 0.2 mL xylazine (100 mg/mL), and 1.8 mL sterile saline. All mice in the I−R and OVX−R groups were also anesthetized to control for the possible impact of anesthesia. A 16 Gy (single fraction) radiation was delivered in mice at the hind limb by a Philips RT250 orthovoltage unit. A specially designed lead shield was used to limit radiation to only the hind limbs. Proper placement of shielding was confirmed using Kodak EDR-2 film and total dose delivered was verified using micro thermo-luminescent dosimeters (micro-TLD).

Ovariectomy verification

Wet uterine weights of mice from the I±R and OVX±R groups were measured immediately post-mortem to verify efficacy of vendor-performed ovariectomy surgeries. Ovary-intact mice had a median wet uterine weight of 0.057 g, which was significantly greater than that of 0.014 g for ovariectomized mice (Wilcoxon rank-sum test, p = 0.0003).

MicroCT

Bone microarchitecture of mice was analyzed with a microCT Scanner (μCT 35, Cone-Beam microCT, Scanco Medical, Switzerland). The distal femoral metaphysis was scanned within a region of 0.3–1.0 mm from the growth plate in order to avoid the primary spongiosa, with a slice thickness of 7 μm resolution (100 slices) at 70 kVp. Using the manufacturer's software, cancellous bone regions of interest (ROIs) were drawn (see

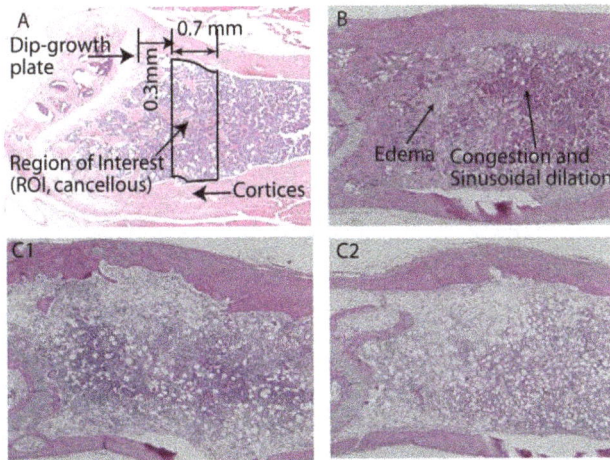

Figure 2. Schematic representation of bone and marrow. A. region of interest in sagittal view of a normal control mouse. B. Sagittal section of bone marrow from an intact mouse 8 days post-irradiation. Note the areas of congestion and sinusoidal dilation characterized by increased density of red blood cell within the expanded vascular spaces; also present are areas of edema characterized by increased volume of pale pink fluid in the interstitial spaces. C. Sagittal sections of bone marrow 30 days after irradiation in intact (C1) and OVX (C2) mice. Note the more intensely purple areas indicative of higher hematopoietic activity in C1 compared with C2, as well as expanded adipose in C2 compared with C1.

Figure 2 A). The cancellous bone is composed of trabecular bone matrix and marrow. The cancellous bone volume fraction (BV/TV %; i.e. the ratio of the segmented trabecular bone volume to the total tissue volume of the region of interest) of the ROI was estimated.

Histology

The left hind limb of each mouse was dissected. Following μCT scanning, the distal femur was collected, fixed in 10% formalin for 24 h, decalcified in Immunocal (a mild formic acid solution; Decal Corp, Tallman, NY) at 4°C until soft, processed and embedded in paraffin wax. Paraffin sections of 4 μm thick were mounted on glass slides for histological analysis. Complete sagittal sections of mouse femur were stained with hematoxylin and eosin (H&E) and were evaluated using standard procedures by a board certified veterinary clinical pathologist experienced in bone marrow evaluation (LS) [18–20]. Briefly, the hemopoietic cellularity (abbreviated as cellularity for the remainder of the manuscript) of the hematopoietic space was visually estimated and scored as a percentage of the total two dimensional area. The numbers of megakaryocytes were estimated as normal, mildly decreased, decreased, or markedly decreased. The ratio of myeloid to erythroid precursors (M:E ratio) was scored as normal, mildly increased, increased, or markedly increased. If the overall cellularity was ≤5%, the numbers of hematopoietic precursors were considered too low to accurately estimate the M:E ratio and no estimate was undertaken. Figure 2 illustrates congestion, sinusoidal dilation, and edema that were observed transiently after radiation (2B), as well as variations in hematopoietic cellularity and % adipose tissue observed on day 30 of the protocol (2C).

The maturation of hematopoietic precursors was assessed as normal or left shifted (i.e., less differentiated), indicating an abnormal number of relatively immature precursors relative to more mature forms. If the overall cellularity was ≤5%, the

progression of maturation could not be accurately assessed and no evaluation was conducted. The presence of morphologic abnormalities including sinusoidal dilation, edema, congestion, inflammation, necrosis, fibrosis, vasculitis and increased hemosiderin was indicated as follows: 0 indicating abnormality was absent, 1+ mild, 2+ moderate, 3+ marked and 4+ severe changes. Endosteal lining cells were classified as normal or plump (i.e., activated).

Marrow fat measurement

The number and percent adipocyte area (as a percentage of field) were determined from a histological section scan by a single observer using Adobe Photoshop CS5 (version 12.0.4). Reported values were then averaged for each treatment group.

Statistical Analysis

For ovary-intact mice, two-way ANOVA with Tukey's post tests was used to evaluate the effects of radiation, time and their interaction on bone marrow hematopoietic cellularity. Megakaryocyte, myeloid: erythroid ratio, sinusoidal dilation, congestion and edema were analyzed using Kruskal-Wallis test for the comparisons across three time points in each of the I-R and I+R arms, and Wilcoxon rank-sum test for the comparisons between two time points in the same arm and between non-irradiated and irradiated arms at the same time point.

Comparisons between ovary-intact and ovariectomized mice were limited to Day 30 because ovariectomized mice had been measured for that time-point only. Wilcoxon rank-sum test was used for the comparisons between radiation treatments for the same type of mice and between different types of mice given the same radiation treatment for megakaryocyte, myeloid:erythroid ratio, congestion and fibrosis.

To understand the interrelationships between hematopoiesis, adipogenesis and bone, two-factor multivariate analysis of variance (MANOVA) was conducted for Day 30 hematopoietic cellularity, marrow fat, and BV/TV. Factors including ovary status, radiation exposure, and their interaction were considered in the MANOVA model. Correlation between every two tissue components was evaluated by partial correlation coefficient. Following the MANOVA, two-way ANOVA was performed for individual tissue components and Tukey's post tests were used for multiple comparisons.

For Kruskal-Wallis and Wilcoxon rank-sum tests, unadjusted p values are reported and subject to adjustment by Bonferroni's method. For Tukey's post tests, adjusted p values are reported. All the analyses were conducted using SAS 9.2 (SAS Institute Inc., Cary, NC, USA).

Results

Time course of the hematopoietic response to radiation in intact female mice

In ovary-intact mice, we established that exposure to radiation resulted in marked hypocellularity of the hematopoietic components of the marrow by Day 3 (mean = 3.2%), with considerable recovery but still very low hematopoietic activity on Day 8 (mean = 12.8%, p = 0.0292 when comparing to Day 3) and marked but still incomplete recovery of hematopoietic activity with normal precursor maturation at Day 30 (mean = 72%, p<0.0001 when comparing to both Day3 and Day 8) (See Figure 3). Over the same time course, there was no change in hematopoietic cellularity in the I−R mice (mean = 95.4%, 94.6% and 96.2% for Day 3, 8 and 30, respectively) (Figure 3). As expected, megakaryocyte numbers were significantly depressed by radiation exposure on Days 3 (median scale = −3) and 8 (median scale = −3), with a trend towards ongoing suppression on Day 30 (median scale = −1) (Table 1). Although too few hematopoietic precursors were available for interpretation in the markedly hypocellular Day 3 post-irradiation marrow, the recovery phase was accompanied by significantly increased myeloid to erythroid ratios (median scale = 2 on Day 8 and = 1 on Day 30) characterized by persistent erythroid hypoplasia (Table 1). Radiation resulted in concurrent vascular abnormalities in the marrow space, including moderate to marked sinusoidal dilation and venous congestion that were mostly resolved by Day 30, and transient edema on Day 8 (Table 2). Endosteal lining cells were transiently plump in 4/5 mice on Day 3 only. Increased hemosiderin (iron pigment) was observed in 3/5 irradiated mice and fibrosis in 2/5 irradiated mice on Day 30 only. These changes were not associated with evidence of inflammation in the marrow space.

Hematopoietic response to radiation and OVX on day 30 post-irradiation

Radiation significantly decreased hematopoietic cellularity in intact mice (p = 0.0002), however it resulted in more severe suppression of hematopoietic cellularity in OVX mice (p<0.0001). The interaction between radiation and ovarian function was close to significance (F = 3.93, p = 0.0661) (See Table 3). Effects were similar on megakaryocytes: radiation exposure significantly decreased megakaryocyte numbers for both ovary-intact and OVX mice (p = 0.0450 and 0.0217, respectively), but the effect was exacerbated by absence of ovarian hormones (I+R vs. OVX+R, p = 0.0255) (Table 4). The myeloid to erythroid ratio was increased due to erythroid hypoplasia in irradiated mice regardless of hormonal status (p = 0.0236 and 0.0182) (Table 4).

There was mild residual congestion due to irradiation in ovary-intact mice (p = 0.0495), but this was not observed in OVX mice (p = 0.1336). Irradiation-induced mild fibrosis was observed in OVX mice (p = 0.0143) but not in ovary-intact mice (p = 0.1336). Ovarian hormones did not play a significant role on the development of congestion and fibrosis with or without irradiation (p = 0.2207–1.0000 respectively) (Table 5).

Impact of radiation and OVX on marrow fat and cancellous bone on day 30

Radiation did not significantly increase the marrow adipose content of intact mice (p = 0.1203), however radiation did significantly increase marrow adipose in OVX mice (p<0.0001). OVX significantly increased marrow adipose content in the absence of radiation (p = 0.0132) and with radiation (p<0.0001) (See Table 3). Correspondingly, the interaction between OVX and radiation significantly influenced marrow adipose level (F = 10.14, p = 0.0062). On the other hand, radiation alone significantly reduced BV/TV% (p = 0.0467), but OVX had no additive effects on BV/TV % (OVX*radiation interaction, F = 1.42, p = 0.2520). Collectively, radiation caused a disproportionate increase in marrow adiposity in OVX mice compared with intact animals, but previous ovariectomy did not influence the effect of radiation on BV/TV%, thus demonstrating a dissociation between the regulation of marrow adipose content and bone volume.

Integration of hematopoiesis, adipogenesis, and bone volume

Overall, hematopoietic cellularity and marrow fat content were negatively correlated (partial correlation coefficient = −0.30,

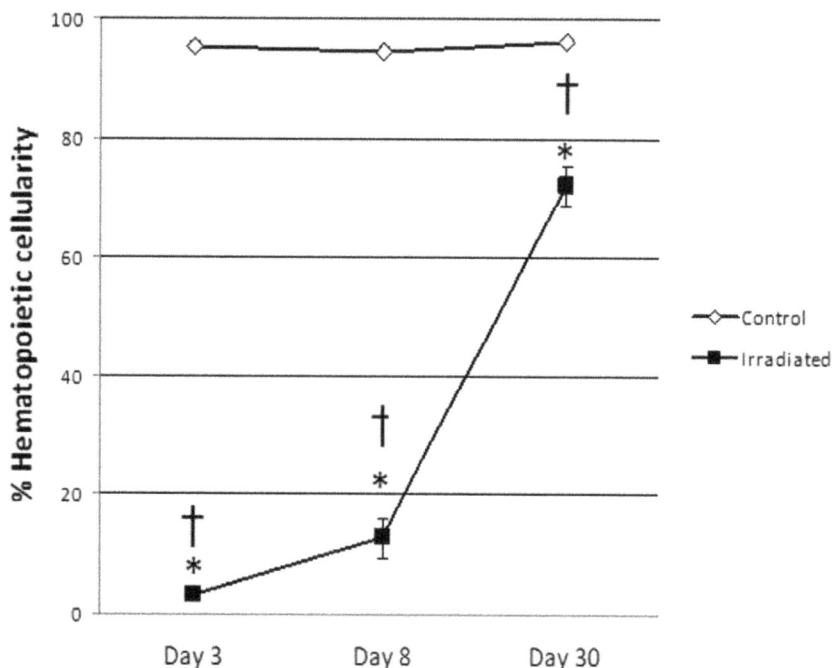

Figure 3. Percent of the marrow space (mean ±SEM) occupied by hematopoietic precursors in intact control (I−R) and irradiated (I+R) mice estimated by visual inspection by a board certified veterinary clinical pathologist (LS) employing standard protocols. Radiation caused marked hypocellularity of the hematopoietic components of the marrow by Day 3, with significant increases but still very low hematopoietic activity on Day 8 and marked but still incomplete recovery of hematopoietic activity with normal precursor maturation at Day 30. There were no changes over time in non-irradiated animals. Two-way ANOVA with Tukey's post-tests: * Irradiated mice had significantly lower cellularity than control mice of the same day, p<0.0001, † Cellularity of irradiated mice increased significantly from Day 3 through Day 30, p: 0.0292 – <0.0001.

Table 1. Megakaryocyte number and myeloid: erythroid ratio in intact control (I−R) and irradiated (I+R) mice estimated by a board certified veterinary clinical pathologist (LS) according to standard protocols.

Treatment	Day	Megakaryocytes					Myeloid:Erythroid ratio				
Control	3	N	N	N	N	N	N	N	N	N	N
	8	N	N	N	N	N	N	N	N	N	N
	30	N	N	N	N	N	N	N	N	N	N
Irradiated	3*	−3	−3	−3	−3	−3	NA	NA	NA	NA	NA
	8*†	−3	−3	−3	−2	−2	+2	+2	+2	+2	+2
	30*†	−1	−1	−1	−1	N	+2	+2	+1	+1	+1

Cells contain the data for individual mice (n = 5/group); N = normal, NA = too few cells to reliably estimate. Numerical scale: −4 severely decreased, −3 markedly decreased, −2 moderately decreased, −1 mildly decreased, +1 mildly increased, +2 moderately increased, +3 markedly increased, +4 severely increased, normal assigned a value of 0 for statistical calculations. Megakaryocyte numbers were significantly depressed by radiation exposure on Days 3 and 8, with a trend towards ongoing suppression on Day 30. Too few hematopoietic precursors were available for interpretation in the markedly hypocellular Day 3 post-irradiation marrow, but the recovery phase was accompanied by significantly increased myeloid to erythroid ratios characterized by persistent erythroid hypoplasia. Wilcoxon rank-sum test:
*Megakaryocytes, Irradiated significantly decreased compared with Control of the same day, Day 3, p = 0.0182; Day 8, p = 0.0236; Day 30, p = 0.0450.
†Myeloid:Erythroid ratio, Irradiation significantly increased when compared with Control, Day8, p = 0.0182; Day 30, p = 0.0236.

p = 0.2616), hematopoietic cellularity and BV/TV% were positively correlated (partial correlation coefficient = 0.12, p = 0.6587), and marrow fat and BV/TV% were negatively correlated (partial correlation coefficient = −0.13, p = 0.6328), however, none of these correlations achieved statistical significance.

To help understand the effect of radiation in the presence or absence of ovarian function on the interrelationships between hematopoiesis, adipogenesis, and bone, we calculated radiation-induced changes in each tissue relative to the other two components for ovary-intact and OVX mice based on Figure 4. First we calculated the differences in least squares means of the three tissue components between non-irradiated and irradiated mice in the ovary intact and OVX groups, respectively. Then we calculated the following 3 ratios for each ovarian function group: difference of % BV/TV over that of % marrow fat, difference of % hematopoietic cellularity over that of % marrow fat, and difference of % BV/TV over that of % hematopoietic cellularity. Mathematically these ratios are the slopes of blue and red lines in Figure 4. They indicate the amount of change in one tissue component per unit change in another tissue component.

Specifically, intact mice demonstrate a 1.2% reduction in bone volume for every % increase in marrow adipose after radiation.

OVX mice only demonstrate a 0.1% decrease in bone volume for every % increase in marrow adipose with radiation treatment. This represents a ten-fold reduction in bone volume loss per % increase in marrow fat when comparing OVX with intact mice (Figure 4, Panel A). Intact mice demonstrate a 0.1% reduction in bone volume for every 1% decrease in hematopoietic cellularity after radiation, however OVX mice show only a 0.02% reduction in bone volume for the same 1% loss of hematopoietic cellularity after radiation. OVX appears to blunt the rate of bone volume loss relative to reduced hematopoietic cellularity after radiation treatment by a factor of 6 (Figure 4, Panel B). Collectively, OVX seems to reduce the responsiveness of bone volume to changes in marrow components, with a greater change in sensitivity to adipose than hematopoiesis. Lastly, intact mice demonstrate a 9.9% reduction in hematopoietic cellularity for every 1% increase in marrow fat after radiation, while OVX results in a 5.1% reduction in hematopoietic cellularity for every 1% increase in marrow fat, approximately a half of the radiation effect for intact mice (Figure 4, Panel C).

Discussion/Conclusions

This study was designed to gain insight into the integrated responses of bone and marrow in a laboratory rodent model of

Table 2. Semi-quantitative assessment of vascular abnormalities in intact control (I−R) and irradiated (I+R) mice estimated by a board certified veterinary clinical pathologist (LS) according to standard protocols.

Treatment	Day	Sinusoidal Dilation						Congestion					Edema			
Control	3	0	0	0	0	0	0	0	0	0	0	0	0	0	0	0
	8	0	0	0	0	0	0	0	0	0	0	0	0	0	0	0
	30	0	0	0	0	0	0	0	0	0	0	0	0	0	0	0
Irradiated	3*†	+3	+3	+2	+2	+2	+2	+2	+1	+1	+3	+1	0	0	0	0
	8*†‡	+2	+2	+2	+2	+2	+3	+2	+2	+2	+2	+2	+2	+1	+1	0
	30	+1	+1	0	0	0	+1	+1	+1	0	0	0	0	0	0	0

Numerical scale: 0 not present, +1 mild, +2 moderate, +3 marked, +4 severe. Radiation caused moderate to marked sinusoidal dilation and venous congestion on days 3 and 8 that was mostly resolved by Day 30, and transient edema on Day 8. Wilcoxon rank-sum test:
*Irradiated (marginally) significantly greater sinusoidal dilation compared with control of the same day, Day 3, p = 0.0507; Day 8, p = 0.0182.
†Irradiated significantly greater vascular congestion compared with control of the same day, Day3, p = 0.0247; Day8, p = 0.0217.
‡Irradiated marginally significantly greater edema compared with control of the same day, Day 8, p = 0.0507.

Table 3. Comparison of group least squares means (± SEM) of hematopoietic cellularity, adiposity, and bone volume in intact (I) and ovariectomized (OVX) mice without radiation (−R) and with radiation (+R) 30 days after radiation treatment.

Treatment group	% Hematopoietic cellularity (SEM)	% Adipose (SEM)	%BV/TV (SEM)
I−R	96.2 (3.0)[a]	1.11 (0.72)[a]	5.61 (0.86)
I+R	72.0 (3.0)[a,c]	3.55 (0.72)[b]	2.63 (0.86)
OVX−R	93.0 (3.4)[b]	4.97 (0.81)[a,c]	4.53 (0.96)
OVX+R	56.0 (3.0)[b,c]	12.14 (0.72)[b,c]	3.66 (0.86)

Within columns, identical letters indicate relevant statistically significant differences between groups at p≤0.001). Radiation significantly reduced hematopoietic cellularity in intact mice, but the effect was more severe in OVX (interaction F = 4.79, p = 0.0439). OVX alone had no effect on hematopoietic activity in the absence of radiation. Radiation significantly increased marrow adipose only in OVX (interaction F = 10.14, p = 0.0062), and OVX increased marrow fat without and with radiation treatment. Radiation significantly reduced BV/TV% (p = 0.0467), but OVX had no additive effect. All statistical analyses were based on two-way ANOVA.

pre- and post-menopausal patients undergoing therapeutic radiation. New research strongly supports bidirectional coregulation of bone and marrow components at the micro-environmental level, attesting to the importance of evaluating these tissues as an integrated unit in order to advance our understanding of the response to injury or physiologic change [5,21]. Our data demonstrated early and transient severe hematopoietic depletion and vascular pathology with later substantial but incomplete recovery 30 days after local irradiation in intact female mice. Furthermore, we showed that the proportionality of more chronic changes post-irradiation among the three tissue components of bone and marrow evaluated (hemopoietic, adipose, and osseous) was distinctly different depending upon the presence or absence of ovarian hormones. Multiple fold increases in the marrow fat fraction due to irradiation were not reflected in equivalent loss of either bone or hematopoietic cellularity in OVX compared with intact mice. OVX appeared to predispose the MSC population toward an adipogenic phenotype; radiation further enhanced adipogenesis in an additive fashion without proportional gross effects on the adjacent bone or hematopoietic cellularity.

As expected, irradiation in intact female mice resulted in significant and persistent decreases in hematopoietic cellularity activity of the bone marrow and increased marrow fat, although subjectively there appeared to be sufficient residual hematopoietic activity to support life in our study animals. These findings are similar to previously reported studies using male Wistar rats [22], which demonstrated early hematopoietic suppression coincident with sinusoidal dilation, and expansion of adipose in the more chronic phase (days 12–180). While specific proportional relation-

ships were not described in detail, the authors did observe that the degree of hematopoietic recovery relative to the degree of adipogenesis varied with the radiation protocol, suggesting that the frequently observed inverse relationship of hematopoiesis and adipogenesis in the marrow does not occur in fixed ratios in all situations. Other studies in mice have specifically demonstrated the detrimental effects of radiation on the in vitro proliferation of both hematopoietic and stromal bone marrow precursor cell populations that were detectable up to six months after explant of marrow stromal cells into culture [23]. Teasing out the relative impact of radiation damage to hematopoietic and mesenchymal precursor cells is confounded by an inability to isolate subcomponents within the complex matrix of the bone marrow microenvironment [24]. In addition, repair of radiation damage may be associated with migration of HSCs as well as MSCs from non-IR treated sites [24,25], further complicating interpretation. Due to our focus on tissue level interaction details in this manuscript, we envision series of future work in this model including mechanistic consideration for the expansion of adipose in the damaged marrow.

The current study found that OVX alone did not significantly reduce hematopoietic cellularity or bone volume while, while marrow fat content was increased. Expansion of the marrow adipose population is often associated with OVX in studies of rats and mice [26–28]. However, these investigators also report concurrent reductions in hematopoiesis or bone mineral density, describing a reciprocal relationship between marrow fat and hematopoiesis and bone. The degree of these changes is time dependent [27], so time and other experimental variables such as

Table 4. Megakaryocyte number and myeloid: erythroid ratio in intact (I) and ovariectomized (OVX) mice receiving either 0 (−R) or 16 Gy radiation (+R) 30 days previously.

Hormone status	Radiation	Megakaryocytes					Myeloid:Erythroid ratio				
Intact	0	0	0	0	0	0	0	0	0	0	0
	16 Gy*‡	−1	−1	−1	−1	0	+1	+1	+1	+2	+2
OVX	0	0	0	0	0	0	0	0	0	0	0
	16 Gy*†‡	−2	−2	−2	−2	−3	+1	+1	+1	+1	+1

Semi-quantitative estimates performed by a board certified veterinary clinical pathologist (LS) according to standard protocols. Cells contain the data for individual mice (n = 5/group). Numerical scale: −4 severely decreased, −3 markedly decreased, −2 moderately decreased, −1 mildly decreased, +1 mildly increased, +2 moderately increased, +3 markedly increased, +4 severely increased, normal assigned a value of 0 for statistical calculations. Wilcoxon rank-sum test:
*Radiation exposure significantly decreased megakaryocyte numbers compared with non-irradiated in both intact and OVX mice (p = 0.0450 and 0.0217, respectively), and
†OVX exacerbated the decrease in megakaryocytes after radiation exposure (I+R vs. OVX+R, p = 0.0255).
‡Myeloid:erythroid ratio was increased by irradiation in both intact and OVX mice (p = 0.0236 and 0.0182, respectively).

Table 5. Congestion and fibrosis in intact and ovariectomized (OVX) mice receiving either 0 or 16 Gy radiation 30 days previously.

Hormone status	Radiation	Congestion					Fibrosis				
Intact	0	0	0	0	0	0	0	0	0	0	0
	16 Gy*	+1	+1	+1	0	0	+1	+1	0	0	0
OVX	0	0	0	0	0	0	0	0	0	0	0
	16 Gy†	+1	+1	0	0	0	+1	+1	+1	+1	0

Semi-quantitative estimates performed by a board certified veterinary clinical pathologist (LS) according to standard protocols. Cells contain the data for individual mice (n = 5/group). Numerical scale: −4 severely decreased, −3 markedly decreased, −2 moderately decreased, −1 mildly decreased, +1 mildly increased, +2 moderately increased, +3 markedly increased, +4 severely increased, normal assigned a value of 0 for statistical calculations. Wilcoxon rank-sum test:
*Radiation exposure significantly increased congestion compared with non-irradiated (p = 0.0495),
†Radiation significantly increased fibrosis compared with non-irradiated (p = 0.0143). Note that ovarian hormonal status did not separately affect either parameter.

age and species or strain may explain variations in the findings. OVX may drive differentiation of the marrow stromal cells towards adipocytes at the expense of osteoblasts, resulting in diminished bone formation [28]. In contrast, other investigators describe enhanced differentiation of marrow stromal cells towards osteoblasts after OVX [29], but that bone loss is due to simultaneous but more robust increased production or activity of osteoclasts, which may actually be partially driven by the ability of osteoblasts to support osteoclastogenesis [26,30,31]. Preliminary histomorphometry in our laboratory indicate that OVX drives down the percent of trabecular bone surface covered by osteoblasts, though not to the same degree as irradiation with 16Gy (data not shown). In addition, we observed a significant increase in osteoclast number following OVX. Some of the effects of ovariectomy may be via canonical estrogen receptor effects on gene transcription [30], however other mechanisms may be mediated by inflammatory cells and cytokines [26,29,31]. The mechanistic connection with expanding adipose may be the role of fat in regulating inflammation via adipokines [26], as well as opposing effects on fat and bone of key regulatory molecules such as PPAR-γ [32].

It should be noted that 30 days after irradiation was equal to 87 days post OVX in the present study (Figure 1). Since bone surfaces are generally quiescent following ovariectomy with time [33], marrow may be expected to respond to radiation to a greater degree when compared with bone, since rapidly dividing cells are more radiosensitive (demonstrated by Figures 3 and 4). Additionally, the ovary intact animals may exhibit more tightly coordinated interactions between the marrow milieu and the adjacent bone, while the lack of ovarian hormones uncouples the two resulting in disproportionate effects between these tissue envelopes as illustrated by Figure 5. New evidence demonstrates more independent regulation of bone and fat under some circumstances [34]. Differential radiosensitivity of the constituent cell populations should be investigated further by more extensive studies in bone and isolated marrow cell survivability.

Our study corroborates the inverse relationship between marrow adipose and bone described by others [32,35], however most noticeably the stoichiometry of the association after radiation therapy is altered significantly by hormonal status. We propose complex interrelationships among the three tissue components of bone and marrow evaluated (hemopoietic, adipose, and osseous) and illustrated this in a multi-dimensional space (Figure 5). OVX and radiation had synergistic effects in promoting marrow adipogenesis and suppressing hematopoiesis. Given the reciprocal relationship between marrow fat and bone, a similar decrement in bone volume was anticipated, and this expectation was reinforced by the disproportionate hematopoietic suppression since normal

osteoblastogenic signals from hematopoietic stem cells might be blunted in this population [36]. Correspondingly, osteoblasts are necessary to maintain the hematopoietic stem cell niche and support hematopoiesis, suggesting that it is reasonable to expect that the effects of radiation on hematopoiesis and bone would closely mirror one another [12,37]. Disproportionate changes in interacting tissue components will need to be further investigated by additional studies with a larger sample size. In addition, cellular and molecular studies are necessary to help understand how ovariectomy influenced the response to radiation in this model. The ability of OVX to disrupt expected relationships between these tissues in response to radiation presents an opportunity to expand the use of this model system to understand the relationships between these closely linked tissues and has clinical implications for the treatment of cancer patients.

Translational importance

Patients with gynecological cancer experience an accelerated and distinct pattern of trabecular bone loss from systemic chemotherapy and local pelvic radiation [1]. The murine model described by this work simulates the effects of pelvic radiation administered to pre- and post-menopausal women who have endometrial or rectal cancers. Bone marrow is considered to be a critical organ as Loren et al recently reported hematological toxicity from pelvic radiation therapy treatment [38,39]. Different radiation modalities such as fractionated radiation therapy and total body radiation are responsible for increased commitment of non-hematopoietic mesenchymal stromal cells towards marrow adipogenesis as well as for increased bone resorption [40–42]. It appears that radiation (and chemotherapy) perturbs the homeostasis of bone and marrow by damaging each individual compartment (bone, hemopoietic and non-hemopoietic). Interaction of these components in presence of radiation with/without ovariectomy is unknown and will begin to unfold through stepwise increased investigations.

The experimental radiation dose is selected to be radiobiologically equivalent to the average prescribed clinical dose. A single fraction 16 Gy is radiobiologically equivalent to high dose of radiation that is given in 2Gy per fraction as hypo-fractionation. Hypo-fractionation helps repairing critical organs which is the basis of radiation therapy. Because a variety of fractionation schema is used among clinical trials, Fowler suggested using the normalized tumor dose (NTD) which is the biological effective dose (BED), normalized to a 2Gy fraction. This is discussed in details by Folwer et al extensively in their 2006 paper [43]. For late normal-tissue complications, 16 Gy (single fraction) irradiation in mice at the hind limb is approximately equivalent to 60 Gy (2 Gy/fraction) radiation dosage delivered to patients in the pelvic region.

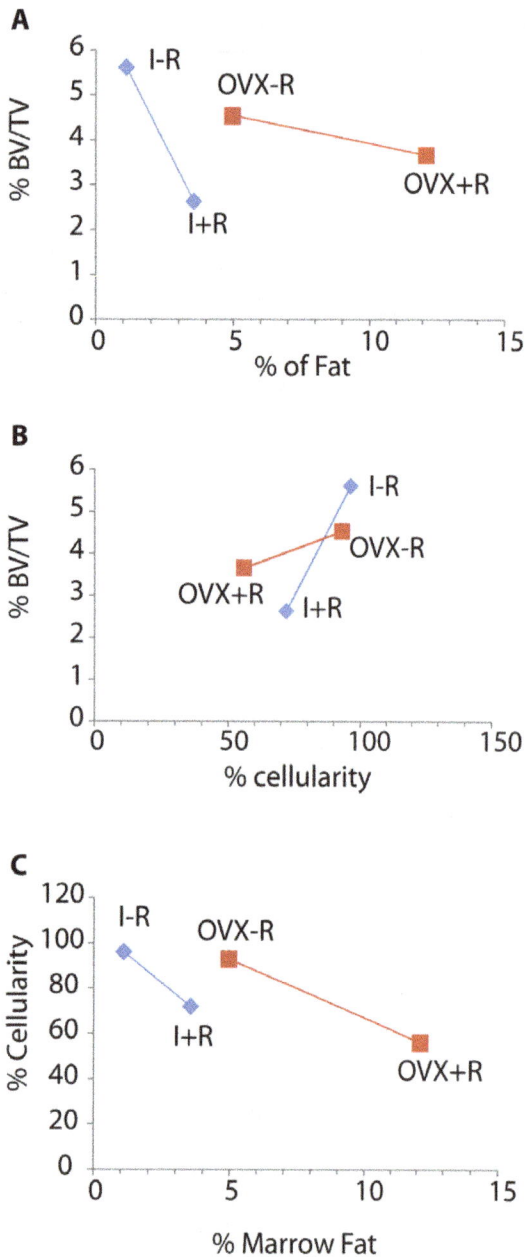

A

B

C

Figure 4. Ovariectomy influences the relationships between bone volume (BV/TV%), adipogenesis (% marrow fat), and hematopoiesis (% cellularity) at Day 30 with or without 16 Gy radiation to the hind limb in mice. Data of every two measurements are represented as least squares mean values for the group. Panel A: OVX results in a 10 fold reduction in the rate of bone volume loss per unit increase in marrow fat after radiation treatment compared with intact mice. Panel B: OVX blunts the rate of bone volume loss relative to reduced hematopoietic cellularity after radiation compared with intact mice by a factor of 6. Panel C: OVX halves the reduction in hematopoietic cellularity compared with increased marrow fat after radiation treatment compared with intact mice.

Briefly, 16 Gy is equivalent to a BED of 101.3 Gy and a NTD of 60.8 Gy, and 60 Gy (2 Gy/fraction) is equivalent to a BED of 100 Gy and a NTD of 60 Gy [using Fowler method [43] assuming α/β to be 3 Gy for late normal-tissue complications] [4]. Approximately 20% of the total murine skeleton (as measured by posthumous dry bone weight) was exposed to radiation. This is

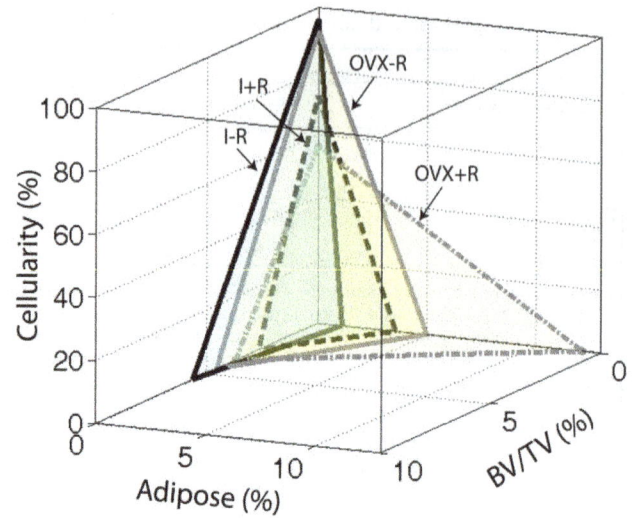

Figure 5. 3-D illustration of interrelationships among the three tissue components of bone and marrow: hemopoietic component measured by cellularity, stromal damage component measured by marrow fat or adipose content, and osseous component measured by the cancellous bone BV/TV%. Cumulative increases in marrow fat after irradiation, in the absence of ovarian function (10 fold) was not reflected by equivalent losses of either cancellous bone or hematopoietic cellularity. The proportionality of changes in these tissue components were maintained among irradiated intact mice.

equal to the percent of total skeleton in the average irradiated pelvic region (20–30% as measured by CT) of a clinical subject. The areas of comparison between our murine model and clinical subjects also have comparable amounts of total skeletal trabecular bone volume. Therefore, as a simplified murine model, a one-time exposure of 16 Gy can be used to accurately simulate clinical irradiation of bone tissue.

Another aspect examined by the present study concerns ovarian status. We have demonstrated that the presence of ovarian hormones may modulate the severity of the radiation effect on bone and marrow. Thus, in the clinic a patient's ovarian status may be important to the ultimate preservation of bone and bone marrow integrity. As shown by Figure 5, the pre-menopausal patient may be at a higher risk for skeletal damage following clinical radiotherapy and should be more closely evaluated for irradiation effects on the skeleton. Additionally, since marrow cellularity (and presumably function) eventually recovers, hematopoietic response to treatment ought to be evaluated long-term.

Conclusions

Therapeutic radiation affects the pattern of bone and bone marrow changes in different ways depending on the ovarian status of the recipient. Radiation results in significant damage to marrow cellularity though it recovers with time. The relationship between marrow adipogenesis and bone loss appears dependent on ovarian function, with the bone loss being greater for a given unit of expansion in marrow fat in the presence than in the absence of ovarian function. Understanding the extent and nature of changes in bone marrow, bone remodeling and related skeletal damage will be beneficial to optimizing potential interventions during or following cancer therapy.

Author Contributions

Conceived and designed the experiments: SH LK. Performed the experiments: SH GF LK KC. Analyzed the data: LS SH KC LK DY CX YZ. Contributed reagents/materials/analysis tools: SH. Wrote the paper: SH LS LK CX DY YZ.

References

1. Hui Susanta K, Khalil Ali, Zhang Yan, Coghill Kathleen, Le Chap, et al. (2010) Longitudinal assessment of bone loss from diagnostic CT scans in gynecologic cancer patients treated with chemotherapy and radiation. American Journal of Obstetrics & Gynecology 203: 353.e351–353.e357.
2. Chen Z, Maricic M, Bassford T, Pettinger M, Ritenbaugh C, et al. (2005) Fracture risk among breast cancer survivors: Results from the Women's Health Initiative Observational Study. Archives of Internal Medicine 165: 552.
3. Baxter N, Habermann E, Tepper J, Durham S, Virnig B (2005) Risk of pelvic fractures in older women following pelvic irradiation. JAMA 294: 2587–2593.
4. Hui SK, Fairchild GR, Kidder LS, Sharma M, Bhattacharya M, et al. (2012) Skeletal Remodeling Following Clinically Relevant Radiation-Induced Bone Damage Treated with Zoledronic Acid. Calcified Tissue International 90: 40–49.
5. Despars G, St-Pierre Y (2011) Bidirectional interactions between bone metabolism and hematopoiesis. Experimental hematology 39: 809–816.
6. Sacchetti B, Funari A, Michienzi S, Di Cesare S, Piersanti S, et al. (2007) Self-renewing osteoprogenitors in bone marrow sinusoids can organize a hematopoietic microenvironment. Cell 131: 324–336.
7. Blake G, Griffith JF, Yeung D, Leung P, Fogelman I (2009) Effect of increasing vertebral marrow fat content on BMD measurement, T-Score status and fracture risk prediction by DXA. Bone 44: 495–501.
8. Rodríguez JP, Astudillo P, Ríos S, Pino AM (2008) Involvement of adipogenic potential of human bone marrow mesenchymal stem cells (MSCs) in osteoporosis. Current Stem Cell Research & Therapy 3: 208–218.
9. Rodríguez JP, Montecinos L, Ríos S, Reyes P, Martínez J (2000) Mesenchymal stem cells from osteoporotic patients produce a type I collagen-deficient extracellular matrix favoring adipogenic differentiation. Journal of cellular biochemistry 79: 557–565.
10. Zhang H, Lu W, Zhao Y, Rong P, Cao R, et al. (2011) Adipocytes Derived from Human Bone Marrow Mesenchymal Stem Cells Exert Inhibitory Effects on Osteoblastogenesis. Current Molecular Medicine 11: 489–502.
11. Aanei CM, Flandrin-Gresta P, Zugun Eloae F, Carasevici E, Guyotat D, et al. (2012) Intrinsic growth deficiencies of mesenchymal stromal cells (MSCs) in myelodysplastic syndromes (MDS). Stem Cells and Development 21(10): 1604–1615.
12. Liu S, Hu P, Hou Y, Li P, Li X, et al. (2011) The Additive Effect of Mesenchymal Stem Cells and Bone Morphogenetic Protein 2 on γ-Irradiated Bone Marrow in Mice. Cell Biochemistry and Biophysics 61: 539–550.
13. Bernardo M, Cometa A, Locatelli F (2012) Mesenchymal stromal cells: a novel and effective strategy for facilitating engraftment and accelerating hematopoietic recovery after transplantation?. Bone Marrow Transplantation 47: 323–329.
14. Meunier P, Aaron J, Edouard C, VIGNON G (1971) Osteoporosis and the replacement of cell populations of the marrow by adipose tissue: a quantitative study of 84 iliac bone biopsies. Clinical Orthopaedics and Related Research 80: 147.
15. Martin R, Zissimos S (1991) Relationships between marrow fat and bone turnover in ovariectomized and intact rats. Bone 12: 123–131.
16. Nuttall M, Gimble J (2000) Is there a therapeutic opportunity to either prevent or treat osteopenic disorders by inhibiting marrow adipogenesis? Bone 27: 177–184.
17. Muruganandan S, Roman A, Sinal C (2009) Adipocyte differentiation of bone marrow-derived mesenchymal stem cells: cross talk with the osteoblastogenic program. Cellular and molecular life sciences 66: 236–253.
18. Elmore SA (2006) Enhanced histopathology of the bone marrow. Toxicologic pathology 34: 666–686.
19. Travlos GS (2006) Histopathology of bone marrow. Toxicologic pathology 34: 566–598.
20. Travlos GS (2006) Normal structure, function, and histology of the bone marrow. Toxicologic pathology 34: 548–565.
21. Bianco P (2011) Minireview: The Stem Cell Next Door: Skeletal and Hematopoietic Stem Cell "Niches" in Bone. Endocrinology 152: 2957–2962.
22. Tong XQ, Sugimura H, Kisanuki A, Asato M, Yuki Y, et al. (1998) Multiple Fractionated and Single-Dose Irradiation of Bone Marrow. Acta Radiologica 39: 620–624.
23. Greenberger J, Anderson J, Berry L, Epperly M, Cronkite E, et al. (1996) Effects of irradiation of CBA/CA mice on hematopoietic stem cells and stromal cells in long-term bone marrow cultures. Leukemia: official journal of the Leukemia Society of America, Leukemia Research Fund, UK 10: 514.
24. Greenberger JS, Epperly M (2009) Bone marrow-derived stem cells and radiation response. Semin Radiat Oncol 19:133–139.
25. Harrison DE, Astle CM (1982) Loss of stem cell repopulating ability upon transplantation. Effects of donor age, cell number, and transplantation procedure. The Journal of experimental medicine 156: 1767.
26. Kim YY, Kim SH, Oh S, Sul OJ, Lee HY, et al. (2010) Increased fat due to estrogen deficiency induces bone loss by elevating monocyte chemoattractant protein-1 (MCP-1) production. Molecules and cells 29: 277–282.
27. Lei Z, Xiaoying Z, Xingguo L (2009) Ovariectomy associated changes in bone mineral density and bone marrow haematopoiesis in rats. International Journal of Experimental Pathology 90: 512–519.
28. Benayahu D, Shur I, Ben-Eliyahu S (2000) Hormonal changes affect the bone and bone marrow cells in a rat model. Journal of cellular biochemistry 79: 407–415.
29. Li JY, Tawfeek H, Bedi B, Yang X, Adams J, et al. (2011) Ovariectomy disregulates osteoblast and osteoclast formation through the T-cell receptor CD40 ligand. Proceedings of the National Academy of Sciences 108: 768.
30. Imai Y, Youn MY, Kondoh S, Nakamura T, Kouzmenko A, et al. (2009) Estrogens maintain bone mass by regulating expression of genes controlling function and life span in mature osteoclasts. Annals of the New York Academy of Sciences 1173: E31–E39.
31. Tyagi AM, Srivastava K, Sharan K, Yadav D, Maurya R, et al. (2011) Daidzein Prevents the Increase in CD4+CD28null T Cells and B Lymphopoesis in Ovariectomized Mice: A Key Mechanism for Anti-Osteoclastogenic Effect. PLoS One 6: e21216.
32. Rosen C, Ackert-Bicknell C, Rodriguez J, Pino A (2009) Marrow fat and the bone microenvironment: developmental, functional, and pathological implications. Critical reviews in eukaryotic gene expression 19: 109.
33. Boyce R, Franks A, Jankowsky M, Orcutt C, Piacquadio A, et al. (1990) Sequential histomorphometric changes in cancellous bone from ovariohysterectomized dogs. Journal of Bone and Mineral Research 5: 947–953.
34. Abdallah B, Kassem M (2012) New factors controlling the balance between osteoblastogenesis and adipogenesis. Bone 50: 540–545.
35. Rosen C, Bouxsein M (2006) Mechanisms of disease: is osteoporosis the obesity of bone? Nature Clinical Practice Rheumatology 2: 35–43.
36. Jung Y, Song J, Shiozawa Y, Wang J, Wang Z, et al. (2008) Hematopoietic stem cells regulate mesenchymal stromal cell induction into osteoblasts thereby participating in the formation of the stem cell niche. Stem Cells 26: 2042–2051.
37. Visnjic D, Kalajzic Z, Rowe DW, Katavic V, Lorenzo J, et al. (2004) Hematopoiesis is severely altered in mice with an induced osteoblast deficiency. Blood 103: 3258–3264.
38. Mell L, Schomas D, Salama J, Devisetty K, Aydogan B, et al. (2008) Association between bone marrow dosimetric parameters and acute hematologic toxicity in anal cancer patients treated with concurrent chemotherapy and intensity-modulated radiotherapy. International Journal of Radiation Oncology, Biology, Physics 70: 1431–1437.
39. Rose BS, Liang Y, Lau SK, Jensen LG, Yashar CM, et al. (2012) Correlation Between Radiation Dose to ^{18}F-FDG-PET Defined Active Bone Marrow Subregions and Acute Hematologic Toxicity in Cervical Cancer Patients Treated with Chemoradiotherapy. International Journal of Radiation Oncology Biology Physics 83: 1185–1191.
40. Clavin NW, Fernandez J, Schönmeyr BH, Soares MA, Mehrara BJ (2008) Fractionated doses of ionizing radiation confer protection to mesenchymal stem cell pluripotency. Plastic and reconstructive surgery 122: 739.
41. Ma J, Shi M, Li J, Chen B, Wang H, et al. (2007) Senescence-unrelated impediment of osteogenesis from Flk1+ bone marrow mesenchymal stem cells induced by total body irradiation and its contribution to long-term bone and hematopoietic injury. Haematologica 92: 889.
42. Wang Y, Liu L, Pazhanisamy SK, Li H, Meng A, et al. (2010) Total body irradiation causes residual bone marrow injury by induction of persistent oxidative stress in murine hematopoietic stem cells. Free Radical Biology and Medicine 48: 348–356.
43. Fowler J (2006) Development of radiobiology for oncology–a personal view. Physics in Medicine and Biology 51: 263.

16

A Survey Study on Gastrointestinal Parasites of Stray Cats in Northern Region of Nile Delta, Egypt

Reda E. Khalafalla*

Department of Parasitology, Faculty of Veterinary Medicine, Kafrelsheikh University, Kafrelsheikh, Egypt

Abstract

A survey study on gastrointestinal parasites in 113 faecal samples from stray cats collected randomly from Kafrelsheikh province, northern region of Nile delta of Egypt; was conducted in the period between January and May 2010. The overall prevalence was 91%. The results of this study reported seven helminth species: *Toxocara cati* (9%), *Ancylostoma tubaeforme* (4%), *Toxascaris leonina* (5%), *Dipylidium caninum* (5%), *Capillaria* spp. (3%), *Taenia taeniformis* (22%) and *Heterophyes heterophyes* (3%), four protozoal species: *Toxoplasma gondii* (9%), *Sarcocyst* spp. (1%), *Isospora* spp. (2%) and *Giardia* spp. (2%) and two arthropod species; *Linguatula serrata* (2%) and mites eggs (13%). The overall prevalence of intestinal parasites may continue to rise due to lack of functional veterinary clinics for cat care in Egypt. Therefore, there is a need to plan adequate control programs to diagnose, treat and control gastrointestinal parasites of companion as well as stray cats in the region.

Editor: Thomas J. Templeton, Weill Cornell Medical College, United States of America

Funding: The funders are the Faculty of Veterinary Medicine and the Department of Parasitology at the University of Kafrelsheikh, Egypt; these funds are part of a general institutional research fund offered by the faculty council to the Department of Parasitology. The funders had no role in study design, data collection and analysis, decision to publish, or preparation of the manuscript.

Competing Interests: The author has declared that no competing interests exist.

* E-mail: Redabast@hotmail.de

Introduction

Gastrointestinal parasites are the main causes of morbidity in domestic cats [1]. In Egypt and other parts of the world these parasites cause great public health problems.

Several factors affect the frequency of a species of parasite in a population. The prevalence of intestinal parasites can vary due to geographical region; presence of veterinary care; habits of the local animal populations; season of the year and the cat population composition. Several epidemiological surveillance studies reported that feral/stray cats present high frequency of parasites [2,3,4,5].

In Egypt, little is known about the parasites of cats. This knowledge allows for improved explanations as to the distribution of parasitism and its significance to the health of humans and animals inhabiting the area under study. So that, the aim of this study is to determine the parasites of stray cats inhabiting the Nile Delta region of Lower Egypt.

Nile Delta of Egypt is that territory situated from south to north between Cairo and the Mediterranean Sea, respectively and from west to east between the Rosetta branch and the Damietta branch of the Nile River, respectively. The population density is very high and estimated by 34 million inhabitants over 25,000 km^2, i.e., with 1,360 residents per km^2 (Cairo population is not counted) [6].

The Nile Delta territory is characterized by a moderate climate. During summer it is moderately hot and dry where the temperature is ranged between 25–35°C while during winter its climate is warm and scanty to moderate rainy. Temperatures range between highs of 35 to 40°C during June to August, and lows of 5 to 10°C between December and January [6].

Materials and Methods

Over the period between January and May 2010, 113 fecal samples of stray cats were collected in a weekly pattern from different sandy spots representing Kafrelsheikh province, defined as the northern part of the Nile Delta region of Egypt. Stray cats could not be caught and therefore could not be identified as to age, sex and breed. They were observed as closely as possible depositing and burying their feces in separate holes in sandy spots. Collection of the fecal samples determined that some samples were freshly deposited whereas others were not. Approximately 100 gm of cat feces were collected from individual holes and the remainder discarded hygienically.

All fecal samples were initially examined macroscopically for the presence of tapeworm proglottids or nematodes. Flotation centrifugation methods were applied using zinc sulphate and saturated salt solution (specific gravity 1.2) as described [7,8,9]. Identification of parasite species was performed based on egg and cyst morphology for the well documented species [10].

Results and Discussion

Description of the fecal parasite infections indicated that the overall infection rate was 91%. The individual prevalence of infections is shown in Table 1. The positively infected samples were infected with protozoa (12%), cestodes (23%), nematodes (21%), trematodes (3%) and arthropods (15%, Table 1 and Figure 1). Figure 2 and Table 2 present the type of the infection as 42%, 35% and 13% were infected with single (mono-infection), two to three (poly-infection) or more species of endoparasites, respectively.

Table 1. Prevalence of gastrointestinal parasites of stray cats in Kafrelsheikh province of Nile Delta region in Egypt (n = 113 fecal samples).

parasites	Infected samples (n = 113)	Prevalence%
Toxoplasma gondii	10	9%
Isospora spp.	2	2%
Giardia spp.	2	2%
Sarcocyst spp.	1	1%
All protozoal infections	**14**	**12%***
Taenia taeniformis	25	22%
Dipylidium caninum	6	5%
All cestode infections	**26**	**23%***
Toxocara cati	10	9%
Toxascaris leonina	6	5%
Ancylostoma tubaeforme	5	4%
Capillaria spp.	3	3%
All nematode infections	**24**	**21%***
Heterophyes heterophyes	3	3%
All trematode infections	**3**	**3%***
Mites eggs	15	13%
Liguatula serrata	2	2%
All arthropod infections	**17**	**15%***

*The total for each type (e.g.; Cestodes, Protozoa, etc) is sometimes lesser than the sum of individual infections.

The reported parasites were seven helminth species: *T. cati* (9%), *A. tubaeforme* (4%), *T. leonina* (5%), *D. caninum* (5%), *Capillaria* spp. (3%), *T. taeniformis* (22%) and *H. heterophyes* (3%), four protozoal species: *T. gondii* (9%), *Sarcocyst* spp. (1%), *Isospora* spp. 2% and *Giardia* spp. (2%) and two arthropod species; *Linguatula serrata* (2%) and mites eggs (13%; Table 1).

This study estimates a 91% prevalence of intestinal parasites in stray cats, and this figure is in general agreement with published

reports of stray cats in northern Iran (90% prevalence; [11]); mid-Ebro Valley, Spain (90%; [5]); and Rio de Janeiro (90%; [12,13]. However, comparison of the present study with published surveys indicated that great differences in prevalence were observed for particular parasite species; perhaps due to regional, environmental or climatic variations.

T. taeniformis was the dominant tapeworm reported in examined fecal samples of stray cats in Nile Delta of Egypt with a prevalence rate of 22% which is lower than that reported in Doha, Qatar (74%, [14]). However, it is more or less in the same range as that recorded in Cairo, Egypt (30%, [15]) and that in Iran (18%, [16]). While the prevalence rate of *T. taeniformis* in the current research is higher than that recorded in Jordan (3.8%, [16]) and in Iran (12% [17]).

D. caninum was encountered with low prevalence (5%) in comparison with other surveys. For example, *D. caninum* was harboured in 51% and 45% of the wildcats, *Felis catus*, necropsied in studies performed in Britain [18] and Egypt [15], respectively.

T. cati was found to be the frequent nematode eggs in the current study, however, the overall *T. cati* prevalence was relatively low (9%) in comparison with the prevalences encountered in Denmark (79%, [19]), in Spain (55%, [2]), in Greece (67%, [19]) and in England (53%, [5]).

Ancylostoma tubaeforme, *T. leonina* and *Capillaria* spp. were the other nematode species found in the present survey, with lower prevalences. For example, *A. tubaeforme*, in other studies, the estimated prevalences were 40% in Israel [20], 39.5% in Belgium [21] and 41% in the Republic of South Africa [22].

Mite eggs and sometimes mites larvae were found in 13% of examined fecal samples as well *Linguatula serrata* larvae were identified only in two samples (2%). In the present study, mite infection in the stray cats was evident and due to the cat's grooming habits, the mite eggs were swallowed and dropped with feaces.

In the current study, the all protozoan infections recovered was 12% which included *T. gondii* (9%), *Isospora* spp. (2%), *Giardia* spp. (2%) and *Sarcocystis* spp. (1%). The most dominant protozoal infection was *T. gondii* in stray cats recorded in the present study was generally within the reported results from the Middle East which revealed a range of Toxoplasmosis in stray and domestic cats from 12.5% to 78.1% [16,23,24,25].

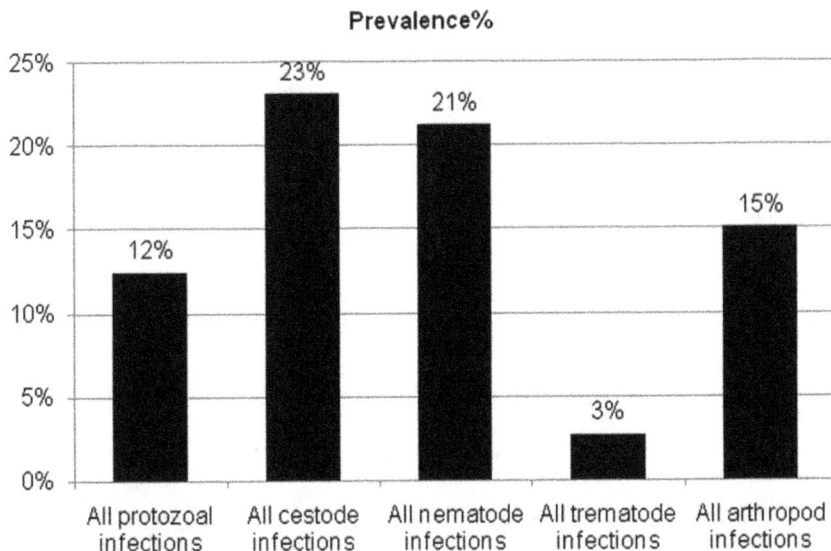

Figure 1. The overall prevalence of different infections in stray cats in northern region of Nile Delta, Egypt.

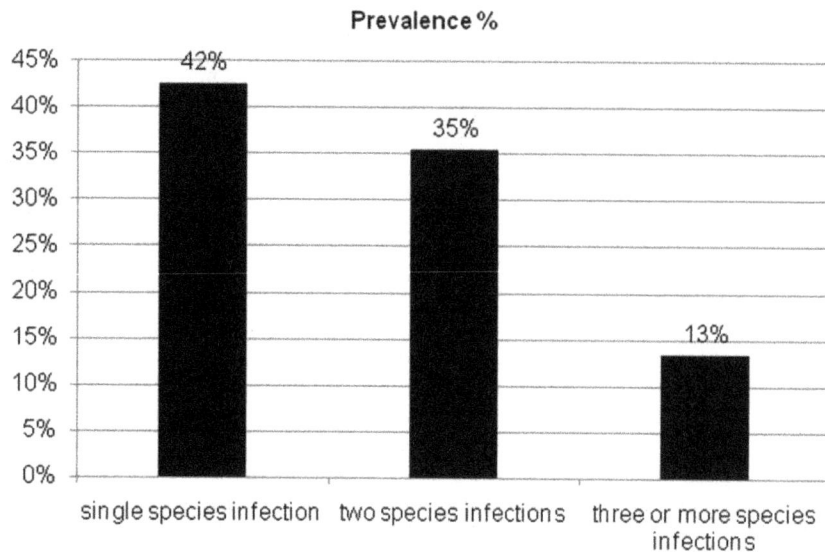

Prevalence %

Figure 2. The prevalence of single species, two species and poly-infections (three or more species) in stray cats in northern region of Nile Delta, Egypt.

Conclusion

High prevalence rate of cats with a wide range of parasitic organisms in the studied area suggests that inhabitants face risk of parasitic infections through contact with infected cats and their excretion. Therefore, both animal and human health education are recommended in the developed communities. As well the veterinarians and physicians should play an important role in increasing the degree of awareness of feline zoonotic parasites, which could be helpful to prevent or minimise zoonotic transmission.

Table 2. Types of different mixed infections with gastrointestinal parasites of stray cats in Kafrelsheikh province of Nile Delta region in Egypt (*n* = 113 fecal samples).

mixed infection	prevalence (*n* = 113)	%
single species infection	48	42%
two species infections	40	35%
three or more species infections	15	13%
All infections	103	91%

Acknowledgments

I wish to express my sincere and grateful thanks to the Department of Parasitology, and to the Faculty of Veterinary Medicine, Kafrelsheikh University, Egypt, for their support.

Author Contributions

Conceived and designed the experiments: RK. Performed the experiments: RK. Analyzed the data: RK. Contributed reagents/materials/analysis tools: REK. Wrote the paper: RK.

References

1. Hendrix CM, Blagburn BL (1983) Common gastrointestinal parasites. Vet Clin North Am 13: 627–646.
2. Calvete C, Lucientes J, Castillo JA, Estrada R, Garcia MJ, et al. (1998) Gastrointestinal helminth parasites in stray cats from the mid-Ebro Valley, Spain. Vet Parasitol 75: 235–240.
3. McColm AA, Hutchison WM (1980) The prevalence of intestinal helminths in stray cats in central Scotland. J Helminthol 54: 255–257.
4. Niak A (1972) The prevalence of Toxocara cati and other parasites in Liverpool cats. Vet Rec 91: 534–536.
5. Nichol S, Ball SJ, Snow KR (1981) Prevalence of intestinal parasites in feral cats in some urban areas of England. Vet Parasitol 9: 107–110.
6. LookLex/Encyclopedia of the Orient: The Nile Delta. Available: http://lexicorient.com/e.o/nile_delta.htm. Accessed 2011 Jun 18.
7. Dryden MW, Payne PA, Ridley RK, Smith V (2005) Comparison of Common Fecal Flotation Techniques for the Recovery of Parasite Eggs and Oocysts. Vet Ther 6(1): 17.
8. Faust EC, D'Antonio JS, Odom V, Miller MJ, Peres C, et al. (1938) A critical study of clinical laboratory techniques for the diagnosis of protozoan cysts and helminth eggs in feces. Am J Trop Med Hyg 18: 169–183.
9. McGlade TR, Robertson ID, Elliot AD, Read C, Thompson RCA (2003) Gastrointestinal parasites of domestic cats in Perth, Western Australia. Vet Parasitol 117: 251–262.
10. Soulsby EJL (1982) Helminths, Arthropoda, and Protozoa of domesticated animals. 7th Ed. London: Baillier, Tindal and Cassel.
11. Sharif M, Daryani A, Nasrolahei M, Ziapour SP (2010) a survey of gastrointestinal helminthes in stray cats in northern Iran. Comp Clin Pathol (2010) 19: 257–261.
12. Barrientos Serra CM, Antunes Uchôa CM, Alonso Coimbra R (2003) Exame parasitologico de fezes de gatos (Felis catus domesticus) domiciliados e errantes da Regiao Metropolitana do Río de Janeiro, Brasil. Rev Soc Bras Med Trop 36(3): 331–334.
13. Labarthe N, Serrao M, Ferreira A, Almeida N, Guerrero J (2004) A survey of gastrointestinal helminths in cats of the metropolitan region of Rio de Janeiro, Brazil. Vet Parasitol 123: 133–139.
14. Abu-Madi MA, Behnke JM, Prabhaker KS, Al-Ibrahim R, Lewis JW (2010) Intestinal helminths of feral cat populations from urban and suburban districts of Qatar. Vet Parasitol 168(2010): 284–292.
15. El-Shabrawy MN, Imam EA (1978) Studies on cestodes of domestic cats in Egypt with particular reference to species belonging to genera Diplopylidium and Joyeuxiella. Journal of the Egyptian Veterinary Medical Association 38: 19–27.
16. Morsy TA, Michael SA, El Disi AM (1980) Cats as reservoir hosts of human parasites in Amman, Jordan. Journal of the Egyptian Society of Parasitology 10: 5–18.

17. Zibaei M, Sadijadi SM, Sarkari B (2007) Prevalence of Toxocara cati and other intestinal helminths in stray cats in Shiraz, Iran. Tropical Biomedicine 24: 39–43.

18. Hutchison WM (1956) The incidence and distribution of Hydatigera taeniaeformis and other intestinal helminths in Scottish cats. J Parasitol 43: 318–321.

19. Haralampidis ST (1977) Simbole sti melete ton parasitin tez gatas. [Vet. Med. Diss.] Laboratory of Parasitology and Parasitic Diseases, School of Veterinary Medicine, Greece: Aristotle University of Thessaloniki.

20. Lengy J, Steiman I, Steiman Y (1969) The current helmintofauna of stray dogs and cats in Israel. J Parasitol 55: 1239.

21. Thienpoint D, Vanparijs O, Hermans L (1981) Epidemiologie des helminthoses du chat en Belgique Frequence d'Ollulanus tricuspis. Rec Med Vet 157: 591–595.

22. Baker MK, Lange L, Verster A, Van Der Plaat S (1989) A survey of helminths in domestic cats in the Pretoria area of Transvaal, Republic of South Africa: I. The prevalence and comparison of burdens of helminths in adult and juvenile cats. J S Afr Vet Assoc 60: 139–142.

23. Abu-Madi MA, Al-Molawi N, Behnke JM (2008) Seroprevalence and epidemiological correlates of Toxoplasma gondii infections among patients referred for hospital-based serological testing in Doha, Qatar. Parasites & Vectors 1: 39.

24. Abu-Zakham AA, el-Shazly AM, Yossef ME, Romeia SA, Handoussa AE (1989) the prevalence of Toxoplasma gondii antibodies among cats from Mahalla El-Kobra, Gharbia Governorate. J Egypt Soc Parasitol, Jun; 19(1): 225–9.

25. Hossain A, Bolbol AS, Bakir TM, Bashandi AM (1986) A serological survey of the prevalence of Toxoplasma antibodies in dogs and cats in Saudi Arabia. Trop Geogr Med 38: 244–245.

17

Phosphorus Metabolic Disorder of Guizhou Semi-Fine Wool Sheep

Xiaoyun Shen[1,4,6], **Jinhua Zhang**[3,5], **Renduo Zhang**[2]*

1 Chongqing University of Science and Technology, Chongqing, China, **2** School of Environmental Science and Engineering, Guangdong Provincial Key Laboratory of Environmental Pollution Control and Remediation Technology, Sun Yat-sen University, Guangzhou, China, **3** Guizhou Normal University, Guiyang, China, **4** Office of Poverty Alleviation of Guizhou Province, Guiyang, China, **5** Guizhou Institute of Pratacultural, Guiyang, China, **6** Pratacultural Ecology Institute, Bijie University, Bijie, China

Abstract

Guizhou semi-fine wool sheep are affected by a disease, characterized by emaciation, lameness, stiffness in the gait, enlargement of the costochondral junctions, and abnormal curvature in the long bones. The objective of this study was to determine possible relationships between the disease and mineral deficiencies. Samples of tissue and blood were collected from affected and unaffected sheep. Samples of soil and forage were collected from affected and unaffected areas. The samples were used for biochemical analyses and mineral nutrient measurements. Results showed that phosphorus (P) concentrations in forage samples from affected areas were significantly lower than those from unaffected areas ($P < 0.01$) and the mean ratio of calcium (Ca) to P in the affected forage was 12:1. Meanwhile, P concentrations of blood, bone, tooth, and wool from the affected sheep were also significantly lower than those from the unaffected group ($P < 0.01$). Serum P levels of the affected animals were much lower than those of the unaffected ones, whereas serum alkaline phosphatase levels from the affected were significantly higher than those from the unaffected ($P < 0.01$). Inorganic P levels of the affected sheep were about half of those in the control group. Oral administration of disodium hydrogen phosphate prevented and cured the disease. The study clearly demonstrated that the disease of Guizhou semi-fine wool sheep was mainly caused by the P deficiency in forage, as a result of fenced pasture and animal habitat fragmentation.

Editor: Christopher James Johnson, USGS National Wildlife Health Center, United States of America

Funding: This work was partly supported by the national science and technology support program (2011BAC09B01), the Natural Science Foundation of Guizhou Province of China ([2012]2184), the cooperation projects of Guizhou Province, Bijie City, and the Kunming Branch of Chinese Academy of Science (2010-04), and the China Agriculture Research System (CARS-40-30). The funders had no role in study design, data collection and analysis, decision to publish, or preparation of the manuscript.

Competing Interests: The authors have declared that no competing interests exist.

* E-mail: zhangrd@mail.sysu.edu.cn

Introduction

Guizhou semi-fine sheep are vital to the production system of the Karst mountain areas of Southwest China. During the past 10 years, Guizhou semi-fine sheep have been affected by a disease, characterized by emaciation, lameness, enlargement of the costochondral junctions, and abnormal curvature in the long bones. Severe cases included permanent recumbency and eventual death. Based on preliminarily epidemiological and clinical data, this locally nutritional and metabolic disease may be associated with mineral imbalance for the animal.

The disorder has been observed throughout the years with peak incidence occurring between July and September and mainly occurred in ewes and lambs. In severe areas, 30% of sheep were affected and the mortality reached 15%. Similar syndromes have been reported in cattle [1,2], water buffaloes [3], pigs [4], dogs [5], camels [6], and wild yaks [7], all of which are related to nutrition imbalance. However, there is no any available information about the disease affecting Guizhou semi-fine wool sheep. Therefore, the objective of this study was to determine the pathogeny of this disease and to establish possible relationships between the disease and mineral deficiencies.

Materials and Methods

Ethics statement

The sheep used in these experiments were cared as per outlined in the *Guide for the Care and Use of Animals in Agricultural Research and Teaching Consortium* [8]. Thirty affected and 30 unaffected sheep were slaughtered with electrical stunning then exsanguination, which was approved by the Institute of Zoology, Chinese Academy of Sciences, Institutional Animal Care and Use Committee (Project A0566). The experiments were conducted in the pasture of Bijie Comprehensive Experiment Station, Agriculture Research System, China. A permit was issued by the station authority (contact information: Ms. Lijuan Li, lzdxsxy@163.com, 8615086346733). The field studies did not involve endangered or protected species.

Study area

The study area was located in a region adjoined by the provinces of Guizhou, Yunnan, and Sichuan (26°56'-27°47' N, 103°56'-104°51' E), with the average elevation 2100 m above the sea level, the annual precipitation 956 mm, and the average atmospheric temperature 9–11°C. The main grassland species include Puccinellia (*Chinam poensis ohuji*), Siberian Nitraria (*Nitraria sibirica pall*), Floriated astragalus (*Astragalus floridus*), Poly-branched astragals (*A. polycladus*), Falcate whin (*Oxytropis falcate*), Ewenki automomous banner (*Elymus nutans*), Common leymus (*Leymus secalinus*), and June grass (*Koeleria cristata*). Most of the plants are herbaceous and good resources for grazing animals.

Epidemiological investigations

A detailed investigation on the epidemiology of the disease in the sheep was carried out in the affected area. Collected data included the history, incidence, character, and regularity of the disease, and the natural ecological conditions. We interviewed many local herdsmen who have been living in the area for many years, asking for background information on the disease. Data about the ecological and environmental conditions and their effects on the disease were obtained from local records and annual reports provided by the local government. Clinical signs were recorded by directly observing herd activities on the pasture.

Sample collections

On July 1 of 2011, 60 Guizhou semi-fine wool sheep were selected for the following experiments, among which 30 were selected from 1650 sheep in affected pasture (26°58.5' N, 104°28.3' E). All the affected animals showed obvious clinical signs, including lameness, weakness, and enlargement of the costochondral junctions. Other 30 unaffected sheep were selected from Hezhang County of Guizhou Province (26°59.5' N, 104°52.3' E), where the disease had not been reported. Clinical examination showed that all of the unaffected animals were in good health, which was used as the control group.

Blood samples of the selected animals were obtained from the jugular vein using 1% sodium heparin as anticoagulant, and stored at −10°C for analysis of trace elements. Serum samples for biochemical analysis were taken in tubes without anticoagulant. The serum samples were separated by centrifugation (G: 10000–12000, time: 5–10 min, and plastic tube type: EF8977) and stored at −10°C in plastic vials. Wool samples were taken from the animal necks, washed, and degreased [9], and then kept on silica gel in a desiccator until analyses. After the affected and unaffected sheep were slaughtered, routinely post-mortem pathological examination was conducted by visually observing the tissues. Samples of ribs, hips, and teeth were collected from the animals to determine minerals in the tissues. The tissue samples were dried at 60–80°C for 48 h and stored on silica gel in a desiccator.

Samples of forage and soil were collected in July of 2011 in the affected areas (26°58.5' N, 104°28.3' E). Thirty forage samples were collected from randomly distributed locations, i.e., from 6 affected areas and 5 samples in each area. To reduce soil contamination, the herbage samples were cut 1–2 cm above the ground level [10,11]. The forage samples were dried at 60–80°C for 48 h and ground to facilitate chemical analysis [12]. At the same locations, 30 soil samples were taken from the surface layer (0–30 cm), using a 30 mm diameter cylindrical corer. Each soil sample was composited by four soil cores collected at the site. The soil samples were dried at 60–80°C for 48 h and passed through a 2 mm sieve. Soil pH values were 6.8 to 7.2. Thirty forage samples were also collected from the unaffected grassland in Hezhang County.

Biochemical examination

Lactate dehydrogenase (LDH), alkaline phosphatase (AKP), γ-glutamyl transferase (γ-GT), creatinine (CRT), calcium (Ca), inorganic phosphorus (IP), total protein (TP), albumin(Alb), and globulin (Glod) were determined using the serum samples and an automatic biochemical analyzer (OLYMPUS AU 640, Olympus Optical Co., Japan). Quality control serum (Shanghai Biochemical

Co) was used to validate the blood biochemistry data. Serum protein electrophoretic studies were performed on cellulose acetate [13]. All serum biochemical values were measured at 20°C.

Analysis of mineral contents

Concentrations of copper (Cu), iron (Fe), zinc (Zn), manganese (Mn), and Ca in samples of the animal tissues (blood, wool, ribs, hips, and teeth), soil, and forage were measured using a Perkin-Elmer AAS5000 atomic absorption spectrophotometer (Perkin-Elmer, Norwalk, Connecticut, USA). Molybdenum (Mo) content was determined using the flameless atomic absorption spectro-photometry (Perkin-Elmer 3030 graphite furnace with a Zeeman background correction). Fluorine (F) content was determined using ion chromatography (Metrohm MIC-7 advanced, Switzerland). Phosphorus was determined by spectrophotometry [12]. The accuracy of the analytical values was checked by reference to certified values of elements in the National Bureau of Standards (NBS) (bovine liver SRM 1577a).

Treatment and prevention

In one severely affected area, 35 affected sheep were selected from 650 animals in the affected pasture for a treatment experiment. Among them, 10 affected sheep (5 males and 5 females) were given disodium hydrogen phosphate (Na_2HPO_4) orally at a dose of 50 g per animal and grazed on fenced pasture. The treatment was repeated once a week between July and September of 2011. The rest of the selected sheep grazed on the affected and fenced pasture without any treatment. Clinical signs were recorded by directly observing the sheep activities on the pasture. Specific attention was paid to signs of lameness, gait stiffness, and abnormal curvature in forelegs.

Statistical analyses

Data were analyzed using the Statistical Package for the Social Sciences (SPSS, version 14.0, Inc., Chicago, Illinois, USA), and presented in the form of mean ± standard error (SE). Significant differences between groups were assessed using Student's *t* test with least significant differences of 1% ($P < 0.01$) or 5% ($P < 0.05$).

Results

Epidemiology

The disorder mainly occurred in mature females and lambs of Guizhou semi-fine wool sheep throughout the year, with a peak incidence between July and September. Pregnant and post-partum females were most commonly affected by the disease. The clinical signs were less obvious in mature males. In severe areas, 30% of sheep were affected and the mortality reached 15%. Besides the symptoms described above, long bones of the affected sheep were broken frequently without apparent stress. However, body temperature, respiratory rate, and heart rate of the affected animals were normal.

Autopsy findings

Visual autopsy examination showed that gross bone lesions of the affected lambs and adults were similar. Almost all bones, particularly the mandible, scapula, ilium, hip bone, and ribs, were affected. The affected bones were porous, brittle, light, susceptible to fracturing, and easier to be cut and sawn. The marrow cavity was enlarged and extended into the epiphysis, and the cortex was thin, spongy, and soft. Spontaneous fractures frequently occurred on ribs and pelves of the affected sheep. Enlargement of joints with apparent bowing of long bone and broadening of the epiphyses were typical. Many old enlarged scars were observed in ribs of affected adult females. Irregular ulcers were sometimes seen on the surface of joints. Kidneys were prominently enlarged and softened with a yellowish appearance, and livers were slightly swollen.

Biochemical results

Serum AKP, LDH, and CRT of the affected sheep were significantly higher than those in the unaffected animals ($P <$ 0.01), while IP levels were about half of those in the control group. The AKP values of the affected animals were two times higher than those of the unaffected sheep (Table 1). Likewise, concentrations of serum α-globulin and β-globulin of the affected sheep were significantly higher than those of the control group ($P <$ 0.01). Serum α-globulin of the affected sheep was significantly lower than those in the control group ($P < 0.01$) (Table 2). There were no significant differences in other biochemical values between the affected and unaffected sheep.

Minerals

Concentrations of P in the soil and forage samples in the affected area were significantly lower than those in the unaffected area ($P < 0.01$) (Table 3). The P concentrations in the forage samples of the unaffected area were 5.4 times higher than those in the affected area. The mean Ca:P ratio in forage of the affected area was 12:1. Other values of the mineral elements were within the normal ranges. In addition, P concentrations in the blood and wool samples and in ribs, hips, and teeth from the affected animals were roughly half of those from the unaffected group (Tables 4 and 5).

Treatment and prevention

Animals treated with Na_2HPO_4 recovered gradually within 10 to 20 d. Generally, appetite improved quickly and signs of lameness in most animals improved within 5 to 10 d after the treatment. However, foreleg deformation recovered slowly and required prolonged treatment. Females and lambs were more vulnerable than males in the treated and untreated sheep. The 10 treated sheep totally survived. Among the 25 of untreated animals, 5 males survived, 2 of 10 females and 2 of 10 lambs eventually died. It was noteworthy that 2 of 10 untreated females died and none of 5 treated females died, while none of untreated and treated males died.

Table 1. Biochemical parameters in serum samples of Guizhou semi-fine wool sheep.

Property	Affected	Unaffected
LDH[a] (μmol/l)	5.86±1.38[b]	3.51±0.62
γ-GT (IU/l)	25.3±3.7	26.2±3.5
AKP (IU/l)	121±17.3[b]	56.2±8.7
CRT (μmol/l)	153±35[b]	116±21
Ca (mmol/l)	2.53±0.21	2.61±0.23
IP (mmol/l)	1.15±0.22[b]	2.28±0.22

[a]LDH = Lactate dehydrogenase; AKP = alkaline phosphatase; γ-GT = γ-glutamyl transferase; CRT = creatinine; Ca = calcium; IP = inorganic phosphorus.
[b]Results between the affected and unaffected Guizhou semi-fine wool sheep were significantly different ($P<0.01$).

Table 2. Serum protein concentrations (g/l) of Guizhou semi-fine wool sheep.

Items	Affected	Unaffected
Total protein	63.7±4.9	65.9±5.3
Albumin	45.3±3.7	46.7±3.6
α-Globulin	3.92±0.5[b]	2.82±0.7
β-Globulin	4.73±0.6[b]	3.12±0.6
γ-Globulin	9.83±0.7 [b]	13.3±1.7
A/G[a]	2.45±0.51	2.43±0.47

[a]A = albumin; G = globulin.
[b]Results between the affected and unaffected Guizhou semi-fine wool sheep were significantly different ($P<0.01$).

Table 3. Mineral element concentrations (ppm) in soil and forage samples collected in the affected and unaffected areas.

Elements	Soil		Forage	
	Affected area	Unaffected area	Affected area	Unaffected area
Cu	16.7±2.9	16.9±2.7	6.9±2.3	6.3±2.7
Mo	1.33±0.37	1.28±0.38	1.16±0.37	1.13±0.38
Fe	4527±371	4332±323	376±31	382±37
Zn	28.7±4.3	28.2±5.1	5.5±1.2	5.3±1.7
Mn	55.7±11.5	53.8±11.2	13.2±3.9	13.3±3.6
Ca	12278±457	12719±419	2866±217	2613±192
P	31.9±6.5[a]	56.5±6.7	239±13[a]	1279±31
F	25.78±5.8	25.23±6.3	21.5±4.9	22.5±5.3
Ca: P	385:1	225:1	12:1	2:1

[a]Results between the affected and unaffected areas were significantly different ($P<0.01$).

Discussion

Several mineral nutrition related diseases of sheep have been studied in the literature. Huang (2001) and Huang and Chen (2002) reported the pathogenesis of Tibet sheep and goats because of sulfur (S) and Cu deficiency in forage in Gansu Province of China [14,15]. Shen (2011) reported a disease of semi-fine wool sheep in Guizhou Province, which was related to S deficiency caused by high Fe in forage. The main signs of the disease included wool-eating, emaciation, losing appetite, pica, and weight loss [16]. Yuan et al. (2011) reported another disease of semi-fine wool sheep in Guizhou Province, which was caused by Cu deficiency mainly due to high S and Mo content in forage [17]. Compared with the diseases above, the disease in this study occurred in a different region, i.e., the adjoined region of Guizhou, Yunnan, and Sichuan Provinces, with different characteristics, and different nutrition deficiency problems. Therefore, it was the first time to report this disease of Guizhou semi-fine wool sheep.

Preliminary epidemiological and clinical observations indicated that Guizhou semi-fine wool sheep suffered a nutritional and

Table 4. Mineral element concentrations in the whole heparinised blood and wool samples of the Guizhou semi-fine wool sheep (The unit for F is in ppb and others in ppm).

Elements	Blood		Wool	
	Affected	**Unaffected**	**Affected**	**Unaffected**
Cu	0.75±0.23	0.76±0.25	5.18±1.23	5.15±1.31
Mo	0.36±0.06	0.37±0.07	0.31±0.05	0.33±0.09
Fe	512.3±22.9	513.6±23.8	333.2±21.6	337.5±17.5
Zn	15.3±2.9	15.7±2.7	87.5±4.8	89.3±3.8
Mn	0.51±0.15	0.58±0.17	5.77±1.16	5.73±1.17
Ca	127.0±13.7	127.3±11.5	1019±41	1097±67
P	253.0±22.4[a]	368.0±32.4	81.9±13.7[a]	157.7±15.7
F	18.7±5.4	19.1±6.1	18.9±4.7	19.7±5.7

[a]Results between the affected and unaffected Guizhou semi-fine wool sheep were significantly different (P<0.01).

metabolic disease associated with P deficiency. Our experimental results showed that the P concentrations in the soil and forage in the affected areas were significantly lower than the unaffected areas. In addition, P levels in serum, wool, bones, and teeth from the affected sheep were markedly lower, and serum AKP level was significantly higher than those of the unaffected animals. The result was consistent with the response criteria in P deficiency disease of wildlife yaks and Bactrian camels [6,7,18]. The oral supplement of Na_2HPO_4 appeared to cure the disease successfully. The above results clearly demonstrated that the disorder problem of Guizhou semi-fine wool sheep was related to the P deficiency in forage, which was attributable to the current herding practices as discussed below.

The local herd practices have a great impact on nutrition imbalance for grazing animals. In 1990s, the pasture and livestock were allocated to individual families in an attempt to improve the local herdsmen's life and productivity. Animals grazed in fixed and limited areas within fenced pasture. As a result, the fenced pasture and habitat fragmentation might create nutrition imbalance problems for animals. Nutrient contents in the soil and forage are spatially distributed. If animals graze in an extensive area, they have chances to graze in poor as well as rich nutrition areas.

Therefore, the nutrition imbalance problem is minimal [19]. In the present study, P concentrations in the soil and forage from the affected areas were significantly lower than those in the unaffected areas. Within the fenced pasture, the sheep grazed in the same pasture with P deficiency during the year. As a result, Guizhou semi-fine wool sheep suffered the disease related to the P deficiency.

For many grass species, the period with relatively high P concentrations (>0.3%) available to grazing animals is pretty short [20–22]. In most years, mature forage contains P <0.15% [4,23]. In general, the sufficient P levels for ruminants are >0.005% in soils and >0.3% in forage [3,24]. However, in the present study, the P levels of the soil and forage in the affected areas were 0.0031% and 0.024%, respectively, which were much lower than the sufficient levels.

Among the factors influencing Ca and P utilization metabolism, a Ca:P ratio of 1:1 to 2:1 is usually recommended for proper utilization of the elements by animals [2,25]. Dietary Ca:P ratios <1:1 or >7:1 should adversely affect growth and feed efficiency of animals [21,26]. In our study, the mean Ca:P ratio in forage from the unaffected area was 2:1. However, the mean Ca:P ratio in forage from the affected area was 12:1, which should have a negative impact on the Ca and P metabolism of the semi-fine wool sheep in the area. To prevent P deficiency in grazing livestock, oral supplement of bone meal, phosphate and mineral mixtures is recommended [1,4].

A number of response criteria have been used to evaluate the P status of animals, including serum levels of P, Ca, and alkaline phosphatase (AKP). Previous research suggests that bone criteria are more sensitive to P than to other elements. A marked hypophosphataemia is also a good indicator of a severe P deficiency, even if serum levels of Ca are unaffected. Phosphorus levels of blood samples are not a good indicator for the P status because P levels can be normal for a long period after animals have been exposed to serious P deficiency [25,27].

Phosphorus deficiency disease should be differentiated from chronic fluorosis in mature animals. The typical characteristic of fluorine toxicity includes mottling and pitting of teeth and enlargements on the shafts of long bones. In this study, the fluorine concentrations in soil and forage were lower than the critical values of 30–40 ppm [28]. The fluorine concentrations in bones, tissues, blood, and wool were within the normal range. Therefore, the disease of Guizhou semi-fine wool sheep was not related to fluorosis. A general opinion is that sheep rarely suffer

Table 5. Mineral element concentrations in bones and teeth of Guizhou semi-fine wool sheep (The unit for Ca and P is in g/kg dry sample and others in ppm).

Elements	Rib		Hip		Teeth	
	Affected	**Unaffected**	**Affected**	**Unaffected**	**Affected**	**Unaffected**
Cu	7.93±2.2	7.64±2.3	5.78±1.56	5.69±1.37	4.82±0.73	4.87±0.76
Mo	1.37±0.61	1.35±0.51	2.57±0.51	2.53±0.61	2.35±0.57	2.48±0.53
Fe	179.9±11.9	173.2±12.7	177.7±14.8	175.3±15.7	157.5±11.1	153.7±12.5
Zn	113.7±11.9	112.7±12.9	98.3±7.8	97.7±7.3	92.8±5.7	91.9±5.1
Mn	6.67±1.31	6.59±1.49	4.53±1.21	4.57±1.13	6.17±0.53	6.13±0.58
Ca	131.9±12.1	137.5±12.2	127.6±17.5	125.6±23.1	177.3±22.6	173.8±23.7
P	37.3±5.7[a]	75.7±12.6	35.1±3.1[a]	78.3±11.6	32.3±6.1[a]	77.6±7.5
F	57.3±13.7	55.7±12.6	65.1±13.1	63.3±11.6	72.3±16.1	77.6±7.5

[a]Results between affected and unaffected the Guizhou semi-fine wool sheep were significantly different (P<0.01).

clinically from P deficiency [29]. However, mature females and lambs are more susceptible to P deficiency than mature males.

Acknowledgments

The valuable review comments from Dr. Neville Suttle and another anonymous reviewer are gracefully acknowledged.

References

1. Blood DC, Radostits OM, Arunde JH, Gay CC (1989) The Veterinary Medicine, 7th ed. Balliere Tindall, London, UK, 1502 pp.
2. Shupe JL (1988) Clinical signs and bone change associated with phosphorus deficiency in beef cattle. American Journal of Veterinary Research. 49:1619–1636.
3. Heuer C, Bode E (1998) Variation of serum inorganic phosphorus and association with hemoglobinuria and osteomalacia in female water buffaloes in Pakistan. Preventive Veterinary Medicine 33: 69–81.
4. McDowell LR (1992) Mineral in Animals and Human Nutrition Academic Press. Inc, New York, USA, 770 pp.
5. Zhang D, Liu Z, Zhang Q (1989) Studies on rickets in police dogs. Journal of Gansu Agricultural University 3:324–327. [In Chinese]
6. Liu Z (2005) Studies on rickets and osteomalacia in Bactrian camels (Camelus bactrianus). The Veterinary Journal 169:444–453.
7. Shen X, Zhang R (2012) Studies on "Stiffness of Extremities Disease" in the Yak (Bos mutus). Journal of Wildlife Disease 48(3):542–547.
8. Federation of Animals Science Societies (2010) Guide for the care and use of agricultural animals in research and teaching. 3rd Edition. FASS, Champaign, Illinois, 169pp.
9. Salmela S, Vuori E, Kilpo JO (1981) The effect of washing procedures on trace element content of human hair. Analytica Chimica Acta 125: 131–137.
10. Arthington JD, Rechcig JE, Yost GP, McDowell LR. Fanning MD (2002) Effect of ammonium sulfate fertilization on bahiagrass quality and copper metabolism in grazing beef cattle. Journal of Animal Science 80 (10):2507–2512.
11. Tiffany ME, Mc Dowell LR, O'connor GA, Martin FG, Wilkinson NS, et al. (2002) Effects of residual and reapplied biosolids on performance and mineral status of grazing beef steers. Journal of Animal Science 80:260–266.
12. Wang K, Xu H, Luo X (1996) Trace Element in Life Science. Metrology Press, Beijing, China, 1040 pp. [In Chinese].
13. Wang J, Liu Z (2004) Veterinary Clinical Diagnosis. Chinese Agricultural Press, Beijing, China, 373 pp. [In Chinese].
14. Huang Y (2001) An experimental study on treatment and prevention of shimao zheng (fleece-eating) in sheep and goats in the Haizi area of Akesai County in ChinaÐ Veterinary Research Communications. 26: 39–48.
15. Huang Y, Chen H (2002) Studies on the pathogenesis of Shimao Zheng in sheep and goats. Veterinary Research Communications. 25: 631–640.
16. Shen X (2011) Studies of wool-eating ailment in Guizhou semi-fine wool sheep. Agricultural Sciences in China. Agricultural Science in China. 10 (10):168–1623.
17. Yuan R, Li L, Wang Q, Du G (2011) Copper deficiency in Guizhou semi-fine wool sheep on pasture in south west China karst mountain area. African Journal of Biotechnology. 10 (74): 17043–17048.
18. Braithwaite GD (1985) Endogenous faecal loss of phosphorus in growing lambs and the calculation of phosphorus requirements. Journal of Agricultural Science. 105: 67–72.
19. Shen X, Du G, Chen Y (2006) Copper deficiency in yak on pasture in western China. The Canadian Veterinary Journal. 47: 902–906.
20. Field AC, Williams JA, Dingwall RA (1985) The effect of dietary intake of calcium and dry matter on the absorption and excretion of calcium and phosphorus by growing lambs. Journal of Agricultural Science. 105(2): 237–243.
21. Karn JF (2001) Phosphorus nutrition of grazing cattle: a review. Animal Feed Science and Technology 89: 133–153.
22. Scott D, Buchan W (1985) The effect of feeding either roughage or concentrate diets on salivary phosphorus secretion, net intestinal absorption and urinary excretion in the sheep. Quarterly Journal of Experimental Physiology. 70: 365–375.
23. Scott D, BuchanW (1987) The effect of feeding either hay or grass diets on salivary phosphorus secretion, net intestinal absorption and on the partition of phosphorus between urine and faeces in the sheep. Quarterly Journal of Experimental Physiology. 72: 331–338.
24. Scott D, Rajaratne AAJ, Buchan W (1995) Factors affecting faecal endogenous phosphorus loss in the sheep. Journal of Agricultural Science. 124: 145–151.
25. Wang Z, Cao G, Hu Z, Ding Y (1995) Mineral element Metabolism and Animal Disease, Shanghai Science-Technology Press, Shanghai, China, 544 pp. [In Chinese].
26. Scott D, McLean AF, BuchanW (1984) The effect of variation in phosphorus intake on net intestinal phosphorus absorption, salivary phosphorus secretion and pathway of phosphorus excretion in sheep fed roughage diets. Quarterly Journal of Experimental Physiology. 69: 439–452.
27. Maduell F, Gorriz JL, Pallardo LM, Pons R, Santiago C (2005) Assessment of phosphorus and calcium metabolism and its clinical management in hemodialysis patients in the community of valencia. Journal of Nephrology 18: 123–137.
28. Huang Y, Liu Z (2001) Toxicopathy and nutritional disorder disease in animals. Gansu Science and Technology Press, Lanzhou. pp.194–199. [in Chinese].
29. Suttle NF (2010) The mineral nutrition of livestock. 4th ed. CABI Publishing Cambridge, USA, 579 pp.

Author Contributions

Conceived and designed the experiments: XS. Performed the experiments: JZ. Analyzed the data: XS JZ. Contributed reagents/materials/analysis tools: XS RZ. Wrote the paper: XS RZ.

18

A Case-Control Study of Risk Factors for Bovine Brucellosis Seropositivity in Peninsular Malaysia

Mukhtar Salihu Anka[1], Latiffah Hassan[1]*, Siti Khairani-Bejo[1], Mohamed Abidin Zainal[2], Ramlan bin Mohamad[3], Annas Salleh[1], Azri Adzhar[4]

1 Department of Veterinary Pathology and Microbiology, Faculty of Veterinary Medicine, Universiti Putra Malaysia, Serdang, Selangor, Malaysia, 2 Department of Agribusiness and information system, Faculty of Agriculture, Universiti Putra Malaysia, Serdang, Selangor, Malaysia, 3 Veterinary Research Institute, Ipoh Perak, Malaysia, 4 Epidemiology and Surveillance Unit, Department of Veterinary Services, Putrajaya, Malaysia

Abstract

Bovine brucellosis was first reported in Peninsular Malaysia in 1950. A subsequent survey conducted in the country revealed that the disease was widespread. Current knowledge on the potential risk factors for brucellosis occurrence on cattle farms in Malaysia is lacking. Therefore, we conducted a case-control study to identify the potential herd-level risk factors for bovine brucellosis occurrence in four states in the country, namely Kelantan, Pahang, Selangor and Negeri Sembilan. Thirty-five cases and 36 controls of herds were selected where data on farm management, biosecurity, medical history and public health were collected. Multivariable logistic regression identified that *Brucella* seropositive herds were more likely to; have some interaction with wildlife (OR 8.9, 95% CI = 1.59–50.05); originated from farms where multiple species such as buffalo/others (OR 41.8, 95% CI = 3.94–443.19) and goat/sheep (OR 8.9, 95%CI = 1.10–71.83) were reared, practice extensive production system (OR 13.6, 95% CI 1.31–140.24) and have had episodes of abortion in the past (OR 51.8, 95% CI = 4.54–590.90) when compared to seronegative herds. Considering the lack of information on the epidemiology of bovine brucellosis in peninsular Malaysia and absence of information on preventing the inception or spread of the disease, this report could contribute to the on-going area-wise national brucellosis eradication program.

Editor: Joao Inacio, University of Brighton, United Kingdom

Funding: This project was funded by the Universiti Putra Malaysia Grant no 01-03-10-0956RU. The funders had no role in study design, data collection and analysis, decision to publish, or preparation of the manuscript.

Competing Interests: The authors have declared that no competing interests exist.

* Email: latiffah@upm.edu.my

Introduction

Bovine brucellosis is a widespread livestock disease with worldwide distribution [1] caused by Gram-negative bacteria of the genus *Brucella*. [2]. In cattle, brucellosis is usually caused by *B. abortus*, but has also been attributed to *B. melitensis* and infrequently to *B. suis* [3,4]. The disease is characterised by infertility, abortion among females, and orchitis and epididymitis in males [5]. Brucellosis causes serious economic losses to farmers and the government through direct production losses as well as additional costs for control and eradication programs [6]. Although bovine brucellosis has been controlled and eradicated in most of the developed nations, it remains a significant problem for both cattle and human health, especially in developing countries [7,8].

As in most Southeast Asia countries, bovine brucellosis has been a problem among livestock for many years in Malaysia [9,10]. The first evidence of the disease was reported at *Institut Haiwan* in Malaysia among imported cattle in 1950 [11], but it was effectively controlled through an intensive testing and slaughter program, accompanied by vaccination of young animals [12]. Sporadic cases of brucellosis continue to occur among local animals and, recently, Malaysian veterinary authorities observed an increasing trend in the seroprevalence of brucellosis among livestock [5,13].

Studies of limited geographic localities to detect bovine brucellosis in Peninsular Malaysia have been carried out [9,12,14]; however, so far none have attempted to identify the risk factors for *Brucella* seropositivity among cattle. Knowledge about important determinants for *Brucella* seropositivity is vital, as these factors can be further explored in strategizing evidence-based disease control measures in the country. In this study, we assessed the role of several putative factors in the occurrence of bovine brucellosis among herds in Peninsular Malaysia and suggest how these factors can be modified to reduce the risk of the infection.

Materials and Methods

Ethics Statement

The study was approved by the Department of Veterinary Services, Putrajaya, Ministry of Agriculture Malaysia. A written consent was sought from every study participant before administering the questionnaire.

Study area and study population

Malaysia is a Southeast Asian country located between 2.3167° North and 111.5500° East. It comprises West Malaysia (Peninsular Malaysia) and East Malaysia (Sabah and Sarawak on Borneo Island) separated by the South China Sea. The study was conducted in Peninsular Malaysia, which is comprised of 11 states and two federal territories and covers an area of 131,598 square kilometres bordering Thailand in the north and Singapore in the south. The country has a tropical climate with warm weather all year round. Rainfall varies throughout the year with an average of 2,400 mm (http://www.met.gov.my). Malaysia has a relatively small cattle population, with an estimated total cattle population in 2010 of 836,910 head [15]. Two main cattle breeds are encountered in Malaysia: Kedah-Kelantan, constituting a high percentage of the total beef cattle, and Local Indian Dairy (LID) cattle, which is the main dairy cattle population. Other breeds are also imported to increase production, including Brahman, Hereford, Aberdeen Angus, Droughtmaster, Bali, among others [16].

For this study we chose four states (Kelantan, Pahang, Selangor, Negeri Sembilan) based on the seroprevalence rates of *B. abortus* in each state in the years prior to the study. The veterinary authorities of Malaysia have been performing systematic and nationwide brucellosis testing and culling as part of the effort to control the infection among livestock in the country. At the time of the study, the estimated cattle population was 128,907 cattle in Kelantan, 47,227 in Negeri Sembilan, 169,312 in Pahang and 31,236 in Selangor from 2,840, 1,212, 4,111 and 1,258 registered livestock premises, respectively [17].

Study design

We performed a case-control study to determine the herd-level risk factors for bovine brucellosis between August 2011 and March 2012. Sampling was performed by selecting states with high seroprevalence of brucellosis based on the nationwide brucellosis serosurveillance data. Within each state, farms were identified via database of the serosurveillance program carried out by the veterinary authority of Malaysia in 2010. The list of herds in dataset of the year 2010 was used as the sampling frame for the herd selection. Stratified sampling within each state was performed to obtain seronegative and seropositive herds. We defined 'case' herds as those cattle herds which, within the previous one year, were found to have at least one seropositive confirmed by both the Rose Bengal Plate Test (RBPT) and the Complement Fixation Test (CFT) as prescribed by the OIE protocol at the Veterinary Research Institute (VRI), while 'control' herds were herds that had no seropositives. The CFT test have a reported sensitivity and specificity of 95% and 100% respectively [18]. From the list of seropositive and seronegative farms in each state, selection of farms were made randomly and lists of the selected farms were delivered to their respective state DVS for their approval, in addition to letters dispatched to individual farms. At the time of our study, some farms were no longer operational, and replacements for them were based on the recommendations of officials from the state DVS.

Sample size was calculated using OpenEpi software version 2.3 (OpenEpi, Atlanta, GA, USA) for an unmatched case-control study with $\alpha = 0.05$, power $= 80$, ratio of cases to controls $= 1.0$, hypothetical proportion of exposure among controls $= 30$ and hypothetical proportion of exposure among cases $= 65$. A total of at least 31 herds each for the cases and control groups were required based on these assumptions. We selected a total of 71 herds (cases n $= 35$, controls n $= 36$) from different states; 20 herds from Kelantan (cases n $= 10$, controls n $= 10$), 16 from Negeri Sembilan (cases n $= 8$, controls n $= 8$), 18 from Selangor (cases n $= 8$, controls n $= 10$) and 17 from Pahang (cases n $= 9$, controls n $= 8$).

Data collection

At each farm visit, state district veterinary officers accompanied the researchers to locate the farms and interview the farmers. The farmers were interviewed using a structured closed-ended questionnaire. The questionnaire sought information on farm demography, farm size, the size of the cattle population in the herd, breed of cattle, origin of the cattle, the system of farm management, biosecurity, medical history of the farm and the health aspect of the farmers.

Data analysis

Descriptive statistics were generated for the study farms/herds in relation to the system of management, farm size, and origin of the cattle. A univariable logistic regression analysis examined the association between case-control status and potential risk factors. Variables were grouped into different categories of general farm characteristics, farm management, biosecurity, medical history of the farm and health aspect of the owners and their staff or family members. The strength of associations between case-control status and potential risk factors was analysed using odds ratio (OR) and 95% confidence interval (CI). Variables significant in the univariable analysis were tested for collinearity using the chi-square test for independence. A multivariable logistic regression was then constructed using a backward unconditional method to identify potential risk factors for bovine brucellosis; interactions were also tested for explanatory variables. Those explanatory variables significantly associated with case/control status in the univariable analysis (p$\leq$0.05) were fitted into the multivariable analysis. Herd size was categorised into <15, 15–30 and>30 head of cattle; the age range of the cattle was categorized into <3, 3–6 and>6 years. The overall goodness of fit was accessed using the Hosmer-Lemeshow test. Information from the questionnaire was entered into a Microsoft excel spreadsheet (Microsoft Corporation) and data was imported into the SPSS version 20 software for statistical analysis (SPSS Inc. Chicago USA).

Results

Description of the study herds

The studied areas contained three management systems: free grazing (extensive system n = 34), feedlot (intensive system n = 19), and semi-intensive (n = 18). Malaysia has a large area cultivated with major crops such as oil palm, rubber, coconut etc. These plantations are integrated with livestock. The government introduced the integration system to improve livestock production and support farmers to eradicate poverty [19]. At the time of the study, Peninsular Malaysia has an estimated cattle population of 778,189 and most of these animals are raised under an integrated system [19,20]. About 47.9% (34) of the farms we studied were extensive/integrated farms, 21 being cases and 13 being controls. Semi-intensive farms comprised 25.4%, with 10 cases and 8 controls, while intensive farms accounted for only 26.8%, comprising 4 cases and 15 controls. Out of the 71 herds in the study, 83.1% (59) herds were beef cattle, while 14.1% (10) were dairy herds and 2.8% (2) practiced both.

Cattle from 64.8% (46) of the herds sampled were from Malaysia, 19% (14) were imported from Australia, 8.5% (6) were from Thailand and the remaining 7% (5) were from other countries. The largest herds were in Kelantan with 800 (112±200) head of cattle, followed by Pahang with 517 (168±142) head, Selangor with 420 (132±112) head and Negeri Sembilan with 270 (127±121) head of cattle. About 94% (67) (34 cases and 33 controls) of farms used an open-housing system while 5.6% (4) (1 case and 3 controls) had closed housing systems. About 53.5% (38)

of the farms sourced drinking water from a river while 28.2% (20) sourced water from the tap. A minority of the farmers 18.3% (13) indicated sourcing water from a pond. Of the studied herds, 90.1% (64) reported doing in-house breeding, while 9.9% (7) indicated doing breeding outside the farm. In response to whether other species of animal were kept on the farm, most of the interviewed farmers reported rearing other species on the farm: 54.9% (39) also rear goats, 10.3% (4) sheep, and 30.8% (13) buffalo, horses or deer.

Among the sampled farms, 49.3% (35) reported cleaning the farm every day while others cleaned less regularly and only 6 (8.5%) reported using disinfectant. About 54.9% of the farmers did not allow visitors into their farm. Well over half (88.7%) of those surveyed have no biosecurity facility on their farm. The majority of the farmers (51, or 71.8%) have no personal protective equipment (PPE) such as gloves, facemask and boots on the farm while only 28.2% (20) use PPE. Most of the farmers (50, or 70.4%) noted the presence of wildlife such as wild boars and tigers around their farms. Of the 71 herds participating in this study, 35.2% (25) possessed no isolation facilities while 64.8% (46) did. About 54.9% (39) of sampled herds had had abortion episodes previously. Only 19.7% (14) of the farmers reported culling seropositive animals while 46.5% (33) indicated treating these animals with unspecified drugs and 46.5% reported selling them.

The result from the univariable logistic regression analysis revealed that the production system, rearing multiple species of animals, the presence of wild life and history of abortion all have significant impact on the bovine brucellosis sero-status of cattle herds in Peninsular Malaysia (Table 1).

Multivariable logistic regression

The multivariable logistic regression results (Table 2) showed the association of various potential risk factors to herd-level seropositivity. The final model indicated that compared to seronegative herds, seropositive herds were significantly more likely to: have some level of interaction with wildlife (OR 8.9, 95% CI = 1.59–50.05), contained mix species of animals such as buffalo, horses, deer or dogs (OR 41.8, 95% CI = 3.94–443.19) and goats/sheep (OR 8.9, 95%CI = 1.10–71.86), practice extensive farming system (OR 13.6, 95% CI = 1.31–140.24) and have had history of abortion (OR 51.8, 95% CI = 4.54–590.90).

The Hosmer-Lemeshow goodness of fit test showed that the model fit the data well ($X2 = 1.960$, d.f. 8, $p = 0.982$). The chi-square test for independence showed no important collinearities between the predictive variables.

Occupational risk and awareness among farmers about brucellosis

About 78% (56) of the farmers participating in the study reported that they had assisted the parturition process of cows on their farm and 71.8% (51) did not use basic PPE such as gloves or boots, especially when cleaning the farms. About 8.5% (6) (3 cases, 3 controls) reported consuming unpasteurized milk from their animals and 19.7% (14) have had episodes of fever, with one of the farmer experiencing undulant fever who was later diagnosed with brucellosis (Table 3)

Discussion

Several factors have been reported to be associated with bovine brucellosis [4,21–24] in other parts of the world, such as the level of hygiene on the farm, the herd size, age of the cattle, sex, system of production, the presence of wildlife, and multiple livestock species within the herd. In this study, we found a significant

association between the cattle production system and *Brucella* seropositivity, where cattle in an extensive system were found to be 13 times more likely to be exposed to *Brucella* infection compared to cattle in an intensive system. The observed increased risk of *Brucella* herd seropositivity based on the system of production confirms earlier findings by several authors [6,23]. In their study, one group found that extensive production systems increased the risk of brucellosis by about 10.6-fold compared to cattle raised in an intensive system. In Malaysia, most cattle are raised in integrated farming systems that combine animal and crop farming simultaneously to enable synergistic interaction and greater overall output in terms of high productivity, profitability, sustainability, environmental safety, recycling, income round the year, adoption of new technology, energy savings, meeting fodder crises and generating more employment [25–27]. The extensive farms in this study practice integrated farming, and in this study we observed poor biosecurity and control of animal movements whereby the majority of the farms in this category had no fence or demarcation. Animals from various herds belonging to different owners freely interact and, in many instances, multiple cattle herds belonging to separate owners can be found on the same premises. This combination of a lack of biosecurity within the herd and poor control of animal movements plays an important role in the epidemiology of many diseases. In the case of brucellosis, an extremely contagious disease, the infection may be easily passed between animals following an abortion episode via pasture or feed contaminated with the organism, inhalation, conjunctiva inoculation, skin contamination, or from contaminated utensils used on infected colostrum for new born calves. Unplanned breeding, which is common in this type of production system, may also occur and sexual transmission plays a major role in the transmission of the disease [28,29]. Most of the respondents (34, 47.9%) from our study confirmed that their animals mingled with other neighbouring cattle herds, and we believe that this maximizes contact between animals and facilitates the spread of the disease between infected and susceptible herds.

Another possible reason for the increased risk of exposure to *Brucella* organisms in the extensive farming system is contact with wildlife. Wild ungulates such as deer, elk and bison have been reported to be infected with *B. abortus* [30] and may serve as reservoirs of the organism transmitting the infection to susceptible cattle. Wild boars have also been incriminated in *B. abortus* infection [31]. We found that farms reporting sightings of wildlife had a 5.5-fold increased risk of *Brucella* seropositivity compared to farms that did not. Our finding is consistent with previous studies reporting the presence of *Brucella* antibodies in wildlife such as wild boars. The observed increased risk within herds that were exposed or interacted with wildlife could be a result of the high percentage of herds from extensive production systems in our study (47.9%), where cattle are allowed to move freely around the plantations and wild boars are also commonly seen roaming the plantations. Wild boars have been established as a reservoir of several infectious diseases [32,33] including brucellosis [34]. In boars, brucellosis is usually caused by *B. suis* biovar 2 [34,35]; however, *B. abortus* has also been isolated [36,37]. In a limited sample size study by Sohayati et al. (2012), the seroprevalence of brucellosis in local wild boars was estimated at 62.5% (n = 8) [38]. The preferred host for *B. abortus* is cattle and other bovidae [39]; however, evidence of cross-infection across species has been reported by Donald (1990) [40] where *B. suis* was isolated from a cow. The presence of wildlife in areas where brucellosis is endemic among livestock is a concern as the wildlife may become infected as a result of spillover from infected cattle and become sustained in

Table 1. Univariable analysis of potential risk factors for bovine brucellosis herd seropositivity in Peninsular Malaysia.

Variable	Category	Cases (n = 35)	Controls (n = 36)	eOR and 95% CI	P-value
Management					
System of production	Intensive	4	15	Ref	Ref
	Semi-intensive	10	8	4.7, 1.11–19.83	0.036
	Extensive	21	13	6.1, 1.65–22.27	0.007
State	Pahang	9	8	Ref	Ref
	N. Sembilan	8	8	0.9, 0.23–3.49	0.866
	Kelantan	10	10	0.9, 0.24–3.24	0.858
	Selangor	8	10	0.7, 0.19–2.69	0.616
Breed	Kedah-Kelantan	7	10	Ref	Ref
	Brahman	3	3	1.4, 0.22–9.26	0.708
	Local Indian Dairy	2	5	0.6, 0.09–3.83	0.564
	Kedah-Kelantan cross	6	3	2.9, 0.53–15.47	0.223
	Mixed	17	15	1.6, 0.49–5.32	0.427
Type	Dairy	2	8	Ref	Ref
	Beef	32	27	4.7, 0.93–24.24	0.06
	Both	1	1	4.0, 0.17–95.76	0.39
Age range of cattle	<3	9	8	Ref	Ref
	3–6	22	21	0.9, 0.30–2.87	0.901
	>6	4	7	0.5, 0.11–2.40	0.393
Herd size	<15	5	5	Ref	Ref
	15–30	2	7	0.3, 0.04–2.11	0.220
	>30	29	23	1.2, 0.30–4.52	0.823
Origin of cattle	Malaysia	21	25	Ref	Ref
	Imported	4	4	1.2, 0.27–5.35	0.820
	Both	10	7	1.7, 0.55–5.25	0.356
Housing	Close-house	1	3	Ref	Ref
	Open-house	34	33	0.3, 0.03–3.27	0.339
Water source	Tap	10	10	Ref	Ref
	Pond	4	9	0.4, 0.10–1.93	0.279
	River	21	17	1.2, 0.42–3.16	0.702
Breeding	In the farm	33	31	Ref	Ref
	Outside the farm	2	5	0.4, 0.07–2.08	0.262
Other species in the farm	No other species	21	11	Ref	Ref
	Buffaloes/Others	13	4	3.1, 1.15–8.09	0.007
	Goat/Sheep	11	11	1.9, 0.63–5.79	0.253
Biosecurity					
How often you clean farm	Daily	7	4	Ref	Ref
	Fortnightly	2	2	2, 0.23–17.33	0.529
	Monthly	1	1	2, 0.11–36.95	0.641
	Weekly	3	3	2.8, 0.90–8.37	0.075
	No cleaning	22	16	2, 0.318–12.59	0.460
Use of disinfectant	No	33	3	Ref	Ref
	Yes	32	3	1, 0.19–5.49	0.971
Visitors	No	16	23	Ref	Ref
	Yes	19	13	2.1, 0.81–5.44	0.126
Washing facilities	No	30	33	Ref	Ref
	Yes	5	3	1.8, 0.40–8.34	0.433
PPE	No	24	27	Ref	Ref
	Yes	11	9	1.4, 0.49–3.88	0.548
Wildlife	No	5	16	Ref	Ref

Table 1. Cont.

Variable	Category	Cases (n = 35)	Controls (n = 36)	eOR and 95% CI	P-value
	Yes	30	20	4.8, 1.54–15.19	0.008
Isolation Facilities	No	14	11	Ref	Ref
	Yes	21	25	0.7, 0.25–1.76	0.406
Medical History					
History of abortion	No	8	24	Ref	Ref
	Yes	27	12	6.8, 2.36–19.29	0.001
Handling abortion	Cull	8	6	Ref	Ref
	Treat	20	13	1.2, 0.33–4.10	0.825
	No response	7	17	0.3, 0.08–1.22	0.094
Clinical sign*	No	2	6	Ref	Ref
	Yes	33	30	3.3, 0.62–17.60	0.160

eOR, exposure odds ratio; Ref, reference categories; CI, confidence interval, PPE, personal protective equipment,
*animal showing at least one of the clinical signs (orchitis, retained placenta, mastitis, weak foetus, decreased milk production, low conception rate).

the wildlife population [34]. Infected wildlife may then serve as a source of *Brucella* infection during wildlife-livestock interactions.

The mixing of different species of animals, especially goats, buffalo and sheep with cattle is an important determinant for *Brucella* transmission in this study and has been reported elsewhere [41–43]. Our result shows that farms with buffalo, deer and horses were 24 times more likely to harbour cattle infected with the *Brucella* organism as compared to farms with only cattle. Similarly, farms with goats/sheep were 5 times more likely to harbour *Brucella* seropositive cattle compared to farms with only cattle. Cross-species infection with other *Brucella* species, especially *B. melitensis*, has been documented in cattle [43,44]. Moreover, other non-cattle ungulates (such as buffalo, deer, and horses), feral swine and dogs may increase the risk of exposure to cattle because the bacteria have been isolated from each of these species [32,45,46] and animals such as buffalo may serve as maintenance hosts for the organism [47] [48]. Animals such as dogs have high mobility and may also serve as carriers of the organism [46,49]. Under experimental conditions dogs can be infected with *B. abortus*, shed bacteria in reproductive discharges, and infect cattle [31].

In countries where extensive farming, especially combined with integrated farming, is widely practiced, the observation of clinical signs such as abortion and stillbirth is more complicated and can prove difficult. In Malaysia, brucellosis in animals has been marked by its indiscernible or unremarkable clinical symptoms, i.e. symptoms such as abortion storm have never been reported. This is probably a result of the unplanned breeding that is commonly practiced in animal production in developing countries [42]. In our study, even though abortion storm has not been reported, sporadic abortion is a significant determinant of bovine brucellosis seropositivity and proves that brucellosis must be included as a differential whenever abortion (even though in low numbers) was observed in a farm. This finding agrees with other studies [50,51]. A study in India found the seroprevalence of brucellosis to be significantly higher in animals with a history of abortion than in those without while a study in Uganda also reported a history of abortion at the herd level to be a significant factor for brucellosis seropositivity. The primary source of the *Brucella* organism in the epidemiology of brucellosis in cattle is the uterine fluid and placenta or aborted foetus expelled by infected cattle during abortion or parturition [52]. Under optimum conditions, the *Brucella* organism can remain for 66 days in moist soil and up to

Table 2. Multivariable logistic regression of potential risk factors for bovine brucellosis herd seropositivity in Peninsular Malaysia.

Variable	Category	Cases (n = 35)	Controls (n = 36)	eOR and 95% CI	P-value
System of production	Intensive	4	15	Ref	Ref
	Semi-intensive	10	8	7.3, 0.88–60.82	0.065
	Extensive	21	13	13.6, 1.31–140.24	0.029
Other species on the farm	No other animals	21	11	Ref	Ref
	Buffalo/others	13	4	41.8, 3.94–443.19	0.002
	Goat/Sheep	11	11	8.9, 1.10–71.83	0.040
History of abortion	No	8	24	Ref	Ref
	Yes	27	12	51.8, 4.54–590.90	0.001
Wildlife	No	5	16	Ref	Ref
	Yes	30	20	8.9, 1.59–50.05	0.013

eOR, exposure odds ratio; Ref, reference categories; CI, confidence interval.

Table 3. Potential risk of *Brucella* infection among cattle farmers.

Variable	Category	Number of farms (%) (n = 71)	Case farms (%) (n = 35)	Control farms (%) (n = 36)
Assist in delivery		56 (78.9)	33(58.9)	23(41.1)
Milk was consumed	Raw	2 (2.8)	1(50)	1(50)
	Boiled	5 (7.0)	2(40)	3(60)
	Never	64 (90.1)	32(50)	32(50)
Symptoms reported by farmers	Fever	14 (19.7)	8(57.1)	6(42.9)
	Undulant fever	1 (1.4)	1(100)	0(0)
	No	56 (78.9)	26(46.4)	30(53.6)
Diagnosed with brucellosis		1 (1.4)	1 (100)	0(0)

185 days in cold soil [51,52]. Although not all abortions are due to brucellosis, abortion is a major clinical sign of the disease in cattle and therefore should be suspected whenever observed [30].

Brucellosis has major public health implications [53], with the disease mainly affecting people who work with livestock or animal products [54]. The findings from our study show that more than 50% of farmers assisted cows during parturition without using the most basic personal protective gear. Studies have shown that assisting animals during parturition increase the risk for brucellosis transmission to humans [55]. Indeed, the findings emphasized the need for basic education and knowledge of brucellosis transmission among farmers. Moreover, although the number of farmers consuming unpasteurised milk is insignificant, those who do have an increased risk for brucellosis. Therefore public health education and promotion on the prevention and control of common zoonotic diseases is certainly necessary for these populations.

Our study should be interpreted with caution because of several limitations. Its major limitation is selection bias, as some of the herds pre-selected were no longer operational upon visiting them. We attempted to reduce this bias by selecting another herd within the same district that had the same *Brucella* status using the sampling frame from the previous serosurveillance conducted by the DVS. Another potential bias is recall bias or selective recall by farmers when they were asked to recall events that may have occurred a few years prior to the study. Selective memory recall is common in case-control study designs because 'cases' may remember information about determinants more vividly and differently than 'controls'. In addition, many farmers do not keep proper documentations and record of animals in their farms, a problem that is pervasive in extensive farms in developing countries. Temporality between cause and effect can also be confusing and difficult to ascertain because of the inherent limitations in case-control study design.

Conclusion

The results of the present study revealed that the production system, presence of wildlife, presence of other non-cattle species on

the same farm and history of abortion were important and significant risk factors associated with bovine brucellosis in Peninsular Malaysia. We believe that among these risk factors, the modifiable factor where changes can be implemented readily and with minimal financial implications would be to improve the biosecurity of farms by placing enclosures in the area through effective fencing. The presence of enclosures will reduce mingling between animals from separate herds and deter wildlife away from animal feed and water sources. We also suggest separating other species of animals from cattle herds to prevent infection from other non-cattle ungulates that may host the organism or result in cross-species *Brucella* infection. Educational program directed at farmers and collaboration between veterinary authorities and herd owners could further improve the management system. The lack of knowledge among farmers on the zoonotic nature of the disease is of concern and veterinary and human medical authorities need to improve public health education among high-risk populations in order to enhance precautionary measures and prevent disease occurrence. Finally, this study provides baseline information for further research on the bovine brucellosis and may be used to modify the level of disease present among herds in Malaysia.

Acknowledgments

The authors acknowledge the Department of Veterinary Services Putrajaya and the Veterinary Research Institute, Ipoh for their assistant and support. We acknowledge the State and district staff of Department of Veterinary Services of Kelantan, Pahang, Selangor and Negeri Sembilan for their helped during farm visits and data collection.

Author Contributions

Conceived and designed the experiments: LH. Analyzed the data: MSA. Wrote the paper: MSA LH. Carried out the study: MSA. Conceived of the study: LH. Approved the final draft of the manuscript: LH. Participated in the design of the study: SKB RBM MAZ AA. Proof reading of the manuscript: SKB RBM MAZ AA. Helped in the survey and data collection: AS. Helped in acquiring the data: AA.

References

1. Abernethy DA, Moscard-Costello J, Dickson E, Harwood R, Burns K, et al. (2011) Epidemiology and management of a bovine brucellosis cluster in Northern Ireland. Prev Vet Med 98: 223–229.

2. Abdussalam M, Fein DA (1984) Brucellosis as a world problem. Dev Biol Stand 56: 9–23.

3. Godfroid J, Cloeckaert A, Liautard J-P, Kohler S, Fretin D, et al. (2005) From the discovery of the Malta fever's agent to the discovery of a marine mammal reservoir, brucellosis has continuously been a re-emerging zoonosis. Vet Res 36: 313–326.

4. Sanogo M, Abatih E, Thys E, Fretin D, Berkvens D, et al. (2012) Risk factors associated with brucellosis seropositivity among cattle in the central savannah-forest area of Ivory Coast. Prev Vet Med 107: 51–56.

5. Anka MS, Hassan L, Adzhar A, Khairani-Bejo S, Mohamad RB, et al. (2013) Bovine brucellosis trends in Malaysia between 2000 and 2008. BMC Vet Res 9: 230.

6. Mekonnen H, Kalayou S, Kyule M (2010) Serological survey of bovine brucellosis in barka and arado breeds (*Bos indicus*) of Western Tigray, Ethiopia. Prev Vet Med 94: 28–35.

7. Apan TZ, Yildirim M, Istanbulluoglu E (2007) Seroprevalence of brucellosis in human, sheep, and cattle populations in Kirikkale (Turkey). Turk J Vet Anim Sci 31: 75–78.

8. Lee BY, Higgins IM, Moon OK, Clegg TA, Mcgrath G, et al. (2009) Surveillance and control of bovine brucellosis in the Republic of Korea during 2000–2006. Prev Vet Med 90: 66–79.

9. Bahaman AR, Joseph P, Bejo SK (2007) A Review of the Epidemiology and Control of Brucellosis in Malaysia. J Vet Malaysia 19: 1–6.

10. Godfroid J, Al Dahouk S, Pappas G, Roth F, Matope G, et al. (2012) A "One Health" surveillance and control of brucellosis in developing countries: Moving away from improvisation. Comp Immunol Microb volume, page?

11. Heng N, Joseph P (1986) Eradication of Brucellosis in cattle in Malaysia and its public health; Petaling Jaya, Malaysia pp. 255–260.

12. Joseph P (1980) Animal brucellosis in Peninsular Malaysia. Tropical Agriculture Research Series No 13 Ministry of Agriculture and forestry, Tokyo, Japan. Tokyo, Japan.

13. DVS (2007) Lapuran Tahunan Jabatan Perkidmatan Haiwan Malaysia. Department of Veterinary Services, Ministry of Agriculture Malaysia.

14. Zainor M, Khairani-Bejo S, Bahaman AR, Zunita Z (2008) Isolation of *Brucella abortus* from aborted bovine fetus. 20th Congress of Veterinary Association Malaysia 15–17 August. Bangi, Putrajaya pp. 69.

15. DVS (2012) Malaysia: Self-Sufficiency In Livestock Products (%), 2003–2012.

16. Johari JA, Jasmi Y (2009) Breeds and breeding program for beef production in Malaysia. 8th Malaysia Congress on Genetics, 4–6 August. Genting Highland, Malaysia pp. 22–29.

17. MOA (2011) Ministry of Agriculture and Agro-Based Industry Malaysia Agrofood Statistics 2011. pp. 3–4.

18. Uzal FA, Carrasco AE, Echaide S, Nielsen K, Robles CA (1995) Evaluation of an indirect ELISA for the diagnosis of bovine brucellosis. J Vet Diagn Invest 7: 473–475.

19. Devendra C (2004) Integrated tree cropsruminants systems: Potential importance of the oil palm. Outlook Agr 33: 157–166.

20. Ismail D (1993) Integrated Production System. In: Hudson RJ, editor. Management of Agricultural, Forestry and Fisheries Enterprises. Canada: UNESCO-EOLSS.

21. Muma J, Godfroid J, Samui K, Skjerve E (2007) The role of *Brucella* infection in abortions among traditional cattle reared in proximity to wildlife on the Kafue flats of Zambia. Rev Sci Tech Off Int Epiz 26: 721–730.

22. Megersa B, Biffa D, Abunna F, Regassa A, Godfroid J, et al. (2011) Seroprevalence of brucellosis and its contribution to abortion in cattle, camel, and goat kept under pastoral management in Borana, Ethiopia. Trop Anim Health Prod 43: 651–656.

23. Megersa B, Biffa D, Niguse F, Rufael T, Asmare K, et al. (2011) Cattle brucellosis in traditional livestock husbandry practice in Southern and Eastern Ethiopia, and its zoonotic implication. Acta Vet Scand 53: 24.

24. Mai HM, Irons PC, Kabir J, Thompson PN (2013) Herd-level risk factors for *Campylobacter fetus* infection, *Brucella* seropositivity and within-herd seroprevalence of brucellosis in cattle in northern Nigeria. Prev Vet Med 111: 256–267.

25. Rota A, Sperandini S (2010) Integrated Crop-Livestock Farming Systems. Livestock Thematic Papers. Tools for Project Design. IFAD, International Fund for Agricultural Development, Rome, Italy.

26. Devendra C (2011) Integrated tree crops-ruminants systems in South East Asia: Advances in productivity enhancement and environmental sustainability. Asian Austral J Anim 24: 587–602.

27. Agricinfo (2011) Farming Systems & Sustainable Agriculture: Benefits or Advantages of Integrated Farming System. My Agriculture Information Bank, 2011. Available: http://www.agriinfo.in/?page=topic&superid=1&topicid=684. Accessed 2014 March 12.

28. FAO (2005) Capacity Building For Surveillance and Control of Zoonotic Diseases; Rome, Italy.

29. Corbel MJ (2006) Brucellosis in humans and animals. Geneva (Switzerland). World Health Organization.

30. Godfroid J, Nielsen K, Saegerman C (2010) Diagnosis of brucellosis in livestock and wildlife. Croat Med J 51: 296–305.

31. CFSPH (2009) Bovine Brucellosis. Available: http://www.cfsph.iastate.edu/Factsheets/pdfs/brucellosis_abortus.pdf. Accessed 2014 March 12.

32. Meng X, Lindsay D, Sriranganathan N (2009) Wild boars as sources for infectious diseases in livestock and humans. Phil Trans R Soc B 364: 2697–2707.

33. Lopes L, Nicolino R, Haddad J (2010) Brucellosis- Risk Factors and Prevalence: A Review. Open Veterinary Science Journal 4: 72–84.

34. Godfroid J (2002) Brucellosis in wildlife. Rev Sci Tech Off Int Epiz 21: 277–286.

35. Watarai M, Ito N, Omata Y, Ishiguro N (2006) A serological survey of *Brucella* spp. in free-ranging wild boar (*Sus scrofa leucomystax*) in Shikoku, Japan. J Vet Med Sci 68: 1139–1141.

36. Hubálek Z, Treml F, Juricova Z, Hunady M, Halouzka J, et al. (2002) Serological survey of the wild boar (*Sus scrofa*) for tularaemia and brucellosis in South Moravia, Czech Republic. Vet Med (Praha) 47: 60–66.

37. Gregoire F, Mousset B, Hanrez D, Michaux C, Walravens K, et al. (2012) A serological and bacteriological survey of brucellosis in wild boar (*Sus scrofa*) in Belgium. BMC Vet Res 8: 80.

38. Sohayati R, Chee WK, Dahlia H, Roseliza R, A A, et al. (2012) Disease from Wild Boar in Malaysia. International Conference on One Health and 24th VAM Congress. Putrajaya, Malaysia pp. 139.

39. De BK, Stauffer L, Koylass MS, Sharp SE, Gee JE, et al. (2008) Novel *Brucella* strain (BO1) associated with a prosthetic breast implant infection. J Clin Microbiol 46: 43–49.

40. Donald SD (1990) Brucellosis in wildlife. In Animal brucellosis (K. . Nielsen & J.R. . Duncan, eds). CRC Press, Boca Raton, Florida, 321–330.

41. Omer MK, Skjerve E, Woldehiwet Z, Holstad G (2000) Risk factors for *Brucella* spp. infection In dairy cattle farms in Asmara, State of Eritrea. Prev Vet Med 46: 257–265.

42. Mcdermott JJ, Arimi SM (2002) Brucellosis in sub-Saharan Africa: epidemiology, control and impact. Vet Microbiol 90: 111–134.

43. Al-Majali AM, Talafha AQ, Ababneh MM, Ababneh MM (2009) Seroprevalence and risk factors for bovine brucellosis in Jordan. J Vet Sci 10: 61–65.

44. Kaoud H, Zaki MM, Shimaa A, Nasr A (2010) Epidemiologyof brucellosis among farm animals. Nature and Science 8: 190–197.

45. Nielsen K, Smith P, Yu W, Nicoletti P, Elzer P, et al. (2005) Towards single screening tests for brucellosis. Rev Sci Tech 24: 1027–1037.

46. Kang S-I, Her M, Heo EJ, Nam HM, Jung SC, et al. (2009) Molecular typing for epidemiological evaluation of *Brucella abortus* and *Brucella canis* isolated in Korea. J Microbiol methods 78: 144–149.

47. Borriello G, Capparelli R, Bianco M, Fenizia D, Alfano F, et al. (2006) Genetic resistance to *Brucella abortus* in the water buffalo (*Bubalus bubalis*). Infect and immun 74: 2115–2120.

48. Alexander KA, Blackburn JK, Vandewalle ME, Pesapane R, Baipoledi EK, et al. (2012) Buffalo, bush meat, and the zoonotic threat of brucellosis in Botswana. PLoS One 7: e32842.

49. Prior MG (1976) Isolation of *Brucella abortus* from two dogs in contact with bovine brucellosis. Can J Comp Med 40: 117–118.

50. Kumar H, Sharma DR, Singh J, Sandhu KS (2005) A study on the epidemiology of brucellosis in Punjab (India) using Survey Toolbox. Rev Sci Tech Off Int Epiz 24: 879–885.

51. Makita K, Fevre EM, Waiswa C, Eisler MC, Thrusfield M, et al. (2011) Herd prevalence of bovine brucellosis and analysis of risk factors in cattle in urban and peri-urban areas of the Kampala economic zone, Uganda. BMC Vet Res 7: 60.

52. Crawford RP, Huber JD, Adams BC (1990) Epidemiology and surveillance. In: Nielsen K, Duncan JR, editors. Animal brucellosis. Boca Raton, Florida: CRC Press. pp. 131–148.

53. Havas KA, Boone RB, Hill AE, Salman MD (2013) A Brucellosis Disease Control Strategy for the Kakheti Region of the Country of Georgia: An Agent-Based Model. Zoonoses Public Health.

54. Memish ZA, Balkhy HH (2004) Brucellosis and international travel. J Travel Med 11: 49–55.

55. John K, Fitzpatrick J, French N, Kazwala R, Kambarage D, et al. (2010) Quantifying risk factors for human brucellosis in rural northern Tanzania. PLoS One 5: e9968.

19

Distinct Transmissibility Features of TSE Sources Derived from Ruminant Prion Diseases by the Oral Route in a Transgenic Mouse Model (TgOvPrP4) Overexpressing the Ovine Prion Protein

Jean-Noël Arsac, Thierry Baron*

Agence nationale de sécurité sanitaire de l'alimentation, de l'environnement et du travail (Anses), Unité Maladies Neuro-dégénératives, Lyon, France

Abstract

Transmissible spongiform encephalopathies (TSEs) are a group of fatal neurodegenerative diseases associated with a misfolded form of host-encoded prion protein (PrP). Some of them, such as classical bovine spongiform encephalopathy in cattle (BSE), transmissible mink encephalopathy (TME), kuru and variant Creutzfeldt–Jakob disease in humans, are acquired by the oral route exposure to infected tissues. We investigated the possible transmission by the oral route of a panel of strains derived from ruminant prion diseases in a transgenic mouse model (TgOvPrP4) overexpressing the ovine prion protein ($A_{136}R_{154}Q_{171}$) under the control of the neuron-specific enolase promoter. Sources derived from Nor98, CH1641 or 87V scrapie sources, as well as sources derived from L-type BSE or cattle-passaged TME, failed to transmit by the oral route, whereas those derived from classical BSE and classical scrapie were successfully transmitted. Apart from a possible effect of passage history of the TSE agent in the inocula, this implied the occurrence of subtle molecular changes in the protease-resistant prion protein (PrPres) following oral transmission that can raises concerns about our ability to correctly identify sheep that might be orally infected by the BSE agent in the field. Our results provide proof of principle that transgenic mouse models can be used to examine the transmissibility of TSE agents by the oral route, providing novel insights regarding the pathogenesis of prion diseases.

Editor: Ina Maja Vorberg, Deutsches Zentrum für Neurodegenerative Erkrankungen e.V., Germany

Funding: The authors have no support or funding to report.

Competing Interests: The authors have declared that no competing interests exist.

* E-mail: thierry.baron@anses.fr

Introduction

Transmissible spongiform encephalopathies (TSEs) are neuro-degenerative diseases that affect both humans and animals. Typical features include characteristic spongiform changes in the brain associated with neuron loss, an absence of inflammatory response, and accumulation in the brain, and sometimes in lymphoid tissues, of an abnormal, partially protease-resistant (PrPres) form of the neuronal prion protein (PrP) encoded by the *prnp* gene of the host [1]. This disease-associated protein is associated with transmissibility of the disease.

The routes by which TSEs occur under natural conditions, have not been fully established. However, scrapie and chronic wasting disease (CWD), in small ruminants and cervids respectively, show horizontal transmissibility under natural conditions [2,3], and many prion diseases are acquired by oral exposure, e.g., bovine spongiform encephalopathy (BSE) [4], transmissible mink encephalopathy (TME) [5], kuru and, most probably, variant Creutzfeldt–Jakob disease (vCJD) in humans [6]. As a result of increased surveillance in the past years, atypical and/or rare TSEs have been identified in cattle (H-type and L-type BSEs) and in small ruminants (Nor98 and scrapie isolates reminiscent of CH1641 experimental scrapie) [7,8,9,10]. The origins of these TSEs remain debated but at least some of them (H-type and L-type BSEs,

Nor98) probably arise sporadically [10,11], such as most cases of Creutzfeldt-Jakob disease (CJD) in humans [12], although particular sequences of the *prnp* gene ($A_{136}H_{154}Q_{171}$ and $A_{136}F_{141}R_{154}Q_{171}$ genotypes) have a major predisposing influence in the case of No98 [13].

Prion diseases pathogenesis has been shown to be heavily dependent on complex interactions between factors specific to the strain of transmissible agent, the route and dose of exposure and the host [13,14]. In this context, experimental transmissions of different TSEs provide useful information about the potential risk of transmission and for understanding disease pathogenesis. We therefore decided to investigate the possible transmissibility by the oral route of a large panel of TSEs derived from prion diseases of ruminants in a transgenic mouse model (TgOvPrP4), after two passages of these sources by the intra-cerebral route [15,16,17,18,19,20]. This choice was made to avoid inoculations of tissues derived from different species (cattle or sheep) with different PrP primary sequences.

In this study our objectives continued our efforts to examine in details the pathogenesis of prion diseases in the TgOvPrP4 transgenic mouse model expressing PrP under the control of a neuron-specific enolase promoter. Our previous studies indeed already showed that, although we failed to detect ovine PrP outside the central nervous system, TgOvPrP4 mice could be successfully infected by intra-peritoneal route with a classical scrapie source [21] and showed PrPres accumulation into lymphoid tissues with some prion strains, including classical scrapie and BSE [21,22].

Materials and Methods

Ethics statement

All mouse transmission experiments were performed in the biohazard prevention area (A3) of the ANSES-Lyon animal facilities, in accordance with the guidelines of the French Ethics Committee (decree 87–848) and European Community Directive 86/609/EEC, with the relevant approval for licensed individuals (LL 69 387 191) to carry out animal experiments (A 69 387 0801) according to a protocol approved (Permit n°98) by the Committee on the Ethics of Animal Experiments (CREEA of the Région Rhône Alpes Auvergne).

TSE sources

All samples used for the 3rd passage (oral and intra-cerebral challenge of TgOvPrP4 mice) consisted of ovine transgenic (TgOvPrP4) mouse brains of the different BSE or scrapie sources obtained after two successive passages by intra-cerebral route.

Inocula were derived from i) natural cases of classical BSE in cattle and classical scrapie in sheep [23], ii) atypical natural TSE isolates collected by active surveillance of scrapie ("CH1641 like", Nor98) [16,24] or of BSE (L-type BSE) [18], iii) experimental samples including classical BSE and CH1641 in $AA_{136}RR_{154}QQ_{171}$ sheep [16,25], transmissible mink encephalopathy (TME) in cattle [18] or scrapie strains passaged in wild-type mice (87V, C506M3) [17].

Transmission studies in mice

The TgOvPrP4 transgenic mice used in the present study express the ovine PrP protein ($A_{136}R_{154}Q_{171}$ genotype) under the control of the neurone-specific enolase promoter, and do not express the murine PrP protein [15].

For intra-cerebral inoculations, experimental groups (n = 6 to 12) of four to six week old female TgOvPrP4 mice were anaesthetized (80 µl of 0.8% ketamin–0.12% xylazine) then inoculated intracerebrally (20 µl per mouse) with a 1% solution (wt/vol) in glucose (5%) of homogenates prepared from brain samples of mice at the terminal stage of the disease during a second passage of the different TSE sources, as previously described [15,16,17,18,19,20,23,25].

Transmissions by the oral route were carried out with experimental groups (n = 6) of four to six week old female TgOvPrP4 mice challenged with 10% brain homogenates in glucose 5% (wt/vol) from intra-cerebrally challenged TgOvPrP4 mice at the terminal stage of the disease during a second passage of the different TSE sources. For intra-gastric administration, mice were housed for 2 hours in bedding- and food-free cages then individually fed (100 µl per mouse) *via* a flexible polypropylene catheter inserted over the tongue about 1 to 2 cm into the oesophagus.

Mice were supplied with food and drink *ad libitum*, then checked at least twice weekly for the presence of clinical signs indicative of TSE. When signs occurred, the mice were monitored daily and were sacrificed with an overdose of anaesthetic solution (200 µl of 0.8% ketamine–0.12% xylazine) if they exhibited any signs of distress or confirmed evolution of clinical signs of prion disease. A few animals were found dead. The whole brain and the spleen from each mouse available for appropriate sampling was frozen

and stored at −80°C until Western blot analysis for PrPres detection.

Western blot analysis of PrPres

Details of the Western blot analyses have been provided in previous publications describing transmission of the TSE sources used in this study. Briefly, brain and spleen from TgOvPrP4 mice inoculated with strain derived from Nor98 scrapie isolate were examined by TeSeE WB (Bio-Rad) following the manufacturer's recommendations, as previously described [19,24]. For other TSE sources, Western blot were performed after PrPres extraction from brain or spleen by ultra-centrifugation, as described [22]. In some experiments, deglycosylation was performed using PNGase F as previously described [16].

PrPres was detected by SHa31 or SAF84 antibodies (4 µg/ml in PBST), recognizing the 148-YEDRYYRE-155 or 167-RPVDQY-172 ovine PrP sequence respectively, and peroxidase-labelled conjugate (Cliniscience) against mouse IgG (1:2,500 in PBST). Bound antibodies were detected by enhanced chemiluminescence (ECL, Amersham). PrPres signals were visualized either on film (Biomax; Kodak) or directly in an image-analysis system (Versadoc; Bio-Rad) and Quantity One software (Bio-Rad).

Results

Transmissibility of TSE sources by the oral route in TgOvPrP4 mice

We examined the transmissibility by the oral route of ten TSE sources from cattle or sheep previously described in the TgOvPrP4 transgenic mouse model, after two serial passages by the intra-cerebral route in this mouse line. The results are summarized in Tables 1 and S1, which show (i) the survival periods of the mice (ii) PrPres detection by Western blot in brains and spleens and (iii) clinical signs of TSE, in comparison to a second and third passage by the intra-cerebral route. Survival periods and PrPres detection in each individual mouse in these experiments are shown in Figure 1.

Regarding clinical signs (Table S1), mice inoculated by oral route generally appeared thin, as they were generally sacrificed or found dead at late ages. Paresis was observed with two classical scrapie sources (a French natural scrapie case or the mouse-adapted C506M3 experimental strain) after oral challenge, whereas this clinical signs is generally observed in mice inoculated by the intra-cerebral route (2nd and 3rd passage) for all the 10 TSE sources. Prostration, another criteria generally observed in mice inoculated by the intra-cerebral route, was observed with the three classical scrapie sources (a French natural scrapie case, the mouse-adapted C506M3 experimental strain or the mouse-adapted 87V experimental strain) but also with the sources derived from experimental bovine TME and the natural Nor98 scrapie isolate. Additionally, clinical signs as dorsal kyphosis, plastic tail and foot clasping were included as signs participating to the definition of the clinical endpoint.

Considering the detection of PrPres in both brains and spleens of the mice (Table 1), the TSE sources derived from classical BSE sources (cattle or ovine BSE) and from two classical scrapie sources (a French natural scrapie case or the mouse-adapted C506M3 experimental strain) were successfully transmitted by the oral route. However, the mean survival periods exceeded 2 years, except in mice that received the source derived from natural scrapie source (mean 564 days post-inoculation (d.p.i.)).

On the other hand, we failed to transmit the six other TSE sources, notably the sources derived from CH1641 and Nor98 scrapie, L-type BSE and bovine-passaged transmissible mink

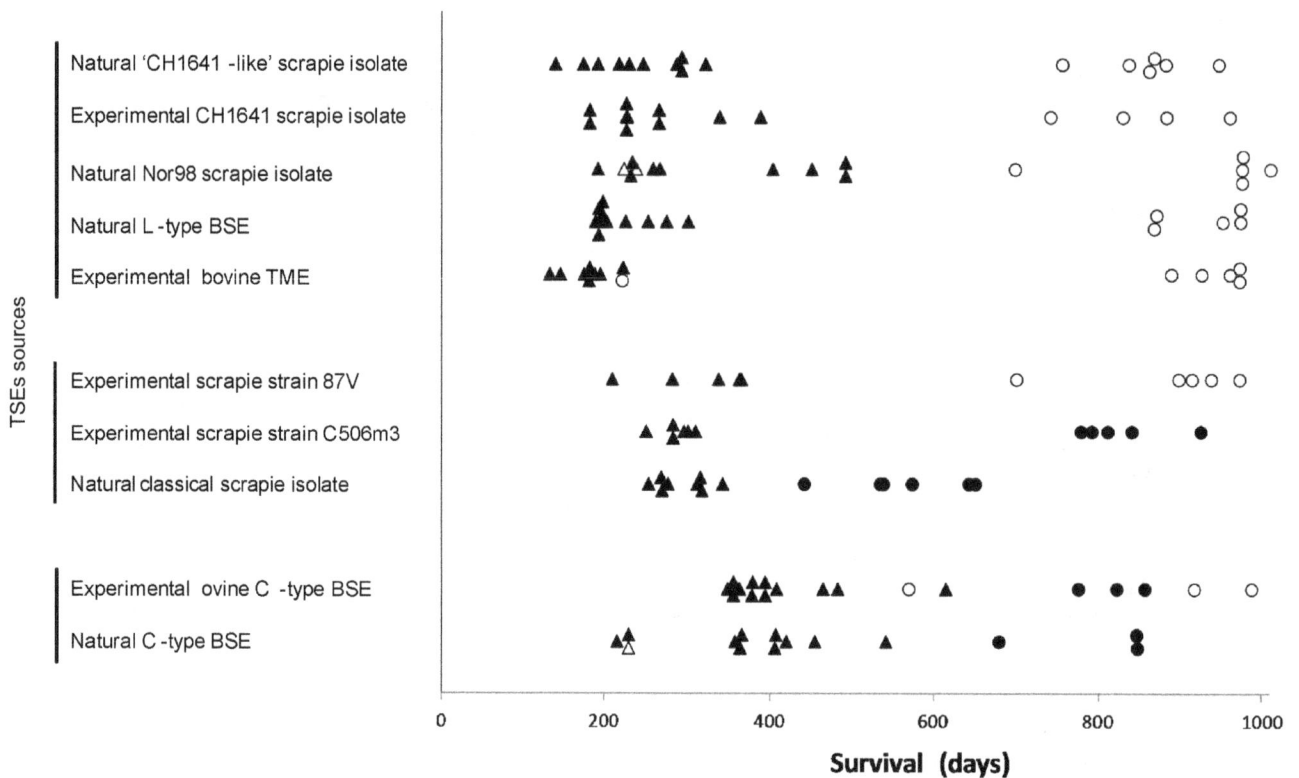

Figure 1. Survival periods and PrPres detection of individual TgOvPrP4 mice challenged by oral *versus* intra-cerebral route. △: intra-cerebral, O: oral. Empty circles or triangles correspond to PrPres negative mice whereas full circles or full triangles represent PrPres positive mice.

encephalopathy (cattle-passaged TME). Interestingly, only two of these TSE sources, derived from cattle (L-BSE and cattle-passaged TME), appeared to be lymphotropic in TgOvPrP4 mice after intra-cerebral inoculation, which was not the case for the four sources derived from scrapie (Nor98, "CH1641-like" natural scrapie, experimental sources CH1641 or 87V).

Changes of PrPres cleavage in the brains of TgOvPrP4 mice orally challenged by BSE

The biochemical features of PrPres were then compared in the brains of mice inoculated by the oral or the intra-cerebral routes (Figure2).

When sources derived from classical BSE and classical scrapie were compared, the characteristic high levels of diglycosylated PrPres ($\sim$70%) were still found in mice orally-challenged with BSE, which were clearly distinct from mice orally challenged with classical scrapie sources (<60%)(Figure2C).

However molecular discrimination of sources derived from BSE and scrapie, based on measuring differences in the apparent molecular mass of the unglycosylated PrPres, was much more difficult. The apparent molecular mass of unglycosylated PrPres in source derived from BSE was clearly much higher in mice infected by the oral route, so that BSE was sometimes indistinguishable from scrapie for this criterion (Figure2B, lanes 5 and 8). Whereas these differences were >1 kDa for the C506M3 strain inoculated by the intra-cerebral route (Figure2B, lane 3), the apparent molecular mass for one mouse inoculated intra-cerebrally with a source derived from classical natural scrapie was low (Figure2B, lane 4), similar to that found for the two BSE sources by this inoculation route (Figure2B, lanes 1 and 2). This same mouse was also the only scrapie-infected mouse in which the proportion of

diglycosylated PrPres was >60% (Figure2C). However, other mice in this experimental group showed a classical scrapie pattern, with a higher apparent molecular mass for the unglycosylated PrPres band and, as in CH1641, C-terminally cleaved PrPres ($\sim$14 kDa for the unglycosylated band) specifically recognised by a C-terminal antibody (SAF84) was detected in all mice (Figure3).

Changes of PrPres glycoform ratios in the spleen of TgOvPrP4 mice orally challenged by scrapie

The biochemical features of PrPres in the spleens of mice inoculated by oral or intra-cerebral routes were similarly compared (Figure4).

Concerning PrPres mobility (Figure4B), it was again less easy to discriminate between sources derived from BSE and scrapie in orally-challenged mice, but to a lesser extent than in the brain since a 0.3–0.5 kDa increase in molecular mass was observed for the unglycosylated PrPres of source derived from BSE (compared to 0.7–0.9 kDa in the brain). As a result, BSE can still be readily discriminated from scrapie by applying this criterion. Interestingly, by intra-cerebral route, for the mouse which showed a PrPres of low apparent molecular mass in the brain after inoculation with a natural scrapie source, scrapie could be readily discriminated from BSE in the spleen, where the apparent molecular mass of PrPres was still high (Figure4B, lane 4).

Examination of the PrPres glycoform ratios revealed an increased proportion of diglycosylated PrPres (approximately 61%–63%) after inoculation with scrapie by both routes (Figure4C), as compared to the PrPres ratios found in the brain, so these glycoform proportions were closer to that of BSE.

Table 1. TSE transmission results by the oral *versus* the intra-cerebral route in TgOvPrP4 ovine transgenic mice.

TSE sources	Survival (analyzed/inoculated)						Brain PrPres			Spleen PrPres		
	2nd i.c.		3rd i.c.		3rd oral		2nd i.c.	3rd i.c.	3rd oral	2nd i.c.	3rd i.c.	3rd oral
Natural 'CH1641-like' scrapie isolate	232±38	(11/12)	253±66	(10/11)	858±62	(6/6)	11/11	10/10	0/6	0/5	0/10	0/6
Experimental CH1641 scrapie isolate	220±31	(11/12)	244±58	(11/12)	853±92	(4/6)	11/11	11/11	0/4	0/5	0/9	0/4
Natural Nor98 scrapie isolate	317±117	(11/12)	ND	(11/12)	927±128	(5/6)	9/11	ND	0/5	0/11	ND	0/5
Natural L-type BSE	202±26	(9/11)	220±39	(11/12)	935±52	(6/6)	9/9	11/11	0/6	3/5	9/9	0/6
Experimental Bovine TME	234±27	(9/11)	178±28	(8/11)	823±296	(6/6)	3/9	8/8	0/6	1/3	4/5	0/6
Experimental scrapie strain 87V	270±55	(10/11)	312±66	(5/6)	884±106	(5/6)	10/10	5/5	0/5	0/7	0/5	0/5
Experimental scrapie strain C506m3	333±26	(12/12)	287±21	(6/6)	829±58	(5/6)	12/12	6/6	5/5	6/6	6/6	5/5
Natural classical scrapie isolate	295±31	(8/11)	ND	(12/12)	564±78	(6/6)	8/8	ND	6/6	7/7	ND	5/5
Experimental Ovine C-type BSE	356±62	(12/12)	412±12	(12/12)	821±143	(6/6)	12/12	12/12	3/6	5/5	6/6	1/5
Natural C-type BSE	354±48	(10/11)	415±61	(8/11)	791±96	(3/6)	10/10	8/8	3/3	5/5	8/8	3/3

Survival periods (means +/– standard deviations) and the number of analyzed mice for the ten TSE sources are shown together with the results of PrPres detection in brain and spleen (number of PrPres positive mice/number of mice examined). The results obtained for the second intra-cerebral passage (2nd i.c.) are shown in comparison with those obtained for the third passage by the oral route (3rd oral) or the intra-cerebral route (3rd i.c.). ND: no data.

Discussion

Our data show that TSE agents inoculated by the oral route can be transmitted in a transgenic mouse model (TgOvPrP4) overexpressing the ovine PrP protein (A_{136} R_{154} Q_{171}) on a murine *pmp-/-* background under the control of the neuron-specific enolase promoter [15]. This extends our previous demonstrations of the transmission of two classical scrapie isolates by intra-peritoneal route in this mouse model [21], which had been unexpected given our failure to detect ovine PrP expression outside the central nervous system. However, transmission of a scrapie source had also been reported in a similar transgenic mouse model expressing the hamster prion protein (NSE HaPrP/MoPrP-/-) and challenged by either the intra-peritoneal or the oral route [26]. This suggested that PrP expression in the peripheral nerves might be sufficient for infection of the brain. Transmission has now been observed with the TgOvPrP4 ovine transgenic model, not only for two sources derived from classical scrapie (a natural scrapie isolate or the C506M3 experimental strain) but also for two sources derived from classical BSE (from cattle or after experimental passage in sheep).

However, it must be emphasized that we did not use brain samples from ruminant isolates (cattle or sheep) but chose to carry out the study using brains from TgOvPrP4 mice intracerebrally inoculated with the prion diseases. We cannot fully exclude possible biological changes after serial intracerebral passages in the ovine transgenic mouse model, including regarding the possible transmission by the oral route. However, this allowed to examine the properties after the same passage history in a same experimental ovinised host and avoid to compare experiments from brain pieces derived from different species (cattle or sheep). Survival periods at primary passage from bovine tissues were already quite long by intra-cerebral from cattle brain tissues, especially for L-BSE (>600 d.p.i.). As a result, life expectancy of the mice could prevent in practice any possibility to identify any transmission of the disease by the oral route.

Nevertheless, the transmission of both sources derived from BSE and scrapie allowed examination of the PrPres molecular differences. For a given sources derived from BSE of either bovine or ovine origin, the apparent molecular mass for PrPres was consistently higher in orally challenged mice, as has already been reported following experimental transmission of BSE in sheep [27]. These slight differences in molecular mass were observed in the brain and to a lesser extent in the spleen. As a result, molecular discrimination between BSE and scrapie, especially in mouse brains, was less straightforward when based on PrPres analyses. This raises concern about our ability to correctly identify sheep that might be orally infected by the BSE agent in the field, from discriminatory analyses of PrPres in the brain [28,29] Indeed the strategy currently used for the discrimination of scrapie and BSE in small ruminants in Europe, is essentially based on the Western blot analyses of the PrPres cleavage in the brain [30].

PrPres molecular changes could suggest a possible emergence of a new strain, although it is also possible that striking molecular changes occur without any detectable strain alteration, as illustrated for instance recently by major changes of glycosylation patterns in BSE transmitted in a porcine transgenic mouse model [31]. As this was revealed by further passage in bovine transgenic mice in this last study, strain typing from our orally infected mice showing altered PrPres features will require further passage by intracerebral route in an appropriate experimental model as it has been well established that the route of infection can strongly influence the apparent phenotype of a TSE strain [32,33].

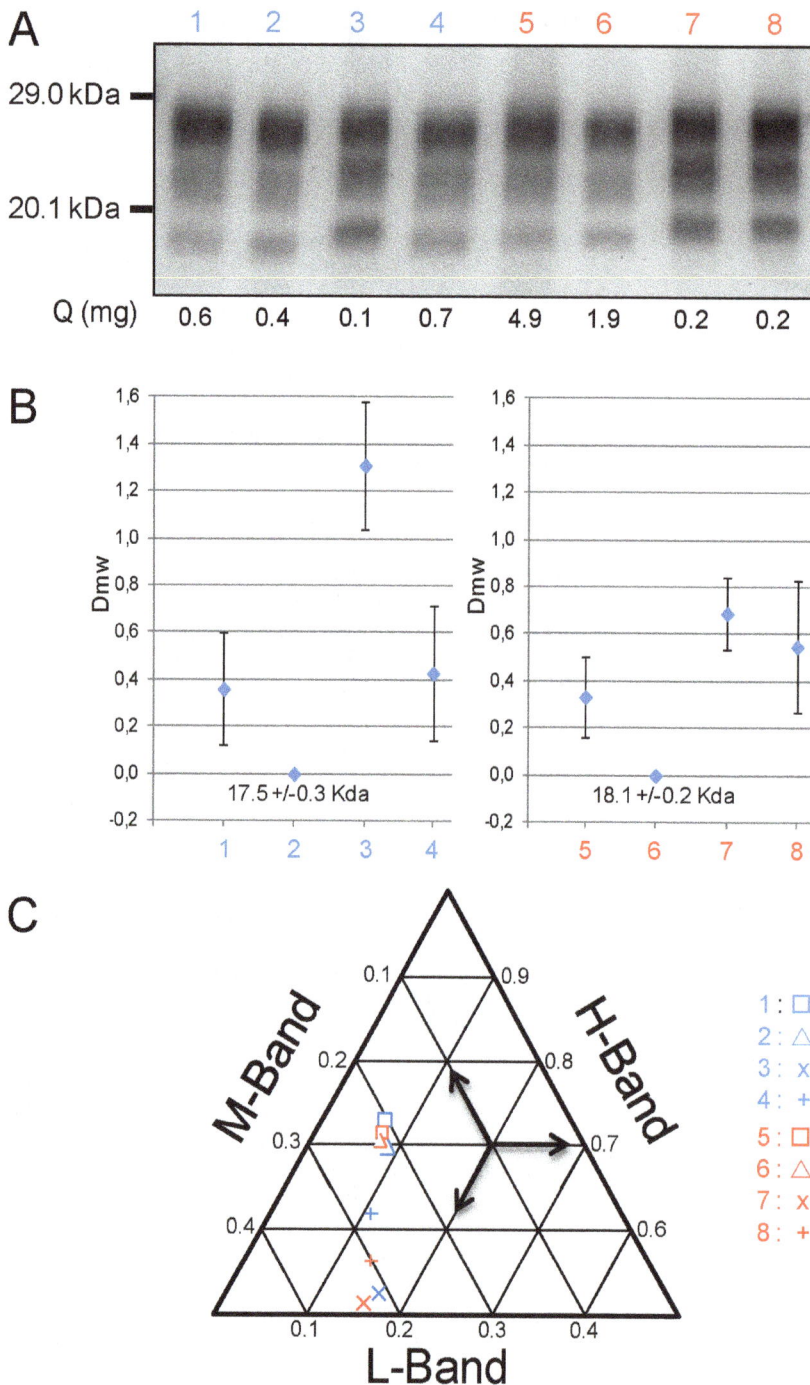

Figure 2. Western blot of brain PrPres in TgOvPrP4 mice infected with classical scrapie or BSE. Mice were challenged by oral (lane 5–8) or the intra-cerebral route (lanes 1–4). A) Western blot detection of PrPres by Sha 31 antibody of different sources derived from classical BSE in cattle (lanes 1, 5), classical BSE in sheep (lanes 2, 6), C506M3 scrapie strain (lanes 3, 7) and natural classical scrapie isolate (lanes 4, 8). The equivalent tissue quantities loaded per lane are indicated at the bottom of each lane. Bars to the left indicate the 29.0 and 20.1 kDa marker positions. B) Differences of the unglycosylated PrPres apparent molecular masses compared to that in mice infected with source derived from ovine BSE by the same inoculation route (means +/− SD of 5 repeated assays). The raw apparent molecular mass of unglycosylated PrPres is indicated for the ovine BSE infected mouse. C) Tern-plot representation of the proportions of diglycosylated (H), monoglycosylated (M) and unglycosylated (L) bands of PrPres for different sources derived from classical BSE in cattle (□), classical BSE in sheep (△), C506M3 scrapie strain (X) and natural classical scrapie isolate (+) (blue: intra-cerebral, red: oral). The means for all repetitions (n = 5) are plotted.

Examination of the molecular features of the PrPres derived from scrapie revealed a modification of the biochemical profile with a PrPres apparent molecular mass and a high proportion of diglycosylated PrPres (>60%) similar to that of BSE-infected mice, but this was the case of a single mouse among those intra-cerebrally inoculated with the strain derived from natural scrapie. This is reminiscent of the emergence of scrapie with CH1641 features that was described after intra-species experimental

A

M (kDa)   19.4   19.0   19.7   18.4   19.4   18.4

B

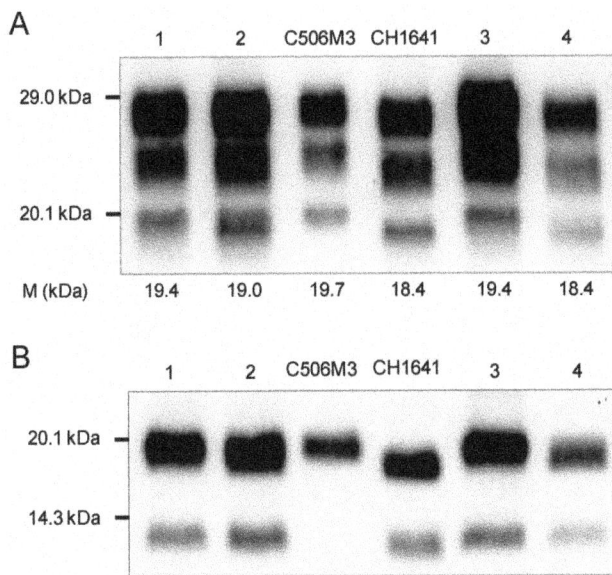

Figure 3. Western profiles in TgOvPrP4 mice infected with source derived from a natural scrapie isolate. PrPres detected, using SAF84 antibody, from four individual TgOvPrP4 mice infected with a natural scrapie isolate [15], at the second passage by the intra-cerebral route (lanes 1–4). PrPres of TgOvPrP4 mice infected with the C506M3 and CH1641 experimental scrapie sources were used as controls. A) The apparent molecular mass measured for the unglyco-sylated PrPres band in this representative Western blot is indicated at the bottom of each lane. Bars to the left indicate the 29.0 and 20.1 kDa marker positions. B) PrPres was analysed after PNGase deglycosylation. Bars to the left indicate the 20.1 and 14.3 kDa marker positions.

transmission in sheep [34]. This is another circumstance when molecular discrimination between scrapie and BSE is more difficult [7,28]. However, in contrast to sources derived from BSE, no significant molecular differences were otherwise observed between mice orally or intra-cerebrally challenged with sources derived from scrapie.

Western blot analysis also revealed slight but consistent differences: the apparent molecular mass of the unglycosylated PrPres protein band in the brain of mice challenged with source derived from ovine BSE, as compared to that derived from bovine BSE by either intra-cerebral or oral route, was consistently lower (0.3–0.4 kDa) whereas the glycoform ratios were the same. These results are similar to those previously described between BSE in cattle and sheep [28], but here, surprisingly, they are observed after passage in a same experimental model expressing the ovine PrP protein. Such differences in PrPres molecular mass were not found in the mouse spleens. The reason why the passage history seems to result in a faint difference in PrPres molecular signature is unclear, and the extent to which this could be associated with possible changes in the pathobiological properties of the BSE agent remains unknown. Such changes have been shown to occur after passage in sheep [35,36,37]. It should also be noted that the attack rate from strain derived from ovine BSE was surprisingly lower and PrPres remained undetected in most (4/5) of the mouse spleens after oral challenge. In addition to possible changes after a passage in sheep, a possible reduction of the capacity of the source derived from ovine BSE agent to propagate by the oral route, following the first two passages that were performed by the intra-cerebral route in a transgenic mouse model characterized by a neuron-specific pattern of expression, cannot be totally excluded.

The previous sources derived from classical scrapie and BSE were the only TSEs examined that were transmissible by the oral route in TgOvPrP4 mice. No transmission by the oral route was achieved with other TSE sources originating from the experimental scrapie sources 87V and CH1641, two natural, "CH1641-like" or Nor98, scrapie isolates, an L-type BSE isolate, or from an isolate of transmissible mink encephalopathy (TME) passaged in cattle. H-type BSE and CWD were not examined as we had been unable to transmit these diseases by the intra-cerebral route in the TgOvPrP4 mouse model [18] (unpublished data). The titers of the inocula used in this study were not determined but transmission had been demonstrated unequivocally by the intra-cerebral route for all the inocula. These results might be partially explained by the pattern of tissue-specific PrP expression in TgOvPrP4 mice, under the control of the neuron-specific enolase promoter, as less neuroinvasive TSEs have been reported to require amplification in the follicular dendritic cells of the lymphoid tissues prior to neuroinvasion via the peripheral nerves [26,38].

It is indeed apparent that the orally transmissible sources derived from classical BSE and scrapie were also able to propagate readily in the spleens of TgOvPrP4 mice, after both intra-cerebral and oral challenges. Among other sources that failed to transmit by the oral route, only L-BSE and bovine TME were lymphotropic by the intra-cerebral route at least during serial passages [18]. As regards the scrapie sources and their transmissibility by peripheral routes, failure to transmit 87V by the oral route had already been reported in sheep, whereas the ME7, 79A and 22A murine strains were transmissible [39]. Very low efficiency in transmitting this 87V strain was also reported in mice by intra-peritoneal route [40]. Also, concerning the ovine scrapie sources, failure to transmit CH1641 scrapie by subcutaneous inoculation was reported in sheep [41]. Oral transmission of Nor98 scrapie has been reported in sheep, but only of the $A_{136} H_{154} Q_{171}$ homozygous $prnp$ genotype [42], thus differing in this respect from TgOvPrP4 mice. The failure of both sources derived from L-BSE and bovine TME to be transmitted by the oral route in TgOvPrP4 is more intriguing. These are the most rapid ruminant TSEs in TgOvPrP4 mice by intra-cerebral route, which makes the results even more significant as transmission of the disease might be expected to occur within the life span of the mice, as observed for sources derived from classical BSE. Moreover we previously reported that L-BSE was readily transmissible from cattle by the oral route in another experimental model, the mouse lemur [43]. In the case of TME, our strain typing studies in several experimental models highlighted similarities with L-BSE and suggested that TME could be the result of a food borne transmission of L-BSE in ranch-raised minks [18,44]. Transmission of these TSEs might involve particular pathways that could be affected in the TgOvPrP4 transgenic mouse model. Besides, our results could be influenced by the protocol used for experimental challenge involving intra-gastric administration, meaning that the inocula were not chewed by the mice, whereas in the case of experiments with L-BSE in lemurs, inocula were mixed to food. Alternatively, we can again consider the hypothesis that oral transmissibility could have been reduced by previous passages by the intra-cerebral route during the two passages in TgOvPrP4 mice, while initial brain samples of ruminants were not analyzed in this first oral route study.

However our results reveal the transmissibility of some TSEs by the oral route in a transgenic mouse model. Interestingly, some of our data suggest a possible influence of the passage history of

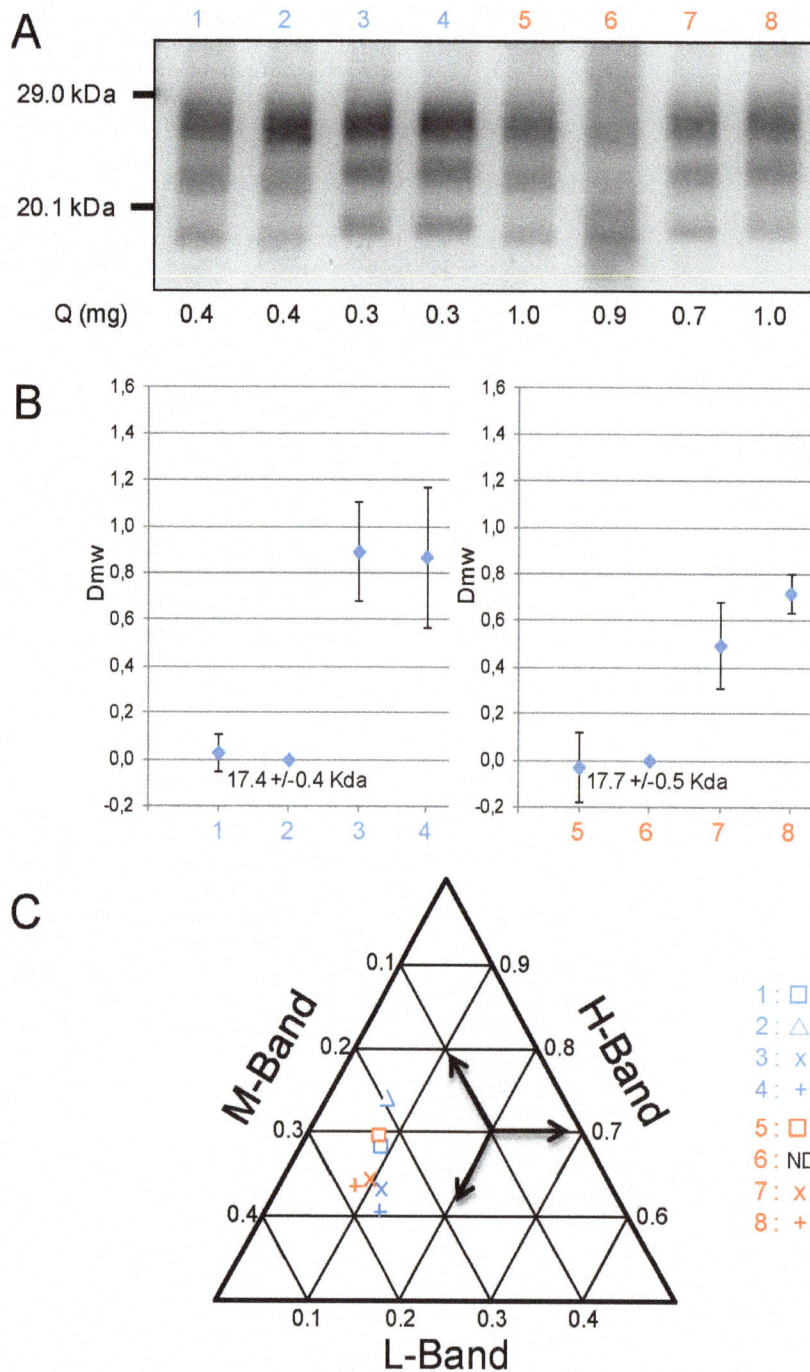

Figure 4. Western blot of spleen PrPres in TgOvPrP4 mice infected with classical scrapie or BSE. Mice were challenged by oral (lane 5–8) or the intra-cerebral route (lanes 1–4). A) Western blot detection of PrPres by Sha 31 antibody of different sources derived from classical BSE in cattle (lanes 1, 5), classical BSE in sheep (lanes 2, 6), C506M3 scrapie strain (lanes 3, 7) and natural classical scrapie isolate (lanes 4, 8). The equivalent tissue quantities loaded per lane are indicated at the bottom of each lane. Bars to the left indicate the 29.0 and 20.1 kDa marker positions. B) Differences of the unglycosylated PrPres apparent molecular masses compared to that in mice infected with source derived from ovine BSE by the same inoculation route (means +/− SD of 5 repeated assays). The raw apparent molecular mass of unglycosylated PrPres is indicated for the ovine BSE infected mouse. C) Tern-plot representation of the proportions of diglycosylated (H), monoglycosylated (M) and unglycosylated (L) bands of PrPres for different sources derived from classical BSE in cattle (□), classical BSE in sheep (△), C506M3 scrapie strain (X) and natural classical scrapie isolate (+) (blue: intra-cerebral, red: oral). The means for all repetitions (n = 5) are plotted.

inocula, including the inoculation routes or host features. These need careful consideration when interpreting data on the pathobiological properties of TSE agents in experimental models. To the best of our knowledge, this is the first report of oral transmission in a transgenic model expressing the prion protein of a species naturally affected by TSEs. It provides proof of principle that such models can constitute useful experimental tools for studies of oral transmission of prion diseases.

Supporting Information

Table S1 Overview of clinical signs observed in TgOvPrP4 ovine transgenic mice after transmission by the oral *versus* the intra-cerebral route. The number of mice euthanized is indicated in each group. The possible presence of paresis, prostration or thinness is specified. ND: no data.

Acknowledgments

We greatly acknowledge the excellent technical assistance of Dominique Canal and Claire Aufauvre. We thank Emilie Antier, Damien Gaillard, Coralie Pulido and Latefa Lakhdar from the Plateforme d'Expérimentation Animale of Anses-Lyon for excellent animal care during the animal experiments.

Author Contributions

Conceived and designed the experiments: JNA TB. Performed the experiments: JNA. Analyzed the data: JNA TB. Wrote the paper: JNA TB.

References

1. Prusiner SB, Groth DF, Bolton DC, Kent SB, Hood LE (1984) Purification and structural studies of a major scrapie prion protein. Cell 38: 127–134.
2. Hoinville LJ (1996) A review of the epidemiology of scrapie in sheep. Rev Sci Tech 15: 827–852.
3. Miller MW, Williams ES (2003) Prion disease: horizontal prion transmission in mule deer. Nature 425: 35–36.
4. Wilesmith JW, Ryan JB, Atkinson MJ (1991) Bovine spongiform encephalopathy: epidemiological studies on the origin. Vet Rec 128: 199–203.
5. Burger D, Hartsough GR (1965) Encephalopathy of mink. II. Experimental and natural transmission. JInfect Dis 115: 393–399.
6. Ghani AC, Donnelly CA, Ferguson NM, Anderson RM (2002) The transmission dynamics of BSE and vCJD. CRBiol 325: 37–47.
7. Hope J, Wood SC, Birkett CR, Chong A, Bruce ME, et al. (1999) Molecular analysis of ovine prion protein identifies similarities between BSE and an experimental isolate of natural scrapie, CH1641. JGen Virol 80 (Pt 1): 1–4.
8. Benestad SL, Sarradin P, Thu B, Schonheit J, Tranulis MA, et al. (2003) Cases of scrapie with unusual features in Norway and designation of a new type, Nor98. Vet Rec 153: 202–208.
9. Casalone C, Zanusso G, Acutis P, Ferrari S, Capucci L, et al. (2004) Identification of a second bovine amyloidotic spongiform encephalopathy: molecular similarities with sporadic Creutzfeldt-Jakob disease. Proc Natl Acad SciUSA 101: 3065–3070.
10. Biacabe AG, Laplanche JL, Ryder S, Baron T (2004) Distinct molecular phenotypes in bovine prion diseases. EMBO Rep 5: 110–115.
11. Biacabe AG, Morignat E, Vulin J, Calavas D, Baron TG (2008) Atypical bovine spongiform encephalopathies, France, 2001–2007. Emerg Infect Dis 14: 298–300.
12. de Pedro-Cuesta J, Glatzel M, Almazan J, Stoeck K, Mellina V, et al. (2006) Human transmissible spongiform encephalopathies in eleven countries: diagnostic pattern across time, 1993-2002. BMC Public Health 6: 278.
13. Outram GW, Fraser H, Wilson DT (1973) Scrapie in mice. Some effects on the brain lesion profile of ME7 agent due to genotype of donor, route of injection and genotype of recipient. JComp Pathol 83: 19–28.
14. Mould DL, Dawson AM, Smith W (1967) Determination of the dosage-response curve of mice inoculated with scrapie. JComp Pathol 77: 387–391.
15. Crozet C, Flamant F, Bencsik A, Aubert D, Samarut J, et al. (2001) Efficient transmission of two different sheep scrapie isolates in transgenic mice expressing the ovine PrP gene. JVirol 75: 5328–5334.
16. Baron T, Biacabe AG (2007) Molecular behaviors of "CH1641-like" sheep scrapie isolates in ovine transgenic mice (TgOvPrP4). JVirol 81: 7230–7237.
17. Bencsik A, Philippe S, Debeer S, Crozet C, Calavas D, et al. (2007) Scrapie strain transmission studies in ovine PrP transgenic mice reveal dissimilar susceptibility. Histochem Cell Biol 127: 531–539.
18. Baron T, Bencsik A, Biacabe AG, Morignat E, Bessen RA (2007) Phenotypic similarity of transmissible mink encephalopathy in cattle and L-type bovine spongiform encephalopathy in a mouse model. Emerg Infect Dis 13: 1887–1894.
19. Arsac JN, Betemps D, Morignat E, Feraudet C, Bencsik A, et al. (2009) Transmissibility of atypical scrapie in ovine transgenic mice: major effects of host prion protein expression and donor prion genotype. PLoS One 4: e7300.
20. Nicot S, Baron TG (2009) Strain-specific proteolytic processing of the prion protein in prion diseases of ruminants transmitted in ovine transgenic mice. JGen Virol 91: 570–574.
21. Crozet C, Lezmi S, Flamant F, Samarut J, Baron T, et al. (2007) Peripheral circulation of the prion infectious agent in transgenic mice expressing the ovine prion protein gene in neurons only. JInfect Dis 195: 997–1006.
22. Baron T, Bencsik A, Morignat E (2010) Prions of ruminants show distinct splenotropisms in an ovine transgenic mouse model. PLoS One 5: e10310.
23. Baron T, Crozet C, Biacabe AG, Philippe S, Verchere J, et al. (2004) Molecular analysis of the protease-resistant prion protein in scrapie and bovine spongiform encephalopathy transmitted to ovine transgenic and wild-type mice. JVirol 78: 6243–6251.
24. Arsac JN, Andreoletti O, Bilheude JM, Lacroux C, Benestad SL, et al. (2007) Similar biochemical signatures and prion protein genotypes in atypical scrapie and Nor98 cases, France and Norway. Emerg Infect Dis 13: 58–65.
25. Crozet C, Bencsik A, Flamant F, Lezmi S, Samarut J, et al. (2001) Florid plaques in ovine PrP transgenic mice infected with an experimental ovine BSE. EMBO Rep 2: 952–956.
26. Race R, Oldstone M, Chesebro B (2000) Entry versus blockade of brain infection following oral or intraperitoneal scrapie administration: role of prion protein expression in peripheral nerves and spleen. JVirol 74: 828–833.
27. Stack M, Gonzalez L, Jeffrey M, Macaldowie C, et al. (2009) Three serial passages of bovine spongiform encephalopathy in sheep do not significantly affect discriminatory test results. JGen Virol 90: 764–768.
28. Stack MJ, Chaplin MJ, Clark J (2002) Differentiation of prion protein glycoforms from naturally occurring sheep scrapie, sheep-passaged scrapie strains (CH1641 and SSBP1), bovine spongiform encephalopathy (BSE) cases and Romney and Cheviot breed sheep experimentally inoculated with BSE using two monoclonal antibodies. Acta Neuropathol 104: 279–286.
29. Vulin J, Biacabe AG, Cazeau G, Calavas D, Baron T (2011) Molecular typing of protease-resistant prion protein in transmissible spongiform encephalopathies of small ruminants, France, 2002–2009. Emerg Infect Dis 17: 55–63.
30. Migliore S, Esposito E, Pirisinu L, Marcon S, Di Bari M, et al. (2012) Effect of PrP genotype and route of inoculation on the ability of discriminatory Western blot to distinguish scrapie from sheep bovine spongiform encephalopathy. JGen Virol 93: 450–455.
31. Torres JM, Espinosa JC, Aguilar-Calvo P, Herva ME, Relano-Gines A, et al. (2014) Elements modulating the prion species barrier and its passage consequences. PLoS One 9: e89722.
32. Langevin C, Andreoletti O, Le Dur A, Laude H, Beringue V (2011) Marked influence of the route of infection on prion strain apparent phenotype in a scrapie transgenic mouse model. Neurobiol Dis 41: 219–225.
33. Vickery CM, Beck KE, Simmons MM, Hawkins SA, Spiropoulos J (2013) Disease characteristics of bovine spongiform encephalopathy following inoculation into mice via three different routes. IntJExp Pathol 94: 320–328.
34. Yokoyama T, Masujin K, Schmerr MJ, Shu Y, Okada H, et al. (2010) Intraspecies prion transmission results in selection of sheep scrapie strains. PLoS One 5: e15450.
35. Espinosa JC, Andreoletti O, Castilla J, Herva ME, Morales M, et al. (2007) Sheep-passaged bovine spongiform encephalopathy agent exhibits altered pathobiological properties in bovine-PrP transgenic mice. JVirol 81: 835–843.
36. Padilla D, Beringue V, Espinosa JC, Andreoletti O, Jaumain E, et al. (2011) Sheep and goat BSE propagate more efficiently than cattle BSE in human PrP transgenic mice. PLoS Pathog 7: e1001319.
37. Plinston C, Hart P, Chong A, Hunter N, Foster J, et al. (2010) Increased susceptibility of human-PrP transgenic mice to bovine spongiform encephalopathy infection following passage in sheep. JVirol 85: 1174–1181.
38. Fraser JR (1996) Infectivity in extraneural tissues following intraocular scrapie infection. JGen Virol 77 (Pt 10): 2663–2668.
39. Siso S, Chianini F, Eaton SL, Witz J, Hamilton S, et al. (2012) Disease phenotype in sheep after infection with cloned murine scrapie strains. Prion 6: 174–183.
40. Bruce ME (1985) Agent replication dynamics in a long incubation period model of mouse scrapie. JGen Virol 66 (Pt 12): 2517–2522.
41. Foster JD, Dickinson AG (1988) The unusual properties of CH1641, a sheep-passaged isolate of scrapie. Vet Rec 123: 5–8.
42. Simmons MM, Moore SJ, Konold T, Thurston L, Terry LA, et al. (2011) Experimental oral transmission of atypical scrapie to sheep. Emerg Infect Dis 17: 848–854.
43. Mestre-Frances N, Nicot S, Rouland S, Biacabe AG, Quadrio I, et al. (2012) Oral transmission of L-type bovine spongiform encephalopathy in primate model. Emerg Infect Dis 18: 142–145.
44. Nicot S, Baron T (2010) Strain-specific barriers against bovine prions in hamsters. JVirol 85: 1906–1908.

20

Clinical Risk Factors Associated with Anti-Epileptic Drug Responsiveness in Canine Epilepsy

Rowena M. A. Packer[1], Nadia K. Shihab[¶1,2], Bruno B. J. Torres[¶3], Holger A. Volk[1]*

1 Department of Clinical Science and Services, Royal Veterinary College, Hatfield, Hertfordshire, United Kingdom, 2 Department of Neurology/Neurosurgery, Southern Counties Veterinary Specialists, Ringwood, Hampshire, United Kingdom, 3 Department of Veterinary Medicine and Surgery, Federal University of Minas Gerais, Belo Horizonte, Minas Gerais, Brazil

Abstract

The nature and occurrence of remission, and conversely, pharmacoresistance following epilepsy treatment is still not fully understood in human or veterinary medicine. As such, predicting which patients will have good or poor treatment outcomes is imprecise, impeding patient management. In the present study, we use a naturally occurring animal model of pharmacoresistant epilepsy to investigate clinical risk factors associated with treatment outcome. Dogs with idiopathic epilepsy, for which no underlying cause was identified, were treated at a canine epilepsy clinic and monitored following discharge from a small animal referral hospital. Clinical data was gained via standardised owner questionnaires and longitudinal follow up data was gained via telephone interview with the dogs' owners. At follow up, 14% of treated dogs were in seizure-free remission. Dogs that did not achieve remission were more likely to be male, and to have previously experienced cluster seizures. Seizure frequency or the total number of seizures prior to treatment were not significant predictors of pharmacoresistance, demonstrating that seizure density, that is, the temporal pattern of seizure activity, is a more influential predictor of pharmacoresistance. These results are in line with clinical studies of human epilepsy, and experimental rodent models of epilepsy, that patients experiencing episodes of high seizure density (cluster seizures), not just a high seizure frequency pre-treatment, are at an increased risk of drug-refractoriness. These data provide further evidence that the dog could be a useful naturally occurring epilepsy model in the study of pharmacoresistant epilepsy.

Editor: Giuseppe Biagini, University of Modena and Reggio Emilia, Italy

Funding: The authors have no funding or support to report.

Competing Interests: Nadia K. Shihab is employed by Southern Counties Veterinary Specialists. There are no patents, products in development or marketed products to declare.

* Email: hvolk@rvc.ac.uk

¶ NKS and BBJT are joint second authors on this work.

Introduction

Epilepsy is the most common chronic neurological condition in humans and dogs, with estimated prevalences of 0.4–1% [1] and 0.6%, respectively [2]. In human medicine, the best improvement in Quality of Life (QoL) for epilepsy patients is achieved when treatment leads to remission (seizure freedom) [3–5]. Indeed, in one study, no significant change in QoL was found after treatment for subjects that did *not* achieve seizure freedom [4]. In addition to anti-epileptic drug (AED) therapy, surgical interventions are utilised to achieve seizure freedom in medically intractable cases [6]. The dog has been considered as a naturally occurring model of human epilepsy [7,8]. There are considerable parallels in the diagnosis of human and canine epilepsy, with similarly high levels of workup, for example and the use of advanced diagnostic imaging and in limited cases, the use of electroencephalography (EEG) [9]. However, in veterinary medicine, most epilepsy trials have primarily focused on reducing seizure frequency, rather than achieving seizure freedom. Indeed, an ≥50% reduction in seizure frequency has been the definition of AED efficacy in the majority of canine epilepsy studies (e.g. [10–17]). This may not be a

satisfactory outcome for the carers (the owners), with nearly one third considering only complete seizure freedom as an acceptable outcome [18]. More than two thirds of dogs with epilepsy will continue to have seizures long-term [19–22] and around 20–30% will remain poorly controlled (<50% reduction of seizure frequency) despite adequate treatment with phenobarbitone (PB) and/or potassium bromide (KBr) [23–25]. Consequently, there is a need to identify those dogs that are likely to have poor outcomes so that owners have realistic, evidence-based expectations of their dog's treatment. This has been an area of focus in human epilepsy, with analyses identifying risk factors for pharmacoresistance and poor outcome (e.g. [26–28]). In contrast, it has been recognised that more epidemiologic studies are needed to further document the nature and occurrence of remission of epilepsy in dogs [29], and identify risk factors associated with positive and negative outcomes. For those dogs that are unresponsive to AEDs, 'alternative' non-pharmacological treatment options need to be developed to improve their quantity and quality of life, for example, dietary and surgical interventions [30].

Remission with or without medication has been observed in canine epilepsy cases, demonstrating that epilepsy in dogs is not *necessarily* a lifelong condition. Remission rates vary between studies, for example in a study of Danish Labrador Retrievers, 24% of dogs were classed as being in remission; with only 1 (6%) of these receiving antiepileptic treatment (drug-induced remission) [21]. In a further Danish study of 63 dogs with epilepsy, the remission rate (both spontaneous remission and remission with treatment) was 15% [22]. In these studies, remission was classified as being seizure free for two years or three years seizure free, respectively. In a Swiss study of Labrador Retrievers, 30% of dogs treated with phenobarbitone became seizure-free, with an average follow-up period of 4.8 years [19]. In a study of the efficacy of phenobarbital compared with KBr as a first line treatment, complete seizure freedom was achieved in 85% and 52%, respectively, of treated dogs [31]. This study only lasted for six months however, and it is possible that the percentage of dogs experiencing seizure freedom would be lower given a longer follow-up period. In addition, higher % treatment success rates may reflect studying animals in first opinion practice environment, where seizure phenotypes are likely to be less severe than animals seen at referral practices.

Several factors related to the natural history of the disease and clinical factors have been implicated in both the experimental and clinical literature as influencing the likelihood of successful treatment with AEDs (either remission or <50% reduction in seizure frequency). For example, recent rodent studies found that early treatment [32] had a positive influence on the likelihood of remission being achieved in certain types of epilepsy. Indeed, in human epilepsy it was thought that patients should be treated with AEDs immediately after a seizure to increase the likelihood of achieving remission. However, evidence that remission rates in countries with and without ready access to AEDs are similar [33] implies that AEDs may act to suppress seizures, but have no influence on achieving remission. In addition, there is increasing evidence from both canine, rodent and human studies, that other aspects of disease e.g. different markers of severity *can* influence drug responsiveness and treatment outcome [19,29,34–36]. This includes a high seizure frequency before treatment, and the presence of cluster seizures and/or status epilepticus. Much of the canine epilepsy literature in this area is derived from single breed studies, thus the aim of this retrospective study was to investigate factors associated with remission in a large population of dogs with epilepsy treated at a multi-breed canine specific epilepsy clinic.

Materials and Methods

Data from dogs treated at a multi-breed canine specific epilepsy clinic at the Royal Veterinary College Small Animal Referral Hospital (RVC SARH) between 2005–2011 was retrospectively collected from RVC's electronic patient records. Clinical data was originally gained via standardised owner questionnaires for epilepsy patients at their first appointment, and longitudinal follow up data was gained via telephone interview with the dogs' owners. All dogs received a uniform diagnostic protocol (including complete blood cell count; serum biochemical profile and dynamic bile acid testing; MRI of the brain, 1.5-Tesla Gyroscan NT, Philips Medical Systems) and a neurological examination to rule out an underlying cause of the seizure activity. Only dogs which were reported in the records to be diagnosed with idiopathic epilepsy, for which a cause was not identified (no remarkable findings on interictal neurological examination, haematology, biochemistry, brain magnetic resonance imaging and cerebrospinal fluid examination), were included in the study. A genetic or hereditary basis cannot be confirmed for every case included in the study, and it is possible that the cause could have been identified

with continuous EEG recording. Only dogs receiving AEDs were included in the study.

Seizures were classified according to the former guidelines of the International League Against Epilepsy, modified for veterinary patients (Berendt and Gram, 1999; Licht et al., 2002). Epilepsy was defined of at least two unprovoked seizures >24 h apart. Cluster seizures were defined as an episode where more than one seizure occurred within a 24 h period, with full recovery of consciousness between seizures. Status epilepticus was defined as seizure activity lasting longer than 10 min without gaining consciousness. Seizure activity lasting less than 10 min without gaining consciousness was classed as a single seizure episode. A consistent history was collected with the help of a questionnaire developed for a previous study [10]. The data collected included: signalment, age presented to the hospital (days), age of dog at the time of the first seizure (days), time until diagnosis (days), duration of the disorder before treatment (days), number of seizures prior to any treatment with an AED, seizure frequency per month before medication, type of seizures experienced, and experience of cluster seizures (yes/no) and status epilepticus (yes/no). Medication administered was recorded, specifically whether phenobarbitone (PB), potassium bromide (KBr) or other 3rd line drugs were prescribed, and response to these drugs recorded as responsive or unresponsive. Follow up time was recorded in days. Treatment success was recorded as:

(i) Seizure-free remission (with or without medication) (1/0)

(ii) ≥50% reduction in seizure frequency (1/0)

Non-responsiveness to an AED was classified as a less than 50% reduction in seizure frequency, despite being within the reference range for the prescribed AED(s) and titrated to the maximum tolerated effective dose. As these data were derived from a clinical population, decision-making leading to the maximum dose of any AED was made by both the clinician and the owner, taking into account adverse effects of the drug and its efficacy. Serum levels of phenobarbitone and/or potassium bromide were checked by the attending clinician, and recorded from the clinical records where available, to ensure the dog was within the reference range for these AEDs and receiving adequate therapy, and to test the effect of this variable.

Ethics statement

This study was approved by the Royal Veterinary College's Ethics and Welfare Committee. The owners of the dogs gave permission for their animals to be used in this study.

Statistical analysis

Differences between outcome variables were tested with a Fisher's exact test for categorical variables with expected values < 10, and the Pearson's chi squared test for expected values >10. The Mann-Whitney U-test was used for continuous variables. Generalised linear mixed models for binary outcomes were then used to identify risk factors in a multivariate analysis for successful treatment outcomes, using the lmer function in R from the lme4 package. Treatment outcomes (i) seizure free remission with or without medication (1/0) and (ii) ≥50% reduction in seizure frequency (1/0) were used as the response variables in models. Follow-up time and serum AED values were tested in the models to verify that they did not have an effect on treatment success. Breed was included as a random effect, with all cross breeds coded plainly as 'cross breed' due to the unknown parentage of many of these dogs. This random effect took into account the genetic non-independence of multiple members of the same breed in the study

Table 1. Association between clinical variables and being in seizure-free remission in canine epilepsy patients.

		Remission		Statistics	
		No (%)	Yes (%)	Fishers exact (2 sided)	P
Sex	Male	75.1	53.6	5.56	0.024
	Female	24.9	46.4		
Neuter status	Neutered	53.2	75.0	4.53	0.038
	Entire	46.8	25.0		
Seizure severity	Status epilepticus	20.0	0.0	0.25	0.802
	No Status epilepticus	80.0	100.0		
	Cluster seizures	62.8	17.9	19.63	<0.001
	No Cluster seizures	37.2	82.1		
		Median (25th–75th percentile)	Median (25th–75th percentile)	Mann Whitney U	P
Age presented to hospital (days)		1080 (720–1800)	1440 (1080–2085)	1933	0.61
Time until diagnosis (days)		180 (62.3–378.8)	90 (15–225)	1204	0.79
Age at onset seizures (days)		720 (441–1286)	1170 (720–1725)	2971	0.026
Duration of disorder before treatment (days)		90 (30–180)	60 (26–120)	578	0.31
Number of seizures before start of treatment		5 (3–8.5)	4 (3–5.3)	1286	0.09
Seizure frequency per month before medication		3 (1–6)	2 (1.25–3.75)	1582	0.39

population, and possible demographic and environmental factors. Predictors including age, sex and neuter status were tested in all models. Multicollinearity was checked for in all models, identified from inflated standard errors in the models, and thus avoided. Model fit was assessed using the deviance and Akaike's information criterion. Data is presented as median with 25th and 75th percentiles and all tests were used two-sided with $P<0.05$ being considered statistically significant.

Results

Population demographics

122 dogs were lost to follow and 344 dogs were included in the analysis, of which 89.5% were pure bred and 10.5% were cross-breeds. The five most common breeds were the Labrador Retriever (14.8%), cross breed (10.5%), Border Collie (9.9%), German Shepherd Dog (8.7%) and the Staffordshire Bull Terrier (5.5%). The majority of dogs were male (70.3%), with 57% of all dogs neutered. The median age (in days) at presentation to the small animal referral hospital was 1260 days (720–2008) (approximately 3.5 years).

Clinical data

The median age at onset of seizures was 780 days (360–1447.5). The median time until diagnosis was 150 days (38–360), with the median duration of the disorder before treatment 67.5 days (30–180). The median number of seizures before the start of treatment was 4.5 (3–7.25) with a median seizure frequency (per month) before medication of 3 (1–5). The median follow up time was 656 days (330–960).

A minority of dogs had experienced status epilepticus (13.1%), whereas nearly half of dogs had experienced cluster seizures (48%). There was a significant association between the presence of status epilepticus and cluster seizures ($X^2 = 8.05$, $P = 0.004$), with 9.8% of dogs experiencing both status epilepticus and cluster seizures. There was no difference between male and female dogs experiencing cluster seizures (48.9% $vs.$ 45.8%; $X^2 = 0.26$, $P = 0.61$); however, more male dogs experienced status epilepticus than female dogs (15.5% vs. 5.2%; $X^2 = 4.12$, $P = 0.041$). At the univariate level (Table 1) dogs without cluster seizures were significantly more likely to go into remission, but there was no difference in dogs with or without status epilepticus.

The most common seizure type was complex-focal seizures with secondary tonic-clonic generalisation (35.7%), followed by generalised tonic-clonic (32.6%), complex-focal (14.1%), and simple-focal seizures with secondary tonic-clonic generalisation (13.7%). The rarest seizure type was simple-focal seizures with only 11 cases (3.8%).

Of the 113 dogs for which PB concentrations were available, they were well within the reference range (29.1 ± 1.60 µg/ml, reference range from our laboratory of 15–45 µg/ml). KBr concentrations were available for 53 dogs and were 1.61 ± 0.11 mg/ml, again well within the reference range from our laboratory of 0.5–1.9 mg/ml.

The majority of dogs were receiving PB at follow up (67.2%), with a further 38.4% of cases receiving KBr, and 27% of all cases receiving PB and KBr in combination. A minority of cases (10.2%) were prescribed a third line AED (e.g. gabapentin, pregabalin, levetiracetam and zonisamide). In addition, 5.4% of cases received

Table 2. Association between clinical variables and ≥50% reduction in seizure frequency in canine epilepsy patients.

		≥50% reduction		Statistics	
		No (%)	**Yes (%)**	**Fishers exact (2 sided)**	**P**
Sex	Male	78.5	64.5	5.54	0.025
	Female	21.5	35.5		
Neuter status	Neutered	50.0	63.2	3.62	0.040
	Entire	50.0	36.8		
Seizure severity	Status epilepticus	21.1	10.2	4.35	0.052
	No Status epilepticus	78.9	89.8		
	Cluster seizures	71.7	33.5	34.01	<0.001
	No Cluster seizures	28.3	66.5		
		Median (25th–75th percentile)	**Median (25th–75th percentile)**	**Mann Whitney U**	**P**
Age presented to hospital (days)		990 (720–1514.8)	1424.5 (840–2094.5)	5795	0.011
Time until diagnosis (days)		183 (72.5–360)	150 (34–360)	4225.5	0.216
Age at onset seizures (days)		720 (360–1125)	968 (447.8–1699)	9893	0.007
Duration of disorder before treatment (days)		37.5 (22.5–142.5)	90 (30–180)	833.5	0.064
Number of seizures before start of treatment		5 (3.3–8.8)	4.5 (3–7.8)	2762	0.276
Seizure frequency per month before medication		3 (1–5)	2 (1–5)	5022.5	0.569

emergency rectal diazepam treatment and 8.1% received pulsed intermittent treatment with levetiracetam.

Risk factors for remission

Fourteen per cent of dogs were in remission on PB treatment. When ≥50% reduction in seizure frequency is used as the outcome measure, success rates are markedly higher with 64.5% of dogs achieving this level of seizure reduction. At the univariate level, several factors were associated with an increased likelihood of achieving remission (Table 1), namely: being female, neutered, no previous experience of cluster seizures and an older age at onset of seizures. The same four factors were also associated with an increased likelihood of achieving an ≥50% reduction in seizure frequency, with the addition of an older age at presentation to hospital (Table 2).

When tested in a multivariate mixed model (Table 3), two categorical variables were significantly associated with the likelihood of remission being achieved; sex and cluster seizures, with female dogs over two times more likely to achieve remission, and dogs with no previous experience of cluster seizures over six times more likely to achieve remission. No effects of neuter status or previous episodes of status epilepticus were found in any model, and were not found to improve model fit (determined by Akaike Information Criterion [AIC] and % correct classification), and as such they were not included in the final model. There were no significant effects of time until diagnosis, duration of time before treatment, the number of seizures before treatment or the seizure frequency per month before medication. No effects of follow up time or serum AED values were found. There were no significant effects of seizure type on the likelihood of remission (p = 0.208);

Table 3. Risk factors for remission in canine epilepsy cases.

Predictor	Odds Ratio (95% CI OR)	SE (coef)	Z	P
Sex				
Female	2.39 (1.01–5.64)	0.44	2.00	0.047
Male	*Ref*			
Cluster Seizures				
No	6.08 (2.35–15.70)	0.49	3.75	<0.001
Yes	*ref*			

Table 4. Risk factors for an ≥50% reduction in seizure frequency in canine epilepsy cases.

Predictor	Odds Ratio (95% CI OR)	SE (coef)	Z	P
Sex				
Female	2.15 (1.12–4.15)	0.33	2.32	0.021
Male	*ref*			
Cluster Seizures				
No	4.66 (2.58–8.39)	0.30	5.14	<0.001
Yes	*ref*			
Age at onset of seizures (days)	1.00 (1.00–1.01)	0.00	2.51	0.013

however the seizure types with the lowest remission rates were simple-focal (0% remission) and complex-focal seizure with secondary tonic-clonic generalisation (14.1% remission).

When an ≥50% reduction in seizure frequency is used as the outcome measure (Table 2 and 4), the same two factors were found to significantly predict the likelihood of achieving remission in a multivariate model (Table 4), with the addition of age at onset of seizures. As age at onset of seizures increases, the likelihood of achieving an ≥50% reduction in seizure frequency increases.

Breeds

Dogs of fifteen different breeds achieved seizure freedom, and dogs of fifty-two breeds achieved an ≥50% reduction in seizure frequency. There was no statistically significant effect of breed on the likelihood of dogs going into remission or having an ≥50% reduction in seizure frequency when tested at the univariate level. Of the breeds with over 10 dogs for which data was available (the Labrador Retriever, Cross Breed, German Shepherd, Border Collie and Staffordshire Bull Terrier), the breed least likely to go into remission or have an ≥50% reduction in seizure frequency was the Border Collie (0% and 40% respectively), followed by the German Shepherd (11% and 35%) and Staffordshire Bull Terrier (0% and 57%). Fishers exact tests revealed only significant effects of being a Border Collie or German Shepherd on the likelihood of entering remission or experiencing an ≥50% reduction in seizure frequency (Table 5). When these breeds were included in multivariate analyses as binary variables, no significant effects were found.

Discussion

The results of this retrospective study provide evidence that the presence of cluster seizures and thus seizure *density* (the temporal pattern of seizure activity) is a more influential risk factor on the likelihood of achieving remission in canine epilepsy than seizure

frequency or the total number of seizures prior to treatment. Nearly half (48%) of dogs in the study population had experienced cluster seizures, of which only 17.9% achieved remission and 33.5% achieved an ≥50% reduction in seizure frequency. This result has previously been found in human epilepsy [37]. The number of epileptic dogs that experience cluster seizures varies between studies, with recent reports between 38% and 64% [20,38]. The breed least likely to achieve remission in this study was the Border Collie, a breed previously demonstrated to have a higher level of cluster seizures than other breeds (84.6% affected) [20], with similar levels reported in other studies (e.g. 94%; [29]). A remission rate of 14.2% was observed in this study, similar to a previous Danish study of canine epilepsy (15%) [22]. These were both mixed study populations; however, in studies of Labrador Retrievers in isolation, higher levels of remission have been observed (24–40%) [19,21]. When >50% reduction in seizure frequency is used as the outcome measure, success rates are markedly higher at 64.5%.

Seizure *density* as well as frequency has been demonstrated to influence the likelihood of remission in humans, with individuals who experience an episode of status epilepticus [39–41], or cluster seizures [37] less likely to go into remission. These results were also seen in a recent study of predictors of pharmacoresistance in rats, where the average seizure frequency per day of 13 rats nonresponsive to medication was 4.31/day, indicating some rats having cluster seizures [36]. This frequency was significantly higher than 20 drug-responsive rats (mean 0.54/day). It is further notable, that of the 13 rats that were unresponsive to medication, a subgroup of six rats (18%) experienced high levels of cluster seizures, with an average of 8.94 seizures per day [36]. Intact male and female dogs have a higher likelihood of having cluster seizures [42] which may have a negative impact on their prognosis. Evidence from canine epilepsy is not clear however, with 89% (8/9) of Border Collies in remission having a history of cluster seizures, status epilepticus, or both [29]. A severe epilepsy

Table 5. Top five breeds most likely to lack drug response.

Breed	% remission	p	% ≥50% reduction	P
Border Collie	0	0.02	40	0.01
German Shepherd	11	0.51	35	0.01
Staffordshire Bull Terrier	0	0.18	57	0.37
Cross Breed	19	0.30	61	0.38
Labrador Retriever	23	0.14	76	0.07

phenotype is often seen in this breed, thus data from a larger population with a diversity of breeds represented would be valuable to gain an insight into this relationship in a wider population with a variety of disease phenotypes.

No evidence was found to support the results of a recent rodent study that found early treatment [32] influenced the likelihood of remission being achieved. There are divergent opinions within the veterinary profession regarding time to treatment after diagnosis of epilepsy, a topic also debated in human medicine [43]. One school of thought advises treatment of seizures as soon as a dog is diagnosed as having recurrent seizures (i.e. after the second seizure episode). However, the impact of AED side effects on QoL may be considerable, with this being the top reason cited by owners for a decreased QoL in their dogs (28% of 25 owners questioned) [44]. As such, the second school of thought considers that there should be a balance between the benefits gained from using AEDs with the potential adverse effects they cause. The results of this study indicated no effect of time to treatment; however, there is mixed evidence regarding its effects on treatment outcome. In clinical studies of epilepsy in dogs, decreased time to treatment has not been observed as a positive influence upon treatment outcome, indeed, one study demonstrated that Labrador Retrievers that were in remission received medication a longer period of time after their first seizure than those dogs which continued to seizure [19]. It should be acknowledged that this result may be biased by animals with a more severe seizure phenotype receiving treatment earlier, due to owner and/or veterinarian concerns. It is currently not veterinary practice to initiate treatment after the first seizure. Early initation of treatment has also proven unsuccessful in several human studies [45–47]. Time to treatment is additionally likely to be influenced by disease severity, for example it was shorter in dogs with episodes of status epilepticus [48], thus being confounding factors in statistical analyses.

A large number of seizures before treatment has been identified as a poor prognostic factor in several previous human studies of epilepsy [34,41,49], with patients experiencing a greater number of seizures prior to initiation of treatment more likely to have refractory epilepsy. In rats, it was recently demonstrated that seizure frequency in the early phase of epilepsy is a strong predictor of refractoriness [36]. This has also been seen in dogs, with refractory dogs having a significantly higher number of seizures prior to presentation and beginning of treatment in Labradors [19] and an initially higher seizure frequency in Border Collies [29]. It has been discussed whether this initial high seizure frequency and subsequent refractoriness may be an effect of kindling (Reynolds, 1995). However, as time to treatment has not been found to be a strong predictor of refractoriness in dogs and humans, initial high seizure frequency has been considered more likely to be the result, rather than the cause of the pathophysiological changes that are later manifested as refractory epilepsy [34,50]. Indeed, in this study and another previous study of canine epilepsy, the number of seizures before treatment was not significantly different between dogs positive vs. negative treatment outcomes [48]. In addition, no effect was found of seizure type upon the likelihood of remission; however, the most common seizure type in dogs that did not achieve remission (39.6%) was complex-focal seizures, also seen in human epilepsy [51,52], adding evidence to the belief that focal seizures are more challenging to treat.

Males were found to be less likely to achieve remission than female dogs. Historically, male dogs are thought to seizure more than female dogs [53], and recent epidemiological studies of idiopathic epilepsy have confirmed a male overrepresentation for this disorder [2,38]. With regard to the impact of sex upon

treatment outcome, little existing data is available. One study noted that female dogs with epilepsy lived longer with the disorder than male dogs, with a median age at death two years greater (8 vs. 6 years, respectively) [22]; however, this outcome measure may be influenced by owner euthanasia decisions, so can only be a proxy of treatment success. In previous studies, male dogs were found to be more highly affected by cluster seizures than female dogs [42]. This result was not found in the current study, and indeed sex and the presence of cluster seizures were found to be independently significant risk factors, thus further investigation is warranted into the effect of sex on treatment outcome.

Age at onset of disease was found to significantly influence the likelihood of achieving an ≥50% reduction in seizure frequency, with dogs experiencing their first seizure at an older age more likely to achieve this level of reduction. This has previously been demonstrated in Border Collies, with the mean age at onset significantly higher in dogs with remission compared to those with active epilepsy [29], and in Labradors, with dogs classed as having excellent or good results (defined as those that were seizure-free, or had an improvement in their seizure frequency, strength and/or duration) having a significantly higher age at onset than uncontrolled dogs [19]. Early age at seizure onset has been previously identified in children to be a predictor of pharmacoresistance [54]. In contrast, in a study of canine juvenile epilepsy (where the first seizure occurs before the age of one year), age at onset had no influence on survival outcome [20].

There are recognised limitations to studying epilepsy in a veterinary referral population [20] due to a bias towards a more severe seizure phenotype, and thus may not be representative of the whole canine epilepsy population. As such, further studies of epilepsy in the first opinion practice population may be warranted, although the level of diagnostic work up may be lower owing to availability of equipment and specialist expertise, and thus confidence in diagnosis may be variable. A further limitation of this study is the varied follow up time of cases. In previous studies, remission was strictly classified as dogs that were seizure free for two or three years [21,22]. In human epilepsy, seizures may re-occur after a period of months of seizure freedom, without alterations to treatment [55]. As such, some of the dogs classified as seizure free in this study may have later experienced seizures. This may be due to a variety of factors including drug tolerance, deterioration of the epilepsy phenotype, acquired drug resistance and poor owner compliance [55]. The median follow up time, however, was 656 days and thus is in line with the follow-up standards of comparable epilepsy studies in the veterinary environment. There are limitations to which variables could be controlled for in this study, introduced by data being collected in a clinical environment with naturally occurring disease in client owned animals. Due to the expense of medication it is possible that clients may decline third line AEDs that may affect the response rate, which may mean the figures here are an underestimate of how many dogs could biologically achieve remission. In addition, EEG is not routinely used in the Canine Epilepsy Clinic data were sourced from, or in veterinary medicine in general at present, and thus there is no confirmation that the 'seizure' episodes reported by owners was indeed seizure activity. A further limitation of this study is that serum AED levels were not available for all dogs; however, clinicians contributing to this dataset routinely checked AED serum levels were within the reference ranges and thus, this is naturally standardised across the sample. Furthermore, not all serum levels were conducted at the same laboratory and therefore could not be analysed in the same dataset. No statistical association between AED levels and treatment outcome were found; however, future studies could include this variable to check this result was not due to the lower power of this sub-sample.

Conclusions

In conclusion, the present provides evidence that it is not merely the absolute *number* of seizures prior to treatment that predicts refractoriness, but their temporal pattern, with those patients experiencing cluster seizures (more than one seizure within a 24 h period) more likely to be pharmacoresistant. Whether this result is an effect of cluster seizures promoting epileptogenesis and causing brain damage that results in seizures resistant to medication, or is actually a reflection of a more aggressive disease phenotype that is harder to treat is unknown, and warrants further investigation. The present study further demonstrates similarities between this naturally occurring model of epilepsy and both experimental

rodent models [36], and human clinical studies [37]. The similarity between clinical environments, high level of diagnostic work up, and shared living environments between humans and dogs further strengthens the use of this readily available animal model.

Acknowledgments

The paper was internally approved for submission (Manuscript ID number CSD_00726).

Author Contributions

Conceived and designed the experiments: NKS BBJT HAV. Performed the experiments: NKS BBJT. Analyzed the data: RMAP. Contributed reagents/materials/analysis tools: RMAP. Contributed to the writing of the manuscript: HAV RMAP.

References

1. Sander JW, Shorvon SD (1996) Epidemiology of the epilepsies. Journal of Neurology, Neurosurgery, and Psychiatry 61: 433–443.
2. Kearsley-Fleet L, O'Neill DG, Volk HA, Church DB, Brodbelt DC (2013) Prevalence and risk factors for canine epilepsy of unknown origin in the UK. Veterinary Record 172.
3. Poochikian-Sarkissian S, Sidani S, Wennberg R, Devins G (2008) Seizure Freedom Reduces Illness Intrusiveness and Improves Quality of Life in Epilepsy. The Canadian Journal of Neurological Sciences 35: 280–286.
4. Birbeck Gretchen L, Hays Ron D, Cui X, Vickrey Barbara G (2002) Seizure Reduction and Quality of Life Improvements in People with Epilepsy. Epilepsia 43: 535–538.
5. Kwan P, Arzimanoglou A, Berg AT, Brodie MJ, Allen Hauser W, et al. (2010) Definition of drug resistant epilepsy: consensus proposal by the ad hoc task force of the ILAE Commission on Therapeutic Strategies. Epilepsia 51: 1069–1077.
6. Ramey WL, Martirosyan NL, Lieu CM, Hasham HA, Lemole Jr GM, et al. (2013) Current management and surgical outcomes of medically intractable epilepsy. Clinical Neurology and Neurosurgery 115: 2411–2418.
7. Löscher W, Schwartz-Porsche D, Frey HH, Schmidt D (1985) Evaluation of epileptic dogs as an animal model of human epilepsy. Arzneimittelforschung 35(1): 82–7.
8. Potschka H, Fischer A, von Rüden E-L, Hülsmeyer V, Baumgärtner W (2013) Canine epilepsy as a translational model? Epilepsia 54: 571–579.
9. Berendt M, Høgenhaven H, Flagstad A, Dam M (1999) Electroencephalography in dogs with epilepsy: similarities between human and canine findings. Acta Neurologica Scandinavica 99: 276–283.
10. Volk HA, Matiasek LA, Luján Feliu-Pascual A, Platt SR, Chandler KE (2008) The efficacy and tolerability of levetiracetam in pharmacoresistant epileptic dogs. The Veterinary Journal 176: 310–319.
11. Platt SR, Adams V, Garosi LS, Abramson CJ, Penderis J, et al. (2006) Treatment with gabapentin of 11 dogs with refractory idiopathic epilepsy. Veterinary Record 159: 881–884.
12. Dewey CW, Cerda-Gonzalez S, Levine JM, Badgley BL, Ducoté JM, et al. (2009) Pregabalin as an adjunct to phenobarbital, potassium bromide, or a combination of phenobarbital and potassium bromide for treatment of dogs with suspected idiopathic epilepsy. Journal of the American Veterinary Medical Association 235: 1442–1449.
13. Dewey CW, Guiliano R, Boothe DM, Berg JM, Kortz GD, et al. (2004) Zonisamide therapy for refractory idiopathic epilepsy in dogs. Journal of the American Animal Hospital Association 40.
14. von Klopmann T, Rambeck B, Tipold A (2007) Prospective study of zonisamide therapy for refractory idiopathic epilepsy in dogs. Journal of Small Animal Practice 48: 134–138.
15. Andrew SE (2008) Immune-mediated canine and feline keratitis. Veterinary Clinics of North America-Small Animal Practice 38: 269–+.
16. Muñana KR, Nettifee-Osborne JA, Bergman RL, Jr., Mealey KL (2012a) Association between ABCB1 genotype and seizure outcome in collies with epilepsy. Journal of Veterinary Internal Medicine 26: 1358–1364.
17. Muñana KR, Thomas WB, Inzana KD, Nettifee-Osborne JA, McLucas KJ, et al. (2012b) Evaluation of levetiracetam as adjunctive treatment for refractory canine epilepsy: a randomized, placebo-controlled, crossover trial. Journal of Veterinary Internal Medicine 26: 341–348.
18. Wessmann A, Volk H, Parkin T, Ortega M, Anderson TJ (2012) Living with canine idiopathic epilepsy: a questionnaire-based evaluation of quality of life. Proceedings of the 24th Symposium ESVN-ECVN. J Vet Intern Med 26: 823–852.
19. Heynold Y, Faissler D, Steffen F, Jaggy A (1997) Clinical, epidemiological and treatment results of idiopathic epilepsy in 54 labrador retrievers: a long-term study. Journal of Small Animal Practice 38: 7–14.
20. Arrol L, Penderis J, Garosi L, Cripps P, Gutierrez-Quintana R, et al. (2012) Aetiology and long-term outcome of juvenile epilepsy in 136 dogs. Veterinary Record 170: 335.
21. Berendt M, Gredal H, Pedersen LG, Alban L, Alving J (2002) A Cross-Sectional Study of Epilepsy in Danish Labrador Retrievers: Prevalence and Selected Risk Factors. Journal of Veterinary Internal Medicine 16: 262–268.
22. Berendt M, Gredal H, Ersbøll AK, Alving J (2007) Premature Death, Risk Factors, and Life Patterns in Dogs with Epilepsy. Journal of Veterinary Internal Medicine 21: 754–759.
23. Trepanier L, Schwark W, Van Schoick A, Carrillo J (1998) Therapeutic serum drug concentrations in epileptic dogs treated with potassium bromide alone or in combination with other anticonvulsants: 122 cases (1992–1996). J Am Vet Med Assoc 213: 1449–1453.
24. Schwartz-Porsche D, Löscher W, Frey H (1985) Therapeutic efficacy of phenobarbital and primidone in canine epilepsy: a comparison. J Vet Pharmacol Ther 8: 113–119.
25. Podell M, Fenner W (1993) Bromide therapy in refractory canine idiopathic epilepsy. Journal of Veterinary Internal Medicine 7: 318–327.
26. Cockerell O, Johnson A, Sander J (1994) Remission of epilepsy: results from the National General Practice Study of Epilepsy. Lancet 346: 140–144.
27. Bonnett LJ, Tudur Smith C, Smith D, Williamson PR, Chadwick D, et al. (2014) Time to 12-month remission and treatment failure for generalised and unclassified epilepsy. Journal of Neurology, Neurosurgery & Psychiatry 85: 603–610.
28. MacDonald BK, Johnson AL, Goodridge DM, Cockerell OC, Sander JWAS, et al. (2000) Factors predicting prognosis of epilepsy after presentation with seizures. Annals of Neurology 48: 833–841.
29. Hülsmeyer V, Zimmermann R, Brauer C, Sauter-Louis C, Fischer A (2010) Epilepsy in Border Collies: Clinical Manifestation, Outcome, and Mode of Inheritance. Journal of Veterinary Internal Medicine 24: 171–178.
30. Martlé V, Van Ham L, Raedt R, Vonck K, Boon P, et al. (2014) Non-pharmacological treatment options for refractory epilepsy: An overview of human treatment modalities and their potential utility in dogs. The Veterinary Journal 199: 332–339.
31. Boothe DM, Dewey C, Carpenter DM (2012) Comparison of phenobarbital with bromide as a first-choice antiepileptic drug for treatment of epilepsy in dogs. J Am Vet Med Assoc 240: 1073–1083.
32. Blumenfeld H, Klein JP, Schridde U, Vestal M, Rice T, et al. (2008) Early treatment suppresses the development of spike-wave epilepsy in a rat model. Epilepsia 49: 400–409.
33. Placencia M, Sander JWAS, Shorvon SD, Roman M, Alarcon F, et al. (1993) Antiepileptic drug treatment in a community health care setting in northern Ecuador: a prospective 12-month assessment. Epilepsy Research 14: 237–244.
34. Kwan P, Brodie MJ (2000) Early Identification of Refractory Epilepsy. New England Journal of Medicine 342: 314–319.
35. Weissl J, Hulsmeyer V, Brauer C, Tipold A, Koskinen LL, et al. (2012) Disease progression and treatment response of idiopathic epilepsy in Australian Shepherd dogs. Journal of Veterinary Internal Medicine 26: 116–125.
36. Löscher W, Brandt C (2010) High seizure frequency prior to antiepileptic treatment is a predictor of pharmacoresistant epilepsy in a rat model of temporal lobe epilepsy. Epilepsia 51: 89–97.
37. Sillanpää M, Schmidt D (2008) Seizure clustering during drug treatment affects seizure outcome and mortality of childhood-onset epilepsy. Brain 131: 938–944.
38. Short AD, Dunne A, Lohi H, Boulton S, Carter SD, et al. (2011) Characteristics of epileptic episodes in UK dog breeds: an epidemiological approach. Veterinary Record 169: 48.
39. Hauser WA (1990) Status epilepticus: epidemiologic considerations. Neurology 40: 9–13.

40. Callaghan BC, Anand K, Hesdorffer D, Hauser WA, French JA (2007) Likelihood of seizure remission in an adult population with refractory epilepsy. Annals of Neurology 62: 382–389.

41. Sillanpää M (1993) Remission of Seizures and Predictors of Intractability in Long-Term Follow-Up. Epilepsia 34: 930–936.

42. Monteiro R, Adams V, Keys D, Platt SR (2012) Canine idiopathic epilepsy: prevalence, risk factors and outcome associated with cluster seizures and status epilepticus. Journal of Small Animal Practice 53: 526–533.

43. Marson AG (2008) When to start antiepileptic drug treatment and with what evidence? Epilepsia 49: 3–6.

44. Chang Y, Mellor DJ, Anderson TJ (2006) Idiopathic epilepsy in dogs: owners' perspectives on management with phenobarbitone and/or potassium bromide. Journal of Small Animal Practice 47: 574–581.

45. Musicco M, Beghi E, Solari A, Viani F (1997) Treatment of first tonic-clonic seizure does not improve the prognosis of epilepsy. Neurology 49: 991–998.

46. Camfield C, Camfield P, Gordon K, Dooley J (1996) Does the number of seizures before treatment influence ease of control or remission of childhood epilepsy? Not if the number is 10 or less. Neurology 46: 41–44.

47. Avanzini G, Depaulis A, Tassinari A, de Curtis M (2013) Do seizures and epileptic activity worsen epilepsy and deteriorate cognitive function? Epilepsia 54: 14–21.

48. Saito M, Muñana K, Sharp N, Olby N (2001) Risk factors for development of status epilepticus in dogs with idiopathic epilepsy and effects of status epilepticus on outcome and survival time: 32 cases (1990–1996). J Am Vet Med Assoc 219: 618–623.

49. Collaborative Group for the Study of Epilepsy (1992) Prognosis of Epilepsy in Newly Referred Patients: A Multicenter Prospective Study of the Effects of Monotherapy on the Long-Term Course of Epilepsy. Epilepsia 33: 45–51.

50. Berg AT, Shinnar S (1997) Do Seizures Beget Seizures? An Assessment of the Clinical Evidence in Humans. Journal of Clinical Neurophysiology Secondary Epileptogenesis 14: 102–110.

51. Regesta G, Tanganelli P (1999) Clinical aspects and biological bases of drug-resistant epilepsies. Epilepsy Research 34: 109–122.

52. Reynolds EH, Elwes RDC, Shorvon SD (1983) Why Does Epilepsy Become Intractable - Prevention of Chronic Epilepsy. Lancet 2: 952–954.

53. Bielfelt SW, Redman HC, McClellan RO (1971) Sire- and sex-related differences in rates of epileptiform seizures in a purebred beagle dog colony. American Journal of Veterinary Research 32: 2039–2048.

54. Cockerell OC, Johnson AL, Sander JW, Shorvon SD (1997) Prognosis of epilepsy: a review and further analysis of the first nine years of the British National General Practice Study of Epilepsy, a prospective population-based study. Epilepsia 38: 31–46.

55. Löscher W, Schmidt D (2006) Experimental and Clinical Evidence for Loss of Effect (Tolerance) during Prolonged Treatment with Antiepileptic Drugs. Epilepsia 47: 1253–1284.

21

Paleomicrobiology: Revealing Fecal Microbiomes of Ancient Indigenous Cultures

Raul J. Cano[1]*, **Jessica Rivera-Perez**[2], **Gary A. Toranzos**[2], **Tasha M. Santiago-Rodriguez**[3], **Yvonne M. Narganes-Storde**[4], **Luis Chanlatte-Baik**[4], **Erileen García-Roldán**[2], **Lucy Bunkley-Williams**[5], **Steven E. Massey**[2]

1 Center for Applications in Biotechnology, California Polytechnic State University, San Luis Obispo, California, United States of America, **2** Department of Biology, University of Puerto Rico, San Juan, Puerto Rico, **3** Department of Pathology, University of California San Diego, San Diego, California, United States of America, **4** Center for Archaeological Research, University of Puerto Rico, Rio Piedras Campus, San Juan, Puerto Rico, **5** Department of Biology, University of Puerto Rico, Mayaguez Campus, San Juan, Puerto Rico

Abstract

Coprolites are fossilized feces that can be used to provide information on the composition of the intestinal microbiota and, as we show, possibly on diet. We analyzed human coprolites from the Huecoid and Saladoid cultures from a settlement on Vieques Island, Puerto Rico. While more is known about the Saladoid culture, it is believed that both societies co-existed on this island approximately from 5 to 1170 AD. By extracting DNA from the coprolites, followed by metagenomic characterization, we show that both cultures can be distinguished from each other on the basis of their bacterial and fungal gut microbiomes. In addition, we show that parasite loads were heavy and also culturally distinct. Huecoid coprolites were characterized by maize and Basidiomycetes sequences, suggesting that these were important components of their diet. Saladoid coprolite samples harbored sequences associated with fish parasites, suggesting that raw fish was a substantial component of their diet. The present study shows that ancient DNA is not entirely degraded in humid, tropical environments, and that dietary and/or host genetic differences in ancient populations may be reflected in the composition of their gut microbiome. This further supports the hypothesis that the two ancient cultures studied were distinct, and that they retained distinct technological/cultural differences during an extended period of close proximity and peaceful co-existence. The two populations seemed to form the later-day Taínos, the Amerindians present at the point of Columbian contact. Importantly, our data suggest that paleomicrobiomics can be a powerful tool to assess cultural differences between ancient populations.

Editor: Bryan A. White, University of Illinois, United States of America

Funding: This study was partially funded by NIH RISE Program (NIH Grant No. 5R25GM061151-12). The authors also would like to thank Mark Brolaski of Mo Bio Laboratories for providing the necessary supplies and support for the extraction of fossil DNA. The funders had no role in study design, data collection and analysis, decision to publish, or preparation of the manuscript.

Competing Interests: The authors have declared that no competing interests exist.

* Email: rcano@calpoly.edu

Introduction

Coprolites are fossilized fecal specimens that give us an opportunity to infer on an extinct organism's diet and intestinal microbiota if the DNA is well preserved. Taphonomic conditions such as a highly biomineralized environment or a rapid decline in the sample's water activity (Aw), induce the fossilization process [1]. It has been widely believed that feces are not well preserved in tropical environments due to the high humid conditions. This may likely be one of the reasons why coprolite studies of indigenous Caribbean and other tropical/subtropical cultures are scarce. However, we obtained human coprolites from Vieques, an island approximately 8 Km off the southeastern coast of Puerto Rico. Located in the Caribbean Sea, 2,020 km from the Equator, the climate in Vieques is generally humid with yearly temperatures ranging from approximately 24 to 28°C.

Puerto Rico is considered an important area for archaeological studies in the Caribbean due to the variety of ancient deposits that

have been found on the island. Over 3,000 ancient settlements have been discovered to date, of which 250 are located in the Island of Vieques and correspond to at least four different ancient cultures that inhabited the island. Among these cultures were the Saladoids and Huecoids, two horticulturalist cultures that coexisted in Vieques (an Island off the coast of Puerto Rico) for over 1,000 years (from 5 AD to 1170 AD) after migrating from South America. Originally from present-day Venezuela, the Saladoids migrated to the island of Vieques by 160 BC and to the main Island of Puerto Rico by 430 BC [2,3,4]. While living in this region they maintained their ancestral heritage, as shown by their signature use of white and red painted pottery. However, they also incorporated different traits that they gradually learned/observed from other cultures present on the island. In contrast, little is known about the origins of the Huecoid culture, but they are believed to be originally from the eastern Andes in present-day Bolivia and Peru and are known to have settled in Puerto Rico by

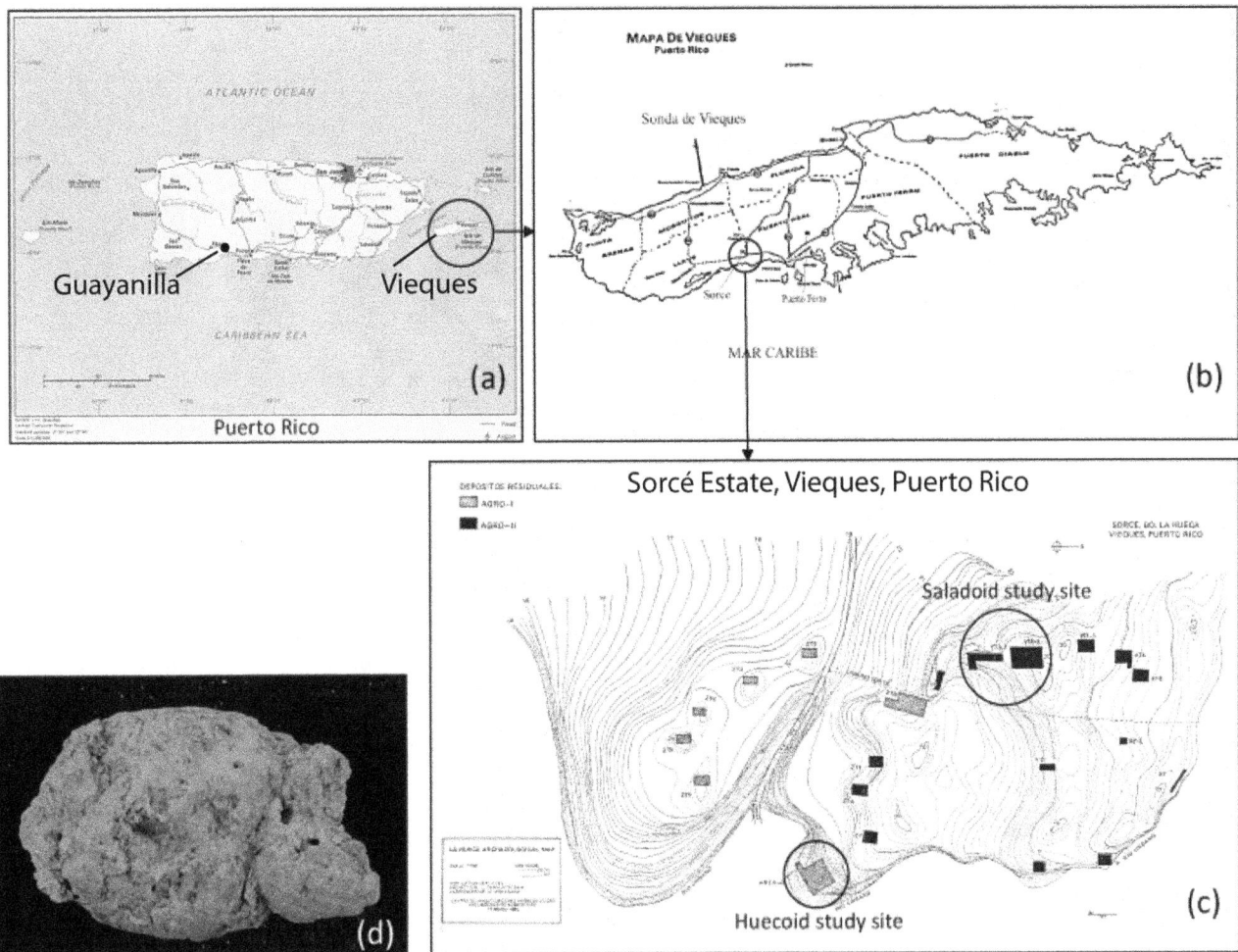

Figure 1. Location and obtainment of coprolites used in this study. Panels (a) and (b) show the sampling sites, located in Sorcé, Vieques, an island off the eastern coast of Puerto Rico. Panel (c) shows the Huecoid and Saladoid archaeological study sites (namely AGRO-I and AGRO-II, respectively). Panel (d) shows a coprolite extracted from these archeological sites.

at least 5 AD. The Huecoids are characterized by their delicate carvings of semiprecious stones and by their resilience to incorporate material or cultural traits from other cultures [5]. The apparent representation of a pair of Andean condors among their amulets suggests to archaeologists their ancestral residence in the Andes. This is also supported by the possible practice of cranial deformation. Both of these cultures greatly impacted other indigenous cultures present on the island, and are thought to have played a part in the development of the predominant culture colloquially referred to as the "Taínos" [6].

Paleomicrobiological studies have shown marked differences between the microbial communities present in Huecoid and Saladoid coprolites [7]. These studies were performed using Terminal Restriction Fragment analysis (TRFL-P), a technique that, although extremely useful for community profiling, has some intrinsic limitations. For example, its total scope extends to the relatively limited database used for downstream analyses. This intrinsic bias implies that microorganisms not in the database will remain hidden to this type of analysis. Also these analyses are often biased towards the most predominant species, leaving out important information on the rare microbiota present in the sample [8]. In light of these limitations, next-generation sequencing (NGS) represents a more appropriate technique for analyzing

these type of samples, mainly due to the high resolving power that characterizes NGS platforms conjointly with bioinformatics tools. Although microbial community profiling when using NGS also has some bias towards the most predominant DNA in the sample, this happens to a lesser extent. Also, NGS is capable of detecting and amplifying previously unidentified/uncultured microorganisms that could be relevant to analysis of the sample's microbial community [9].

The principal aim of this study was to compare these two ancient populations and corroborate whether they present marked differences in their fecal microbiomes due to diet and/or cultural factors. In order to achieve this, we compared the microbiota found in the cores and cortices of coprolites from both cultures using NGS.

Materials and Methods

Sample Description

Coprolites were found in two excavations directed by the archaeologists Dr. Luis A. Chanlatte-Baik and Yvonne M. Narganes-Storde. One excavation site was located at the Sorcé Estate in La Hueca, Vieques, Puerto Rico, the second in Tecla, Guayanilla, PR (**Figure 1**). A total of thirty-four coprolites were used in this study. All thirty-four samples were used for parasitological studies (Huecoid n = 12; Saladoid n = 22). Five of the Saladoid samples used were from Sorce, Vieques and the remaining from Tecla, Guayanilla. In addition, fifteen of the coprolites screened for parasites were also used for microbiome analyses (**Table 1**). Coprolites were provided for this study by Luis Chanlatte-Baik and Yvonne Narganes at the Center for Archaeological Research at the University of Puerto Rico, Rio Piedras Campus. All necessary permits for the collection of samples used in this study were obtained from the Center for Archaeological Research at the University of Puerto Rico, Rio Piedras Campus., complying with all relevant regulations. Repository information, including the nomenclature for precise identification of each specimen containing geographical location, excavation site and archaeological depth for coprolites used in both the DNA and parasitological analyses are described in **Table 1**. Coprolites dated from 180 A.D. to 600 A.D., as indicated by previous ^{14}C dating of material obtained from the same or an equivalent archaeological excavation quadrant and depth of each coprolite (e.g. charcoal and mollusk shells) [10] (**Table 1**). [14]C dating was conducted by Teledyne Isotopes (Westwood, NJ) and BETA Analytic, Inc. (Miami, FL) using standard methods.

Sample Handling and Processing

Coprolites selected for DNA analyses were cut in half; one portion was used for DNA extraction and the other for parasitological studies. All sample processing and DNA extractions for the microbiome analyses were performed in an Ancient DNA laboratory where DNA extraction is conducted in class II hoods assigned exclusively for ancient DNA use. Hoods were exposed to UV light for at least 20 minutes before and after every use. Lab coats designated exclusively for ancient DNA use were routinely decontaminated overnight with commercial chlorine (Clorox). Other aseptic measures include the routine decontamination of the working space with chlorine, the use of sterile, baked and autoclaved DNA-free instruments to extract the DNA, as well as gloves. Controls were done *ad-libitum* for the absence of extraneous DNA.

DNA extraction

To minimize the presence of environmental DNA, approximately 3 mm of the outermost exterior shell of the coprolites was first removed using sterilized brushes as described previously [7]. Approximately 0.25 g of cortex and core samples were separated from each coprolite in the above hoods and DNA was extracted using the PowerSoil DNA Isolation Kit following the manufacturer's instructions (Mo Bio Laboratories, Carlsbad, CA).

Table 1. Description of coprolite samples employed in study.

Sample ID	Specimen Number[1]	Culture	Sampling Area	Radiocarbon date
1a	SV_YTA-1_I-5_6– 60 cm	Saladoid	Cortex	335–395 A.D.
1b			Core	
2a	SV_YTA-2_J-22_80 cm	Saladoid	Cortex	270–385 A.D.
2b			Core	
3a	SV_YTA-2_M-25_40 cm	Saladoid	Cortex	230–385 A.D
3b			Core	
4a	SV_Z-W_2.0 m	Huecoid	Cortex	1300–220 A.D.
4b			Core	
5a	SV_YTA-2_I-24_1-1.2 m	Saladoid	Cortex	Circa 385 A.D.
5b			Core	
6a	SV_Z-M_1.2 m	Huecoid	Cortex	Circa 450 A.D.
6b			Core	
7a	SV_YTA-2_I-15_1 m	Saladoid	Cortex	285–375 A.D
7b			Core	
8a	SV_Z-W_1.8 m	Huecoid	Cortex	Circa 245 A.D.
8b			Core	
9a	SV_Z-W_ 1.6 m	Huecoid	Cortex	Circa 385 A.D.
9b			Core	
10a	SV_Z-C_1.8 cm	Huecoid	Cortex	Circa 245 A.D.
10b			Core	
11b	SV_Z-20_2.0 m	Huecoid	Core	Circa 245 A.D.
12b	SV_Z-X_60 cm	Huecoid	Core	470–600 A.D.
13b	SV_Z-L_70 cm	Huecoid	Core	Circa 385 A.D.
14b	SV_ Z-T_S-1_0.9 m	Saladoid	Core	Circa 385 A.D.
15b	SV_YTA-2_H-21_1.2 m	Saladoid	Core	230–385 A.D

[1]Prefix SV indicates the sampling site was in the Sorcé Estate (S) the Island of Vieques (V) Puerto Rico. The remaining characters refer to the specific excavation site from which the specimens were obtained (e.g., YTA-1_I-5-6_) and archaeological depth (e.g., 60 cm).

DNA amplification and sequencing

Fifteen coprolites encompassing paired samples of cortex and core (for a total of 30 samples) were sequenced using the Ion Torrent PGM System for sequencing (Life Technologies Corp.) of 16S rRNA gene reads and the Roche 454 FLX Titanium instrument for detection of 18S rRNA genes.

The 16S rRNA gene V4 variable region was amplified using the PCR primers 515f (GTGCCAGCMGCCGCGGTAA)/806r (GGACTACHVGGGTWTCTAAT) [11]. This particular region was selected in order to target both bacteria and archaea present in the samples. PCR amplifications were conducted using a single-step 30 cycle PCR using the HotStarTaq Plus Master Mix Kit (Qiagen, USA) under the following conditions: 94°C for 3 minutes, followed by 28 cycles of 94°C for 30 seconds, 53°C for 40 seconds and 72°C for 1 minute, after which a final elongation step at 72°C for 5 minutes was performed. Sequencing was performed at Molecular Research Laboratory, (www.mrdnalab.com), (Shallowater, TX, USA) on an Ion Torrent PGM following the manufacturer's guidelines. Similarly, the fungal 18S rRNA gene was amplified using SSUfungiF (TGGAGGGCAAGTCTGGTG) / SSUFungiR (TCGGCATAGTTTATGGTTAAG) (Hume et al., 2012). A single-step 30 cycle PCR using HotStarTaq Plus Master Mix Kit (Qiagen, Valencia, CA) was used under the following conditions: 94°C for 3 minutes, followed by 28 cycles of 94°C for 30 seconds; 53°C for 40 seconds and 72°C for 1 minute; after which a final elongation step at 72°C for 5 minutes was performed. All amplicon products from each samples were mixed in equal concentrations and purified using Agencourt AMPure beads (Agencourt Bioscience Corporation, MA, USA). Samples were sequenced utilizing the Roche 454 FLX Titanium instrument and reagents according to manufacturer's guidelines

Ancient and Extant Sequence analyses

Sequences of extant Amazonian indigenous cultures were obtained from the Short Read Archive (SRA) database (Accession numbers: ERX115092, ERX115316, ERX115218, ERX115130, and ERX115095). The sequences were microbiomes obtained from amplification of the V4 region of the 16S rRNA gene. These sequences were downloaded in FASTA format and used for all comparative studies as described below.

Raw sequence data were prepared for microbiome analysis using QIIME [12]. A total of 3.4 million multiplexed reads from both the 454 and PGM runs were assigned to samples based on their corresponding barcode using *split_libraries.py* using default filtering parameters. 16S rDNA sequences from coprolites were analyzed, individually or merged with modern stool microbiomes. Coprolite 16S rDNAdemultiplexed sequences were sorted based on sample ID using the QIIME script *extract_seqs_by_sample_id.py* and grouped into core and cortex subsets for further analysis. (**Table 2**). *De novo* Operational Bacterial and fungal operational taxonomic units (OTUs) were selected using *pick_de_novo_otus.py* workflow, obtaining a total of n = OTUs. For *18S* data set from QIIME-formatted Silva 111 reference database for Quast et al 2013; (http://www.arb-silva.de/) genetic reference database for eukaryotes for OTU picking and taxonomy assignments (*assign_taxonomy.py*) was used. *16S* and *18S* taxonomy was defined by ≥97% similarity to reference sequences. The phylogenetic composition of the micro-communities present in the samples was characterized using *summarize_taxa_through_plots.py* up to the genus (L7) level.

Alpha and beta diversity

Alpha diversities and rarefaction curves of communities found in coprolite cores and cortices were computed using the *alpha_rarefaction.py* workflow with a custom parameters file that included Shannon statistical analysis. Alpha diversity metrics such as Chao1, which estimates the species richness, Observed_Species, which counts the unique OTUs in a sample and PD_Whole_Tree, which is based on phylogeny, were used for this analysis. Beta diversity distance matrices, UPGMA trees and PCoA plots were computed using *jackknifed_beta_diversity.py*, with default parameters. Distance matrices between sample types were also computed using Primer E v6 software. For comparative purposes, these data were analyzed in parallel with extant fecal microbiomes

Statistical Analysis

Comparisons between coprolite core and cortex microbiomes were made using Procrustes and Adonis analysis (per mutational multivariate analysis of variance using distance matrices). For Adonis, an unweighted UniFrac distance matrix was used using the QIIME script *compare-categories.py* For Procrustes analysis, the beta diversity of the coprolites' cortices and respective cores were compared using QIIME 1.8. The principal coordinate matrices from unweighted UniFrac PCoA plots from core and cortex samples were transformed using the *transform_coordinate_matrices.py* script and the resulting matrices compared using the script *compare_3d_plots.py*.

Comparison of the microbiomes from coprolites of Saladoid and Huecoid origin were done using the *compare_categories.py* script of QIIME 1.8. For this comparison both the Adonis and Permanova methods were conducted using the unweighted UniFrac distance matrix generated by *beta_diversity_through_plots.py* with 999 permutations.

Microscopic analysis for Parasite Eggs

A total of 34 coprolites were used to search for parasites in both cultures. One gram of each coprolite was rehydrated in 14 mL of an aqueous solution of trisodium phosphate 0.5% for 72 h [13]. Samples were shaken vigorously, screened through a 1,500 µm mesh separating all macroscopic material from the sample. To the resultant filtrate, 1 ml of 10% acetic acidic-formalin solution per 10 g of filtrate was added (10:1) to avoid bacterial and fungal growth [14]. The filtered sample was allowed to settle for 72 h after which ten microscope slides were prepared. 50 µL of sediment from each sample was deposited on a slide and mixed with a drop of glycerin. A cover slip was placed on top and the slide was scanned in a serpentine manner covering the whole slide[15,16]. Each parasite egg and larvae found was photographed and measured at 40× and 60× with a calibrated ocular micrometer. For the lack of a taxonomic key to identify parasite eggs, morphological characters such as projections, shape, and presence of larva inside were used for identification. Other non-parasitic organisms were also photographed. All parasite studies were done at the University of Puerto Rico, Mayagüez, Campus.

Results

16S rRNA gene sequences for the coprolites studied ranged from 11,834–281,055 with a median of 26,308 and 151,135 for core and cortex samples respectively (**Table 2**). Fungal 18S rRNA gene sequences ranged from 1,510 to 10,485 with a median of 3,037 for core samples and 4,595 for cortical samples (**Table 2**). Alpha rarefaction plots showed a sampling depth of 5,000, representing approximately 75% of the sample with lowest species count (**Figure 2**). Alpha diversity metrics were consistently higher for *16S* than *18S* in all samples. Diversity indices are depicted in **Table 3**.

Table 2. Coprolite sequence statistics.

16S SSU

	Coprolite Core			Coprolite Cortex		
	SampleID	Seq Count	Mean Length	SampleID	Seq Count	Mean Length
	1b	112,710	207±87	1a	281,055	210±87
	2b	235,943	204±85	2a	112,178	219±83
	3b	97,550	227±80	3a	153,768	212±85
	4b	302,010	206±86	4a	66,082	218±79
	5b	15,788	159±83	5a	311,595	213±86
	6b	30,782	227±81	6a	222,080	220±85
	7b	226,285	222±82	7a	148,502	206±84
	8b	248,994	212±86	8a	254,785	213±84
	9b	23,862	207±88	9a	114,920	222±83
	10b	18,049	189±96	10a	104,132	219±82
	11b	26,308	225±87	11a	ND	ND
	12b	15,002	213±81	12a	ND	ND
	13b	11,834	221±80	13a	ND	ND
	14b	23,487	208±87	14a	ND	ND
	15b	18,073	201±85	15a	ND	ND
MEDIAN		26,308		MEDIAN	151,135	

18S Fungi SSU

	Coprolite Core			Coprolite Cortex		
	SampleID	Seq Count	Mean Length	SampleID	Seq Count	Mean Length
	1b.ssu	1,930	457±106	1a.ssu	10,485	463±107
	2b.ssu	3,187	458±106	2a.ssu	3,242	434±101
	3b.ssu	2,295	450±111	3a.ssu	2,021	449±104
	4b.ssu	5,191	462±107	4a.ssu	1,895	410±102
	5b.ssu	5,088	458±106	5a.ssu	5,587	421±98
	6b.ssu	1,510	452±105	6a.ssu	4,761	446±103
	7b.ssu	2,577	469±105	7a.ssu	5,273	445±103
	8b.ssu	8,119	468±109	8a.ssu	9,753	449±112
	9b.ssu	2,886	471±108	9a.ssu	4,429	453±99
	10b.ssu	3,411	460±107	10a.ssu	1,991	440±112
	MEDIAN	3,037		MEDIAN	4,595	

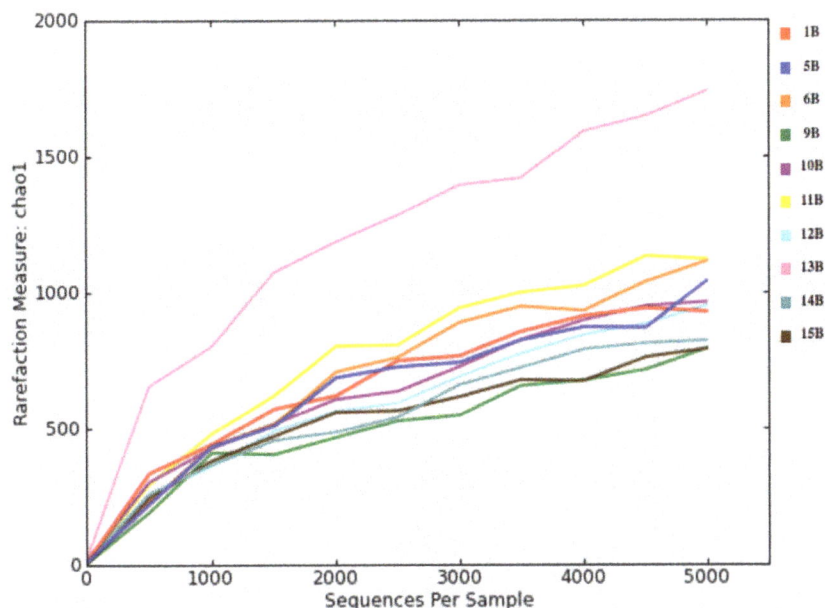

Figure 2. Rarefaction plots the 16S rRNA gene microbiome of the coprolite samples. Rarefaction plots for Huecoid (4B, 6B, 8B, 10B, 11B, 12B, 13B) and Saladoid (1B, 2B, 3B, 5B, 7B, 9B, 14B, 15B) coprolites are shown. Plots were generated using the chao1metic of QIIME 1.8 *alpha_rarefaction.py* with a sampling depth of 5,000. All 15 samples were obtained from the core region (B) of each coprolite.

Statistical Analysis

Procrustes analyses of core and cortex samples were conducted as a control study to assess the fecal microbiome in the coprolites and to see any differences from obvious soil contaminants. Procrustes results showed differing beta diversities when comparing the cortices of the samples to their corresponding cores (**Figure 3**). Cortices showed higher proportions of soil-associated microbes (e.g. 65% Actinobacteria and 11% Firmicutes) compared to the coprolite cores (49% Actinobacteria and 6% Firmicutes). Based on these results, all further studies were conducted using core samples exclusively

Similarly, Adonis analysis showed a significant difference between core and cortex microbiomes with an R^2 of 0.191 (p = 0.001). Adonis and Permanova analyses showed significant differences between the microbiomes of Huecoid and Saladoid coprolites. The Adonis test yielded an R^2 value of 0.287 and a p value of 0.001. Similarly, the Permanova analysis resulted in a Pseudo-F value of 1.98 (p = 0.001).

Fecal microbiome in each culture

16S rDNA analysis. Figure 4 illustrates the differences in taxonomic composition of the Huecoid and Saladoid fecal microbiota. Extant Amazonian fecal microbiome was included for comparative purposes. The proportions of key microorganisms showed major variations between cultures, suggesting possible differences in their diets. While the Burkholderiales, Sphingomonadales and Lactobacillales were more represented in both the Huecoid and Saladoid cultures, the Neisseriales and Bacteroidales were more represented in the Amazonian gut.

Table 4 compares the percent similarities (A) and differences (B) in the fecal microbiomes of the Huecoid and Saladoid. For instance, Bacteroidetes were found to be 13% of the Saladoid fecal microbiota, in comparison Bacteroidetes in the Huecoid comprised approximately only 3% of the microbiota. As there are limitations in targeted *16S* and *18S* sequencing and the limited data available in gene databases, some of the microbiota could

only be confidently identified at a phylum or class level, while others were identified at the Order and Family level.

Figure 5 illustrates the Principal Coordinate Analysis (PCoA) of the bacterial communities found in Huecoid and Saladoid coprolite samples. PCoA of 16S rDNA sequences generated two distinct clusters, where samples originating from the same culture grouped together. Clustering of the samples may have been mainly due to the microbes described in **Table 4**.

18S rDNA Analysis. Figure 6 illustrates the PCoA results of the18s rDNA in Huecoid vs. Saladoid fecal microbiota. PCoA of 18SrDNA sequences showed two distinct clusters for the Huecoid and Saladoid samples. Figure 7 summarizes the relative abundance of fungi in coprolite samples. In general, proportions of Ascomycota were similar between both cultures. However, greater proportions of Basidiomycetes were detected in Huecoid coprolites (Figure 7a). *Saccharomyces spp.* and *Debaryomyces spp.*, were found to be more common in Huecoid feces, whereas *Candida spp.* and *Malasezia spp.* abundances were much higher in Saladoid feces (**Figure 7b**).

Extant vs. extinct fecal microbiotas

Figure 8 compares the Saladoid and Huecoid microbiota to that of fecal microbiota from extant indigenous cultures. Panels (a) and (b) show PCoA of the three groups using PC1 with PC2 and PC3 with PC2. PC1 and PC2 (panel a) show all three groups separating on PC1, representing 51.29% of the variation. The PC3 vs. PC2 plot (panel b) illustrates the differences in microbiome composition that exist among individual samples.

Bacteroidetes were found in higher proportions in modern stool (9.03%) compared to the coprolite samples (0.49%) (**Figure 8**). Similarly, Firmicutes, Clostridiales (specifically Ruminococcaceae, Peptostreptococcaceae, Lachnospiraceae and Eubacteriaceae, among others) made up 81.00% of the modern stool microbial community, while only 18.00% of the coprolite microbiota. In contrast, Actinobacteria were more numerous (48.50% of the microbial community) in coprolites when compared to modern

Table 3. Alpha Diversity Metrics for Coprolite Microbiomes.

Sample ID	Shannon		PD_Whole_Tree		Chao1		Observed_Species	
	16S-V4	Fungi SSU	16S-V4	Fungi SSU	16S-V4	Fungi SSU	16S-V4	Fungi SSU
1a	9.943	4.372	557.945	7.745	14000.189	329.923	10867	234
1b	9.964	3.517	434.365	2.621	11793.849	101.111	8286	56
2a	9.625	2.483	397.655	3.527	11256.698	104.250	7577	68
2b	8.839	2.513	357.141	1.935	9232.645	74.375	6993	53
3a	8.852	2.662	265.672	2.069	6953.633	75.111	5060	54
3b	8.578	3.518	214.855	1.969	5759.892	121.667	4067	70
4a	9.027	ND	224.176	ND	6032.968	ND	4066	ND
4b	9.926	3.189	589.744	2.794	15360.207	128.000	11915	97
5a	10.213	4.623	631.177	6.248	15850.235	243.410	12764	185
5b	8.807	2.360	157.685	1.698	4624.760	91.625	2698	60
6a	9.022	2.436	368.085	2.561	9811.314	87.769	7084	70
6b	6.171	1.995	75.281	0.377	1760.210	21.000	1111	11
7a	9.340	3.525	374.334	5.605	9543.409	167.625	7210	130
7b	8.912	1.046	342.978	1.316	8869.651	66.000	6756	31
8a	10.245	1.951	608.415	3.815	15947.904	248.882	12098	134
8b	9.805	1.033	500.801	3.125	12884.610	180.615	9918	101
9a	8.851	3.358	405.891	4.074	11308.664	252.154	7663	125
9b	8.756	2.257	445.816	1.397	11669.569	72.429	8986	53
10a	8.534	1.701	313.578	1.963	8843.658	105.500	5817	62
10b	8.486	2.394	318.719	2.226	8173.095	80.714	5947	61

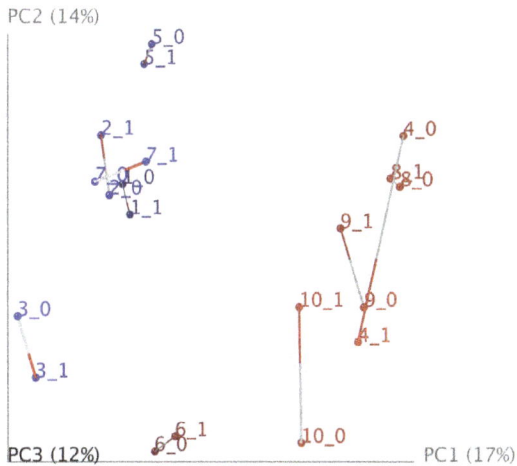

Figure 3. Procrustes analysis compares the 16S microbiome found in the cores and respective cortices of coprolite samples. Samples 6,10, 4, 9 and 8 are of Huecoid origin. Samples 1, 2, 3, 5 ND 7 are of Saladoid origin. Samples identified with number "0" were obtained from coprolite cores and those with the number "1" are from cortical surfaces of the coprolite.

stool samples (2.35%). Specifically, Actinomycetales and Rubrobacterales were found to make up 28.00–33.00% and 10.00–12.00%, respectively, of the detected microbiome.

Eukaryotic Parasites in Coprolites

Eukaryotic enteric parasites were detected in both Huecoid and Saladoid cultures (**Table 5**). There were differences, however, in parasite loads and parasite species between the two cultures. There were twice as many infected Saladoid coprolites as there were Huecoid. *Ascaris lumbricoides* and *Trichuris trichura,* were found in both cultures but with greater number among the Saladoids. *Enterobius vermicularis* and Cestodes were found also in both cultures. Hookworms were found only in Saladoid coprolites. Also, a *Paragonimus westermani* infection may have been detected in a Huecoid coprolite. The overall % positives were much higher in the Saladoid coprolites. *Dipylidium caninum* was observed in 13% of the Saladoid samples, and interestingly not in the Huecoid. Similarly, the genera *Trichostrongylus, Diphyllobotrium* as well as hookworms were found associated only with Saladoid coprolites. As part of the DNA analyses, we found fish parasites (*Goussia spp.*), which were detected exclusively in Saladoid coprolites.

Discussion

Though it has been assumed (correctly in some cases), that excreta is rapidly degraded in humid tropical environments, the

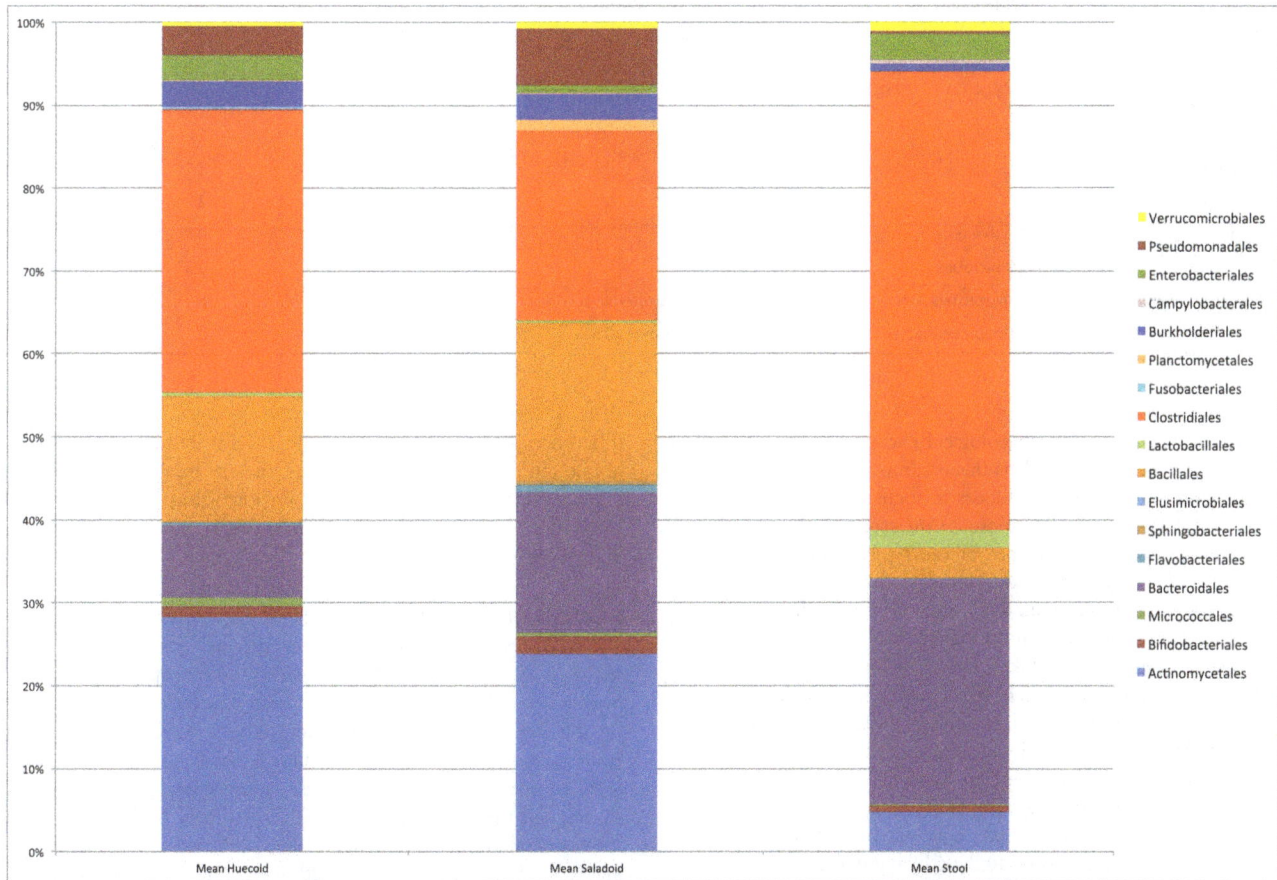

Figure 4. Taxonomic comparison of Huecoid and Saladoid Microbiomes. Figure was generated using summarize_taxa_through_plots.py workflow of QIIME 1.8. Results are illustrated at the Order level. Extant Amazonian stools microbiome was included for comparisons. Mean values for each culture represent taxa obtained from 8 Huecoid coprolite cores, 7 Saladoid samples, and 5 adult, extant Amazonian stools.

Table 4. Similarities (A) and differences (B) found in the microbial fecal communities of the Huecoid and Saladoid cultures.

Taxonomy			Huecoid (%)	Saladoid (%)
Phylum	*Class*	*Order*		
(A) % Taxa Similarities				
Actinobacteria	Nitriliruptoria	-	0.1	0.1
Actinobacteria	Thermoleophilia	-	48.6	53
Bacteroidetes	Flavobacteriia	-	0.1	0.4
Proteobacteria	Gammaproteobacteria	Xanthomonadales	0.2	0.1
Proteobacteria	Deltaproteobacteria	Entotheonellales	0.1	0.3
Proteobacteria	Deltaproteobacteria	Syntrophobacterales	0.3	0.1
Proteobacteria	Deltaproteobacteria	Myxococcales	0.1	0.1
Proteobacteria	Betaproteobacteria	MND1	0.4	0.4
Proteobacteria	Betaproteobacteria	Burkholderiales	0.2	0.5
Proteobacteria	Betaproteobacteria	Burkholderiales	0.3	0.3
Proteobacteria	Alphaproteobacteria	Sphingomonadales	0.1	0.1
Proteobacteria	Alphaproteobacteria	Rhizobiales	0.2	0.4
Proteobacteria	Alphaproteobacteria	Rhodospirillales	0.7	0.1
Planctomycetes	Planctomycetia	Gemmatales	0.5	0.4
Chloroflexi	SAR202	-	0.2	0.5
Chloroflexi	-	-	0.9	0.5
Planctomycetes	Planctomycetia	Pirellulales	0.4	0.1
Nitrospirae	Nitrospira	Nitrospirales	3.5	4.7
Firmicutes	Bacilli	Bacillales	4.7	4.7
Crenarchaeota	Thaumarchaeota	Nitrososphaerales	0.7	0.6
(B) % Taxa Differences				
Chloroflexi	Ellin6529	-	8.7	14
Bacteroidetes	-	-	13.3	2.9
Planctomycetes	-	-	4.1	2.7
Actinobacteria	Actinobacteria	-	1.2	0.4
Actinobacteria	Acidimicrobiia	-	1.2	3.3
Proteobacteria	Gammaproteobacteria	Enterobacteriales	1.2	0
Proteobacteria	Gammaproteobacteria	Pseudomonadales	1.4	3

finding of coprolites in archaeological excavation sites located in Puerto Rico clearly contradicts this assumption. Additionally, it is very uncommon for archaeologists to focus on finding coprolites during archaeological excavations in the tropics as many are not familiar with the morphologies of the typical human or animal coprolite. If we take into consideration that feces are excreted (about 500–1,500 g/person/day), excreta should be one of the most abundant organic archeological findings at human and animal dig sites, if care is taken to search for them [17].

Microbiologically, excreta have its own biota, which, exempting periods of enteritis or other gastrointestinal diseases, and should be relatively constant in diversity and composition. Fecal microbiota are a subset of the microorganisms present in the gastrointestinal tract that are shed during defecation, and as such give much information about an individual's core gut microbiome as well as allochthonous bacteria associated with ingested food, water and very likely, air. Thus, the analysis of fossilized fecal material using NGS can be an important tool in archaeological studies to determine the prevalence of certain microorganisms, pathogenic (such as parasites, for example) and non-pathogenic alike. In terms of the overall composition of the fecal microbiome, however,

differences may exist both in taxon distribution and relative abundance as a result of cultural or dietary habits. In fact, it has been clearly determined in a previous study that the fecal microbiota of these particular Antillean cultures is highly dependent on ethnicity [7].

Analysis of the core vs. cortex of coprolites

Procrustes and Adonis analyses showed marked differences between the cores and cortices of the coprolites. Larger proportions of soil microbes (e.g. Actinobacteria) were observed in the cortices of the coprolites, which were likely due to environmental contamination, whereas smaller proportions were seen in the corresponding cores. In addition, cortices mostly shared soil microbes, possibly due to proximal burial sites, while the core microbiomes of each culture differed greatly from one another. This suggests that, although the outer parts of the coprolites were contaminated with the soil that surrounded the samples, the inner core of the coprolites remained largely intact. This is the principal reason for our downstream analyses to be conducted using only the core of the samples.

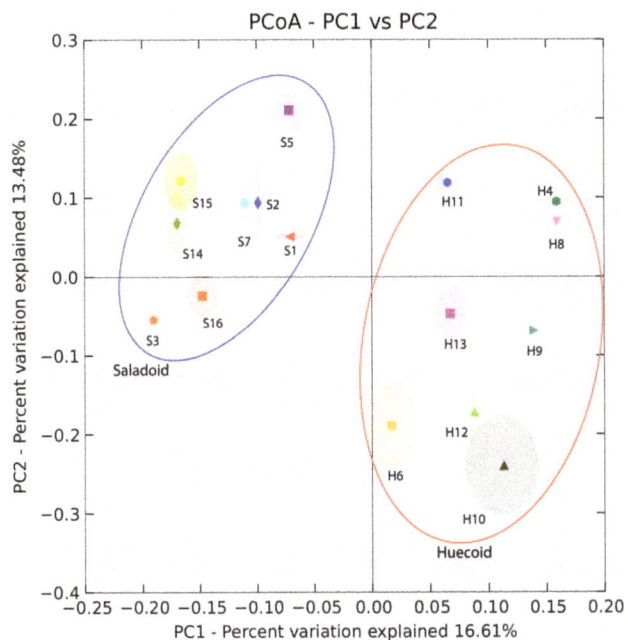

Figure 5. Principal Coordinate Analysis (PCoA) of the Bacterial Communities present in Huecoid and Saladoid Coprolites. Unweighted UniFrac and weighted UniFrac principal coordinates were generated and plotted using QIIME 1.8. Samples with the prefix S are from Saladoid coprolite cores and those with the prefix H were from Huecoid coprolite cores.

Figure 6. Principal Coordinate Analysis (PCoA) of the Fungal Communities present in Huecoid and Saladoid Coprolites. Unweighted UniFrac and weighted UniFrac principal coordinates were generated and plotted using QIIME 1.8. Samples with the prefix S are from Saladoid coprolite cores and those with the prefix H were from Huecoid coprolite cores.

Analysis of Huecoid and Saladoid coprolites

Both the Adonis and Permanova assays showed significant differences in the microbiome composition of coprolites from Huecoid and Saladoid sites. These analyses were performed only on samples obtained from the cores of the coprolites, thus eliminating possible differences due to environmental contamination of cortical material. These results support the hypothesis that Huecoid and Saladoid cultures, even though coexisted in the Island of Vieques, they had different cultural characteristics, most likely as a result of dietary practices.

Key observed differences in each culture's core microbiomes: Inferences on diet

Variations observed in common gut-associated bacteria, such as Proteobacteria and Enterobacteriaceae, which were more abundant in Saladoid and Huecoid samples, respectively, suggest variations in diet or host genetics. Variations in the abundance of intestinal Proteobacteria have been associated to differences in host diet previously [20]. Differences in Bacteroides abundances were also evident between both cultures, and have been associated to a high protein diet [21]. According to the large quantities of fish bones, bivalve and crab shells found in these archaeological deposits, both cultures seemed to ingest a great amount of seafood. However, although fish bones are associated with both cultures [22], we detected freshwater fish-associated amoebic parasites (*Goussia spp.*) exclusively in Saladoid coprolites, suggesting that this particular culture may have consumed raw fish regularly. In addition, previous studies detected *Vibrio sp.* and *Debaryomyces spp* in Saladoid coprolites, further supporting this hypothesis [7]. The presence of *Paragonimus westermani* in a Huecoid coprolite implies the consumption of fresh water invertebrates, or some type of aquatic plants, the secondary hosts for this species. It is known

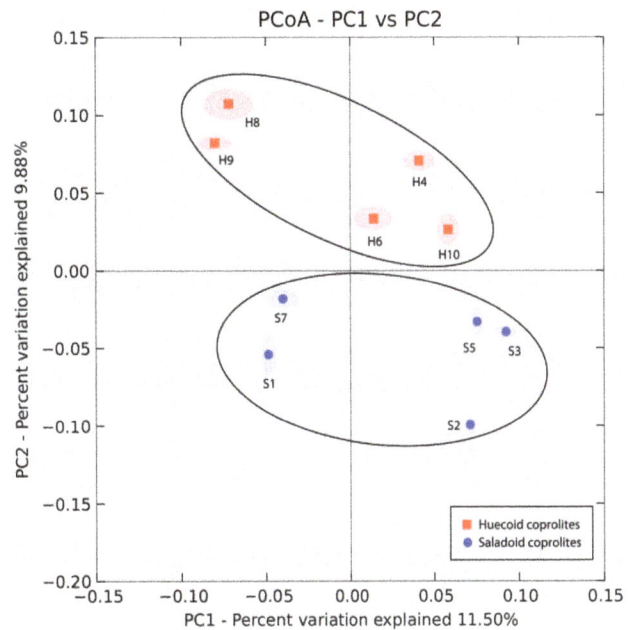

that humans become infected by the consumption of raw food contaminated with these parasites. However, it is important to point out that this parasite is commonly confused morphologically with *Diphyllobothrium latum,* a fish-infecting parasite [23]. Interestingly, *Zea mays* (maize) was detected in coprolites from Huecoid origins, consistent with archaeological work showing its presence at the La Hueca site [24] and confirming its early presence in the Caribbean. Our results suggest that this culture may have helped introduce some of these maize strains to the Antilles during their migrations. Since they were detected in large proportions, Ascomycetes and Basidiomycetes also appear to have been important dietary elements of these cultures. However, it seems that the Huecoids had a preference for Basidiomycota fungi. Although these conclusions are highly hypothetical and perhaps speculative, we believe this is a good starting point if we are to compare future studies such as the one carried out here.

Enteric Parasite infections

The greater parasite load observed in Saladoid coprolites suggests a difference in living arrangements, whereby the population was more likely to be exposed to fecal material and thus parasite transmission. Parasite analyses were done microscopically in a separate laboratory, however the results also show major differences between the taxonomic compositions present in both cultures. A wider variety of parasitic species was detected in the Saladoids, which could also be associated to the way this culture handled their food (as previously mentioned). It is also known that both cultures had dogs as pets, particularly the Saladoids. We detected the canine parasite *Dipylidium caninum* in Saladoid samples, also suggesting pet ownership and perhaps very close contact. However, little if anything is known about the interactions of the Huecoids with dogs. Dogs have a tendency to eat human feces, and this may be one manner in which the parasites are passed from person to person, with the dogs being the

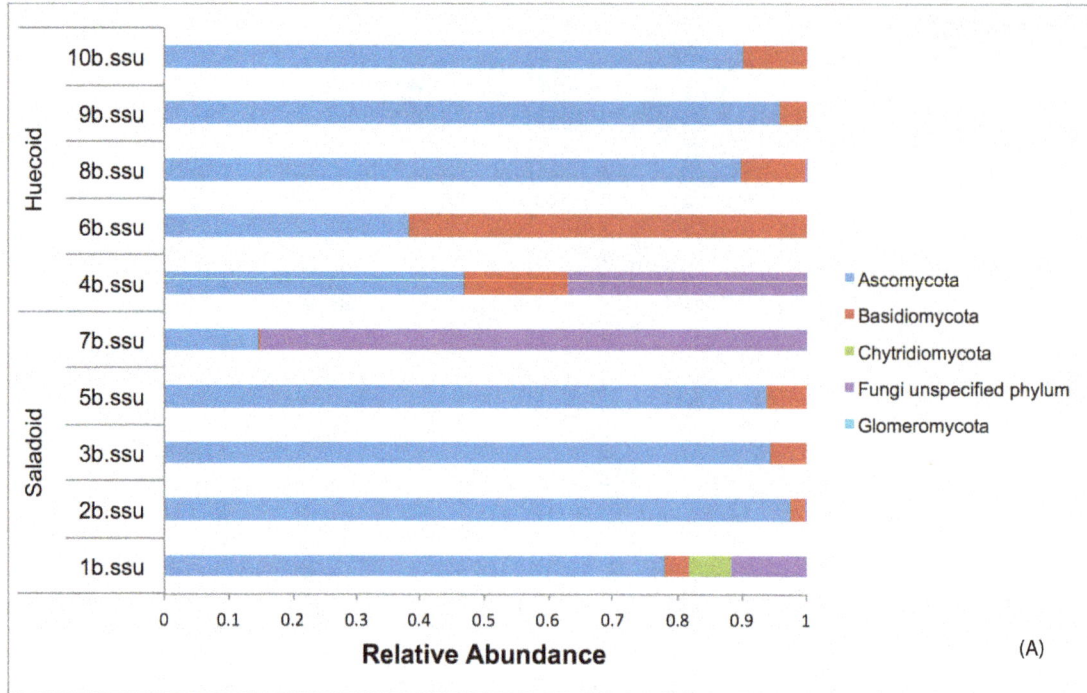

(A)

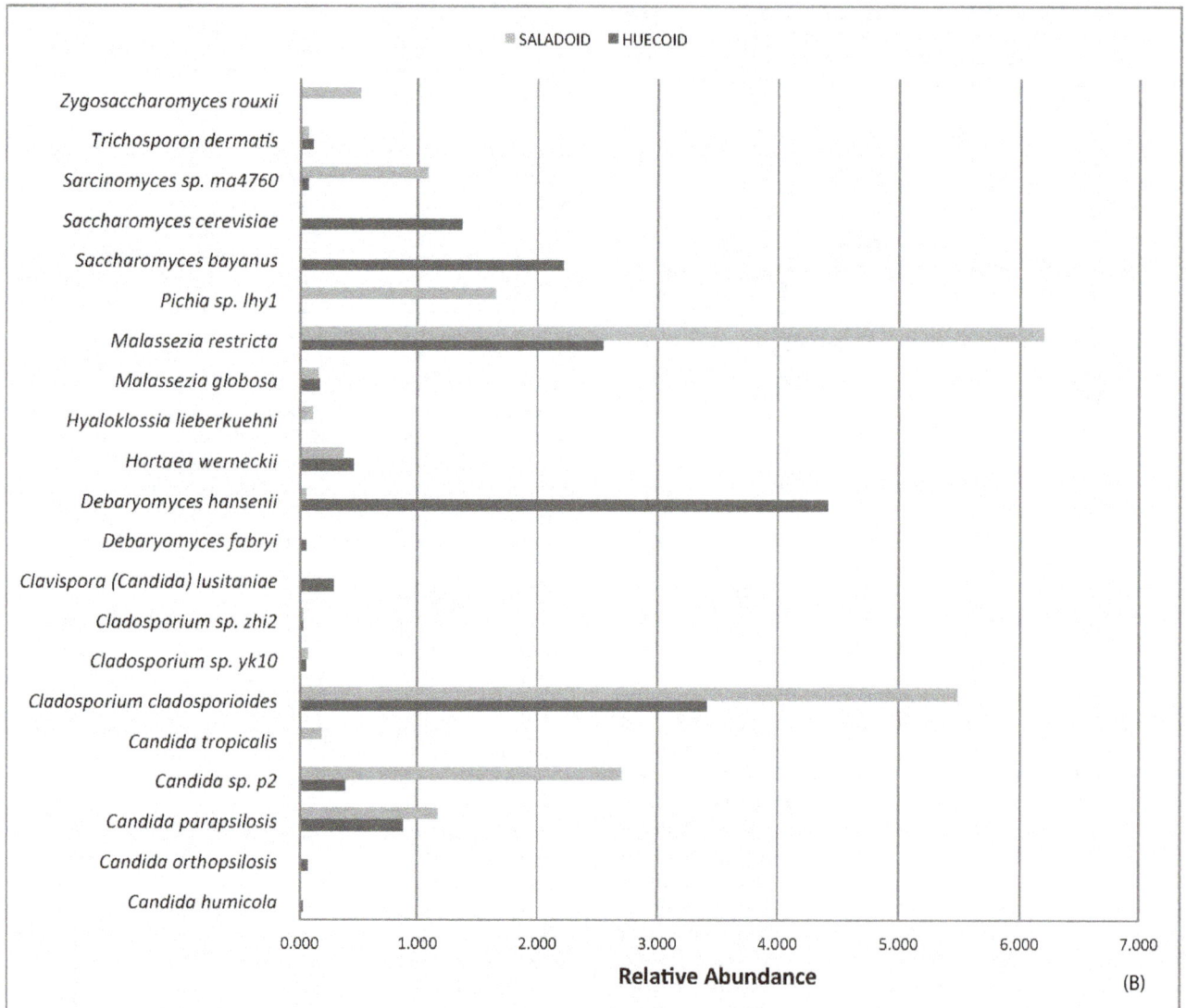

(B)

Figure 7. Relative abundance of fungi in coprolite samples. Panel (a) shows the proportions of fungi detected in Huecoid and Saladoid samples. Panel (b) shows the comparison of the proportions of yeasts detected in both cultures.

vectors. The presence of *Dipylidium caninum* supports this hypothesis, as does the high prevalence of most intestinal parasites detected in the Saladoid coprolites. In addition, present-day ethnic groups in the Amazon basin maintain close relations with dogs and even share their living space with these animals, and although highly speculative, the presence of zoonotic parasites in the Saladoid coprolites is intriguing, and requires further analysis. It is also intriguing that well-formed coprolites had such a high prevalence of enteric parasites, since many of these pathogens result in enteritis in present-day populations, which would not be amenable to the formation of coprolites. It is thus possible that multiple infections with parasites were common, and yet these infections failed to cause enteritis.

The observed differences, both in the core fecal microbiota and the detected remnant food, suggest major variations in the diets of these extinct cultures. This is further supported by the diversity and relative abundances of the parasites detected in each culture. The Saladoid and Huecoid deposits in Vieques are separated by a

distance of 15–150 m [7], which suggests that the observed variations in fecal microbiota are not of geographical origins but more likely due to cultural and dietary differences.

Modern Amazonian stool vs. ancient Antillean stool: Considering the effects of taphonomic conditions

The microbiota detected in the coprolites was associated with those found in modern stool, but mainly differed in the proportions observed for each phylum. We observed two main phyla of Gram-positive bacteria in our samples (Actinobacteria and Firmicutes) and two main phyla of Gram-negative bacteria (Bacteroides and Proteobacteria).

As suggested by other studies, Gram-positive bacteria tend to have a high resistance towards dry conditions, so the presence of such a diverse array of these microorganisms preserved in these coprolites was expected [25,26]. Actinobacteria are notorious for their resistance to arid conditions; this resilience towards

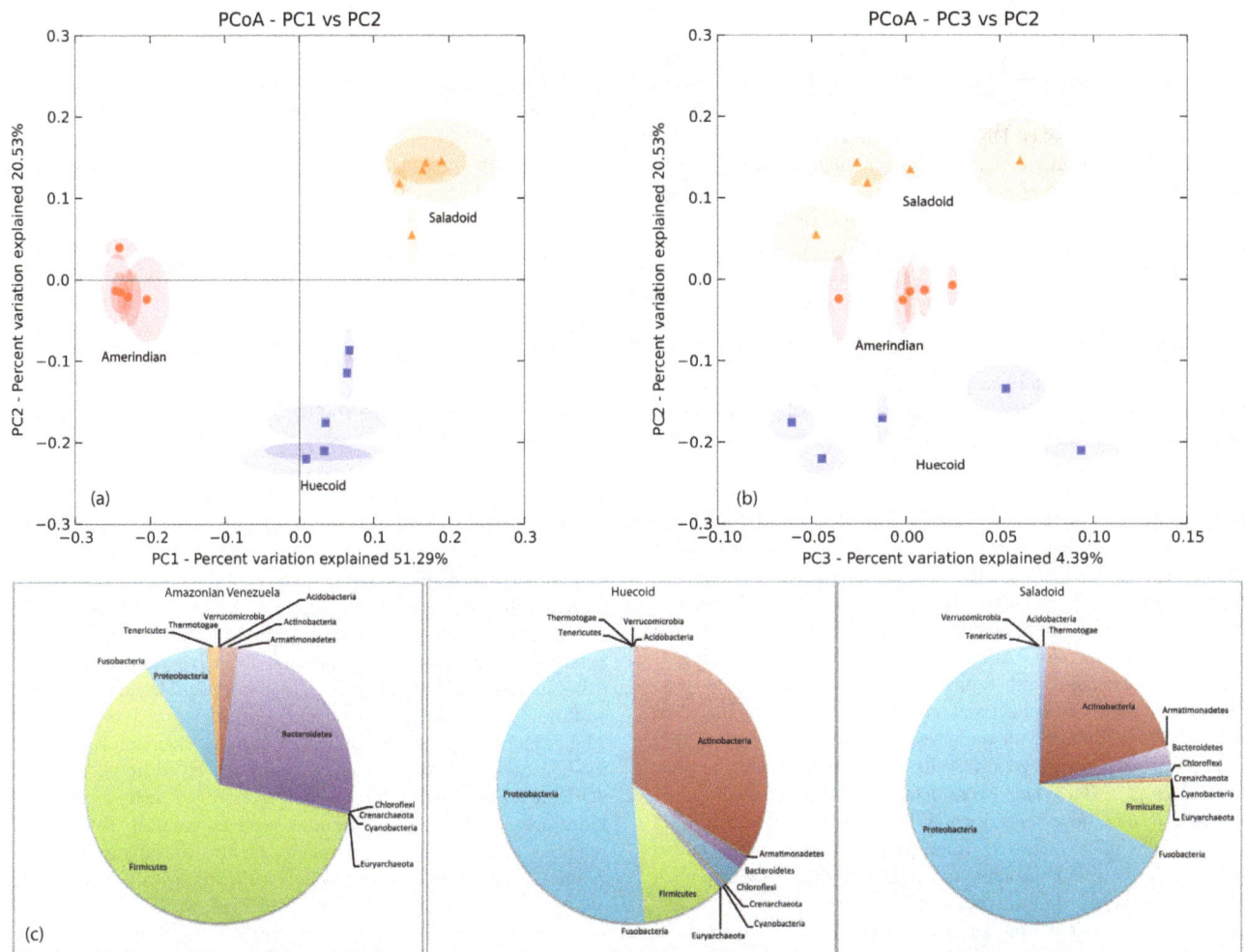

Figure 8. Comparison of Saladoid and Huecoid microbiota to the fecal microbiota of representative, extant indigenous cultures. Panel (a) shows the PCoA of coprolites and the fecal microbiota from extant indigenous cultures plotting PC1 vs. PC2. Panel (b) shows the PCoA of coprolites and the fecal microbiota from extant indigenous cultures plotting PC3 vs. PC2. Panel (c) shows the pie charts of taxa represented in coprolites and extant indigenous cultures.

Table 5. Enteric parasites as detected by microscopy.

Parasite Species	Huecoid (n = 8)		Saladoid (n = 7)	
	% Positive	Average Number Present	% Positive	Average Number Present
Ascaris lumbricoides (unfertilized)	25	56.5	43	27.0
Ascaris lumbricoides (fertilized)	25	151.5	43	44.7
Trichuris trichiura	25	57.7	57	79.3
Enterobius vermicularis	37.5	57.7	43	37.3
Trichostrongylus sp.	ND	ND	43	28.3
Hookworms	ND	ND	29	28.0
Diphyllobothrium sp.	ND	ND	14	26.0
Dipylidium caninum	ND	ND	14	30.0
Unknown Cestode	25	55.5	43	49.3
Paragonimus westermani	13	23.0	ND	ND
Unknown Trematode	ND	ND	14	26.0

taphonomic conditions makes them more likely to be detected in high abundances in archaeological samples [27]. In terms of what can or cannot be detected, we can only assume that over centuries or millennia, most, if not all of the microbiota in the coprolites has been inactivated and, unless there is rapid dehydration, the cells will be lysed and the free DNA will be rapidly degraded. It has been observed that naked DNA will remain relatively undegraded for very short periods of time in aquatic environments [18,19], however, DNA conserved intracellularly in (for example), dormant microorganisms may most likely be better preserved against taphonomic conditions than naked DNA. Again, the mere presence of coprolites indicate that there was rapid dehydration, and thus protection of the nucleic acid material from any extracellular nucleases.

Compared to modern stools, the percentage of Firmicutes detected in the coprolites was much lower. Firmicutes are known to have a low G/C content in their genomes, possibly allowing for faster DNA degradation throughout the fossilization process when compared to bacteria with high [G/C], as in the case of the Actinobacteria, (Taxonomy Browser, NCBI). Interestingly, in spite of Clostridium being spore-formers, the proportion of Firmicutes in coprolites was much lower than detected in the modern stool. However, this may be linked to previous observations suggesting a higher presence of vegetative cells when Clostridium is located in the human gut as compared to soil environments, where the conditions are stressful [28]. In addition, these cells are highly sensitive to oxygen and rapidly die when exposed to oxic conditions. Also, some bacterial spores tend to germinate when they come in contact with the gastrointestinal environment [29] thus leading to more vegetative cells rather than spores.

Low levels of Bacteroides were detected in coprolites compared to modern stool, however, this could be due to the strict anaerobes high sensitivity to oxygen. Interestingly, when compared to modern feces the coprolites showed a higher proportion of Proteobacteria in the microbial community. Though initially counter-intuitive, it is now known that dormancy is a common strategy for long term survival when Gram-negative microorganisms are faced with nutrient and water starvation, exposure to radiation and drastic changes in temperature. Nutritional stress, for example, has been shown to induce the transcription of stress proteins, which ultimately convey the cell a higher resistance towards variations in these abiotic factors [28,30]. This starvation-

induced multi-stress resistance, and other bacterial dormancy mechanisms have been characterized, including a spontaneously initiated dormancy as well [31]. This dormancy state appears to be reversible in some cases [32,33,34] (though the mechanisms for resuscitation remain largely unknown), and could have played a factor in the recent isolation of viable microorganisms from coprolite samples [35].

Although these latent bacteria could account for the diversity of Gram-negative bacteria observed in the coprolites, another possibility could be that the relative half-life of these microorganisms is much higher than that of those no longer detectable in the sample. Depending on their half-life, low abundance taxa (or rare species) could have been eliminated from the sample whilst taxa initially present in higher concentrations could still be detectable after preservation for a thousand years.

Differences in coprolite microbiota and the 'Huecoid problem'

The discovery of the Huecoid culture in the 1970s by Chanlatte and Narganes led to formulation of the 'Huecoid problem', the question whether the Huecoids were ethnically distinct from the Saladoids or were simply a Saladoid subgroup. Classical archeology has provided much evidence for cultural distinctness between the two groups, but has not led to a resolution of the problem. There are many material ways in which the Huecoid and Saladoid cultures may be separated [36]. Technological differences include marked differences in pottery and lapidary carvings and more subtle differences in stone tools such as Adzes and Celts. The Saladoids apparently preferred to make their adornments in mollusk conch, in contrast the Huecoids preferred stone. Evidence of dietary differences includes the absence of turtle remains in Huecoid settlements implying they were taboo [22]. Evidence of religious differences are abundant. Firstly, burial practices are distinct, with Saladoid interments occurring within their settlements, while Huecoid burials have yet to be encountered. Iconography is distinct, unique Huecoid symbolism is seen with birds interpreted as condors, carrying human heads, not represented in Saladoid lapidary or ceramics [24]. The range of materials from which Huecoid lapidary was fashioned is much more diverse than Saladoid as are the decorative themes. Huecoid settlements have been associated with increased ritual activity, indicated by an increased incidence of implements associated with what appears to be an early version of the cohoba ritual [37,38]. Thus, the Huecoids have been described as 'religious specialists', with a spiritual role servicing the majority Saladoid community [24] (see Pagan-Jimenez 2007 for a summary). However, while physical evidence of cultural distinctness is abundant, the true role of the Huecoids remains elusive. Ancient DNA studies might hold the key to answering the 'Huecoid problem'. In our study, we have addressed the question from a unique angle, that is, of using paleomicrobiomics. Our results clearly show that the gut microbiota, prokaryotic and fungal, were distinct between the two cultures. While there exists a possibility that these differences might reflect differences in mammalian host genetics [39,40], which would indicate ethnic uniqueness, we interpret the differences to be mainly due to diet, and, perhaps to interaction with pets, as in the case of enteric parasites.

Given the apparent difference in diet indicated by differences in the intestinal microbiota, this allows us traction into the Huecoid problem. There are very few examples of groups that are differentiated by diet and live in conjoined settlements, but are still part of the same ethnic identity. Thus, it is hard to find a modern parallel of the scenario proposed by Rouse that the Huecoids were a Saladoid subgroup [41]. This does not rule out some unique arrangement within Saladoid society, and so while we would propose that both archaeological and paleomicrobiomic data strongly suggest a distinct ethnic identity to the Huecoids, this awaits confirmation.

Conclusions

We successfully extracted and sequenced DNA from archaeological fecal samples in order to assess possible differences in the fecal communities of individuals from Saladoid and Huecoid indigenous cultures. Our data show that, contrary to common belief, the formation and preservation of coprolites and DNA contained in these coprolites under humid, tropical environments for thousands of years is possible. Not only is the DNA still present, it was also detected by PCR amplification and sequenced successfully. We also demonstrate a clear difference between the fecal microbiota of these two cultures, and therefore variations in

terms of their diet and/or genetic heritage. Similar to previous results, our data also supports the hypothesis stating that the Huecoids and Saladoids originated and migrated independently from their respective origins, as opposed to having a common ancestry.

This study is one of the first in its kind and we hope will point to the importance of coprolites as important cultural markers and thus any archaeological dig should include the search and preservation of any coprolites found at the sites. This study underlines the importance of such samples for future paleomicrobiological studies. The results have several implications. First, it confirms that coprolites are not completely degraded in humid, tropical environments and thus can be formed under suitable taphonomic conditions. Second, it implies that dietary and/or host genetic differences in ancient populations may be reflected in differences in gut microbiome composition and it confirms that the two indigenous cultures were indeed distinct. Third, it demonstrates that paleomicrobiomics could be a powerful tool to assess dietary, health, genetic and cultural differences between ancient populations. Finally, it implies that these two cultures retained distinct technological/cultural differences during a period of close proximity and peaceful co-existence and suggests that the two populations, at least at this location, may have contributed to form the latter day Taínos, the Amerindians present at the point of Columbian contact.

Acknowledgments

This study was partially funded by NIH RISE Program (NIH Grant No. 5R25GM061151-12). We also would like to thank Mark Brolaski of Mo Bio Laboratories for providing the necessary supplies and support for the extraction of fossil DNA.

Author Contributions

Conceived and designed the experiments: RJC SEM. Performed the experiments: RJC JRP EGR YNS LCB. Analyzed the data: RJC SEM GAT YNS TSR LBW. Contributed reagents/materials/analysis tools: RJC SEM GAT. Contributed to the writing of the manuscript: RJC SEM TSR JRP. Obtained permissions for collecting coprolites: YNS LCB.

References

1. Sharma N, Kar RK, Agarwal A, Kar R (2005) Fungi in dinosaurian (Isisaurus) coprolites from the Lameta Formation (Maastrichtian) and its reflection on food habit and environment. Micropaleontology 51: 73–82.

2. Narganes Y (1991) Secuencia cronológica de dos sitios arqueológicos de Puerto Rico (Sorcé, Vieques y Tecla, Guayanilla); Proceedings of the Thirteenth International Congress fo the International Association for Caribbean Archaeology. Curaçao. Pp. 628–646.

3. Rodriguez-Ramos R (2010) Rethinking Puerto Rican Precolonial History. Tuscaloosa: University of Alabama Press.

4. Narganes Y (2007) Nueva cronología de varios sitios de Puerto Rico y Vieques; Proceedings of the Twenty-First Congress of the International Association for Caribbean Archaeology; Trinidad.pp. 275–294.

5. Chanlatte LA, Narganes YM (2002) La CulturaSaladoide en Puerto Rico y su rostro multicolor. Museo de Historia, Antropología y Arte: Universidad de Puerto Rico, Recinto de Río Piedras. pp. 55.

6. Crespo E (2010) Ancient Bones Tell Stories: Osteobiology of Human Remains from Tribes. In: Curet A, Stringer LM, editors.Tribes, People, Power and Rituals at the Center of the Cosmos. Tuscaloosa, AL: University of Alabama Press.

7. Santiago-Rodriguez TM, Narganes-Storde YM, Chanlatte L, Crespo-Torres E, Toranzos GA, et al. (2013) Microbial communities in pre-columbian coprolites. PLoS One 8: e65191.

8. Dunbar J, Ticknor LO, Kuske CR (2001) Phylogenetic specificity and reproducibility and new method for analysis of terminal restriction fragment profiles of 16S rRNA genes from bacterial communities. Applied and Environmental Microbiology 67: 190–197.

9. Hert DG, Fredlake CP, Barron AE (2008) Advantages and limitations of next-generation sequencing technologies: A comparison of electrophoresis and non-electrophoresis methods. Electrophoresis 29: 4618–4626.

10. Chanlatte LA, Narganes YM (2005) Cultura La Hueca. Museo de Historia, Antropologia y Arte: Universidad de Puerto Rico, Recinto de Rio Piedras. pp. 101.

11. Caporaso JG, Lauber CL, Walters WA, Berg-Lyons D, Lozupone CA, et al. (2011) Global patterns of 16S rRNA diversity at a depth of millions of sequences per sample. Proceedings of the National Academy of Sciences of the United States of America 108: 4516–4522.

12. Caporaso JG, Kuczynski J, Stombaugh J, Bittinger K, Bushman FD, et al. (2010) QIIME allows analysis of high-throughput community sequencing data. Nature Methods 7: 335–336.

13. Callen EO, Cameron TWM (1960) A prehistoric diet as revealed in coprolites. New Science 8: 35–40.

14. Goncalves MLC, Araujo A, Ferreira LF (2003) Human intestinal parasites in the past: New findings and a review. Memorias Do Instituto Oswaldo Cruz 98: 103–118.

15. Han ET, Guk SM, Kim JL, Jeong HJ, Kim SN, et al. (2003) Detection of parasite eggs from archaeological excavations in the Republic of Korea. Memorias Do Instituto Oswaldo Cruz 98: 123–126.

16. Fugassa MH, Denegri GM, Sardella NH, Araujo A, Guichon RA, et al. (2006) Paleoparasitological records in a canid coprolite from Patagonia, Argentina. Journal of Parasitology 92: 1110–1113.

17. Saito T, Hayakawa T, Nakamura K, Takita T, Suzuki K, et al. (1991) Fecal Output, Gastrointestinal Transit-Time, Frequency of Evacuation and Apparent Excretion Rate of Dietary Fiber in Young Men Given Diets Containing Different Levels of Dietary Fiber. Journal of Nutritional Science and Vitaminology 37: 493–508.

18. Alvarez AJ, Yumet GM, Santiago CL, Toranzos GA (1996) Stability of manipulated plasmid DNA in aquatic environments. Environmental Toxicology and Water Quality 11: 129–135.

19. Alvarez AJ, Yumet GM, Santiago CL, Hazen TC, Chaudhry R, et al. (1996) In situ survival of genetically engineered microorganisms in a tropical aquatic environment. Environmental Toxicology and Water Quality 11: 21–25.

20. Schwartz K, Chang H, Olson LK (2012) Metabolic Profiles of Ketolysis and Glycolysis in Malignant Gliomas: Possible Predictors of Response to Ketogenic Diet Therapy. Neuro-Oncology 14: 55–55.

21. Wu GD, Chen J, Hoffmann C, Bittinger K, Chen YY, et al. (2011) Linking Long-Term Dietary Patterns with Gut Microbial Enterotypes. Science 334: 105–108.

22. Narganes-Storde Y (1982) Vertebrate faunal remains from Sorce, Vieques, Puerto Rico. MA. Athens, GA: University of Georgia.

23. Garcia SL, Bruckner DA (1993) Liver and Lung Trematodes. Diagnostic Medical Parasitology: ASM Press. pp. 309–321.

24. Pagan-Jimenez JR (2007) De antiguos pueblos y culturas botanicas en el Puerto Rico indigena. American Archeology: Paris Monographs.

25. Pal A, Pehkonen SO, Yu LE, Ray MB (2007) Photocatalytic inactivation of Gram-positive and Gram-negative bacteria using fluorescent light. Journal of Photochemistry and Photobiology a-Chemistry 186: 335–341.

26. Chastanet A, Fert J, Msadek T (2003) Comparative genomics reveal novel heat shock regulatory mechanisms in Staphylococcus aureus and other Gram-positive bacteria. Molecular Microbiology 47: 1061–1073.

27. Zaremba-Niedzwiedzka K, Andersson SGE (2013) No Ancient DNA Damage in Actinobacteria from the Neanderthal Bone. PLoS One 8.

28. Lennon JT, Jones SE (2011) Microbial seed banks: the ecological and evolutionary implications of dormancy. Nature Reviews Microbiology 9: 119–130.

29. Casula G, Cutting SM (2002) Bacillus probiotics: Spore germination in the gastrointestinal tract. Applied and Environmental Microbiology 68: 2344–2352.

30. Kaprelyants AS, Gottschal JC, Kell DB (1993) Dormancy in Non-Sporulating Bacteria. Fems Microbiology Letters 104: 271–286.

31. Carneiro S, Ferreira EC, Rocha I (2011) A Systematic Modeling Approach to Elucidate the Triggering of the Stringent Response in Recombinant E. coli Systems. 5th International Conference on Practical Applications of Computational Biology & Bioinformatics (Pacbb 2011) 93: 313–320.

32. Koltunov V, Greenblatt CL, Goncharenko AV, Demina GR, Klein BY, et al. (2010) Structural Changes and Cellular Localization of Resuscitation-Promoting Factor in Environmental Isolates of Micrococcus luteus. Microbial Ecology 59: 296–310.

33. Cano RJ, Borucki MK (1995) Revival and Identification of Bacterial-Spores in 25-Million-Year-Old to 40-Million-Year-Old Dominican Amber (Vol 268, Pg 1060, 1995). Science 268: 1265–1265.

34. Cano RJ, Borucki MK (1995) Revival and Identification of Bacterial-Spores in 25-Million-Year-Old to 40-Million-Year-Old Dominican Amber. Science 268: 1060–1064.

35. Appelt S, Armougom F, Le Bailly M, Robert C, Drancourt M (2014) Polyphasic Analysis of a Middle Ages Coprolite Microbiota, Belgium. PLoS One 9.

36. Chanlatte-Baik LA (2013) Huecoid Culture and the Antillean Agroalfarero (Farmer-Potter) Period. In: Keegan WF, Hofman CL, Ramos RR, editors.Handbook of Carribbean Archaeology. Oxford: Oxford University Press.

37. Rodriguez M (1997) Religous beliefs of the Saladoid people. In: Wilson SW, editor. The Indigenous People of the Caribbean Gainesville University Press of Florida.

38. Wilson SM (2007). he Archeology of the Caribbean: Cambridge University Press.

39. Kashyap PC, Marcobal A, Ursell LK, Smits SA, Sonnenburg ED, et al. (2013) Genetically dictated change in host mucus carbohydrate landscape exerts a diet-dependent effect on the gut microbiota. Proceedings of the National Academy of Sciences of the United States of America 110: 17059–17064.

40. Lu K, Mahbub R, Cable PH, Ru HY, Parry NMA, et al. (2014) Gut Microbiome Phenotypes Driven by Host Genetics Affect Arsenic Metabolism. Chemical Research in Toxicology 27: 172–174.

41. Rouse I (1992) The Tainos: rise and decline of the people who greeted Columbus. New Haven: Yale University Press.

22

Association of Veterinary Third-Generation Cephalosporin Use with the Risk of Emergence of Extended-Spectrum-Cephalosporin Resistance in *Escherichia coli* from Dairy Cattle in Japan

Toyotaka Sato[1¤], Torahiko Okubo[1], Masaru Usui[1], Shin-ichi Yokota[2], Satoshi Izumiyama[3], Yutaka Tamura[1]*

1 Laboratory of Food Microbiology and Food Safety, Department of Health and Environmental Sciences, School of Veterinary Medicine, Rakuno Gakuen University, Ebetsu, Japan, **2** Department of Microbiology, Sapporo Medical University School of Medicine, Sapporo, Japan, **3** Nemuro District Agriculture Mutual Aid Association, Nakashibetsu, Japan

Abstract

The use of extended-spectrum cephalosporins in food animals has been suggested to increase the risk of spread of *Enterobacteriaceae* carrying extended-spectrum β-lactamases to humans. However, evidence that selection of extended-spectrum cephalosporin–resistant bacteria owing to the actual veterinary use of these drugs according to criteria established in cattle has not been demonstrated. In this study, we investigated the natural occurrence of cephalosporin-resistant *Escherichia coli* in dairy cattle following clinical application of ceftiofur. *E. coli* isolates were obtained from rectal samples of treated and untreated cattle (n = 20/group) cultured on deoxycholate-hydrogen sulfide-lactose agar in the presence or absence of ceftiofur. Eleven cefazoline-resistant isolates were obtained from two of the ceftiofur-treated cattle; no cefazoline-resistant isolates were found in untreated cattle. The cefazoline-resistant isolates had mutations in the chromosomal *ampC* promoter region and remained susceptible to ceftiofur. Eighteen extended-spectrum cephalosporin–resistant isolates from two ceftiofur-treated cows were obtained on ceftiofur-supplemented agar; no extended-spectrum cephalosporin–resistant isolates were obtained from untreated cattle. These extended-spectrum cephalosporin–resistant isolates possessed plasmid-mediated β-lactamase genes, including *bla*CTX-M-2 (9 isolates), *bla*CTX-M-14 (8 isolates), or *bla*CMY-2 (1 isolate); isolates possessing *bla*CTX-M-2 and *bla*CTX-M-14 were clonally related. These genes were located on self-transmissible plasmids. Our results suggest that appropriate veterinary use of ceftiofur did not trigger growth extended-spectrum cephalosporin–resistant *E. coli* in the bovine rectal flora; however, ceftiofur selection *in vitro* suggested that additional ceftiofur exposure enhanced selection for specific extended-spectrum cephalosporin–resistant β-lactamase-expressing *E. coli* clones

Editor: Axel Cloeckaert, Institut National de la Recherche Agronomique, France

Funding: This study was supported in part by a Grant-in-Aid from the Japanese Ministry of Agriculture, Forestry, and Fisheries and a grant from the Program for Developing the Supporting System for Upgrading Education and Research from the Japan Ministry of Education, Culture, Sports, Science, and Technology. The funders had no role in study design, data collection and analysis, decision to publish, or preparation of the manuscript.

Competing Interests: The authors have declared that no competing interests exist.

* E-mail: tamuray@rakuno.ac.jp

¤ Current address: Laboratory of Human Retrovirology, Leidos-Frederick, Inc., Frederick National Laboratory for Cancer Research, Frederick, Maryland, United States of America

Introduction

β-Lactam antimicrobials are used worldwide in clinical settings. Extended-spectrum cephalosporins (ESCs; third- and fourth-generation cephalosporins such as cefpodoxime [CPD], ceftazidime [CAZ], and cefepime [FEP]) are broad-spectrum antimicrobials that have been listed by the World Health Organization (WHO) as critically important for human health [1]. However, the clinical occurrence of ESC-resistant *Enterobacteriaceae* has increased [3,4]. Numerous bacterial infections in food-producing animals and humans are treated with first- or second-generation cephalosporins such as cefazoline (CFZ), cefalexin (LEX), and cefuroxime (CXM), and ESCs such as ceftiofur (CTF) and CPD. In the WHO ranking of antimicrobials according to their importance in

human medicine, the ESCs that are also used in veterinary medicine are listed at the highest rank (critically important antimicrobial agents) on the basis of 2 criteria: (1) the agent or class is the sole therapeutic option or one of few alternatives available to treat serious human disease; and (2) the antimicrobial agent or class is used to treat diseases caused by organisms that may be transmitted via nonhuman sources or diseases caused by organisms that may acquire resistance genes from nonhuman sources [5]. ESCs used in humans and animals are of the same general class and share the same mode of action, even if they differ chemically [6]. Thus, the appearance of ESC-resistant bacteria can be attributable to mechanisms common between humans and animals (mainly by the acquisition of extended-spectrum β-lactamase genes and AmpC-type β-lactamase genes such as bla_{CTX-M} and bla_{CMY}), and interspecies transmission of ESC-resistant bacteria can occur [7,8]. ESC-resistant *Enterobacteriaceae* are found in food animals and their products [7,9–12]. Therefore, discussing issues related to the use of ESCs in veterinary medicine necessitates scientific evidence regarding the joint role played by ESCs in human and veterinary medicine.

CTF is a third-generation cephalosporin that is commonly used in veterinary medicine worldwide [13–15]. In Japan, CTF has been approved for use in cattle as a second-line drug for the treatment of pneumonia and as a first-line drug in serious infectious diseases in dairy cattle. *E. coli* is a commensal bacterial species in cattle feces [16]; some *E. coli* strains act as enteric pathogens in humans and/or are resistant to antimicrobials. [17]. Therefore, it is essential to characterize the *E. coli* with naturally occurring ESC resistance in bovine rectal flora because of the veterinary use of CTF, which may select for antimicrobial resistance. Previous studies have suggested an association between CTF use and the occurrence of ESC-resistant *E. coli* in cattle [2,13–15]. However, it is not known if *E. coli* with naturally occurring ESC resistance is selected for by appropriate veterinary ECS use because many studies have involved artificial intragastric inoculation with extended-spectrum β-lactamase–producing *E. coli* mutants and most do not record antimicrobial use or clinical criteria, such as, detail methods for ECS use, dose, or washout for every cow. All of these factors are important to consider when evaluating for a causal relationship between ECS use and naturally occurring ECS resistance.

In this study, to evaluate the risk of selection of ESC-resistant bacteria related to veterinary treatment with a suitable third-generation cephalosporin, we tried to isolate *E. coli* with naturally occurring ESC resistance from the rectal flora of CTF-treated or untreated dairy cattle after the washout period.

Materials and Methods

Bacterial Samples

We collected 20 dairy bovine rectal feces samples from dairy cattle treated with Excenel (cows 1–20; CTF sodium injection; Pfizer, New York City, USA). Ethical authority was not required according to the Epidemiological and Animal Ethical Research Committee of Rakuno Gakuen University because CTF treatment in this case was performed as part of general clinical treatment, compliant with the Veterinarians Acts and the Pharmaceutical Affairs Law defined by the Ministry of Agriculture, Forestry, and Fisheries in Japan. Briefly, cattle received intramuscular injections of $1–2$ $mg \cdot kg^{-1} \cdot day^{-1}$ CTF for 3 days for serious infectious diseases such as refractory pneumonia, puerperal fever, and hoof disease. This represented the first CTF treatment for these animals, and none had received any other antimicrobials for at least 3 months before sampling. Rectal feces samples were collected after the 8-day washout period, at which point the remaining CTF concentration in the organs and products have no effect on human health, according to the Pharmaceutical Affairs Law defined by the Ministry of Agriculture, Forestry, and Fisheries. The untreated controls included 20 dairy cattle (numbers 21–40) that did not receive any other antimicrobials for at least 3 months and no CTF use for at least 1.5 years before sampling. We did not sample non-treated cattle from herds that contain CTF-treated cattle. All samples were collected from independent farms in Betsukai (Hokkaido, Japan), the most productive dairying area in Japan (at least 100 cattle per farm). We had permission from the farms to collect fecal matter from their private property and CTF use in this study.

Table 1. β-lactam antimicrobial susceptibilities and detection of β-lactamase genes in AMP-resistant isolates in non-supplemented agar.

| Cow number | Number of strains/tested colonies | CTF treatment | MIC (μg/mL) | | | | | | β-lactamase gene |
			AMP (≥32)[a]	AMP /CVA	CFZ (≥32)	CXM (≥32)	CTF (≥8)	CTF/CVA	
5	10/10	+	>128	64/32	64–128	32	1	1/0.5	−1(CtoT)/−18(GtoA)/−42(CtoT)/−82(AtoG)*
7	1/10	+	>128	64/32	128	32	2	2/1	−1(CtoT)/−18(GtoA)/−42(CtoT)/−82(AtoG)*

[a]Breakpoint; *Mutations in the chromosomal *ampC* promoter region.

Table 2. β-Lactam susceptibilities and detection of β-lactamase genes in cephalosporin-resistant isolates in CTF-supplemented agar.

Cow number	Number of strains	CTF treatment	MIC (μg/mL) AMP (≥32)[a]	AMP/CVA	CFZ (≥32)	LEX (≥32)	CXM (≥32)	CTF (≥8)	CTF/CVA	CPD (≥8)	CAZ (≥16)	FEP (≥32)	Inc. type	β-lactamase gene
7	9	+	>128	8/4	>128	>128	>128	>32	1/0.5	>128	2	16	N, FIA, FIB	bla_{CTX-M-2}
7	1	+	128	64/32	>128	32	32	8	8/4	>128	32	≤0.125	I1-Iγ, FIB	bla_{CMY-2}
13	8	+	>128	8/4	>128	>128	>128	>32	1/0.5	>128	1-2	4-8	I1-Iγ	bla_{CTX-M-14}

[a] Break point.

Isolation of E. coli

Fecal samples (1 g) were dissolved in 9 mL of 0.85% sterile saline solution; 100 μL was immediately spread on deoxycholate-hydrogen sulfide-lactose (DHL) agar (Nissui, Tokyo, Japan) supplemented with 4 μg/mL CTF and incubated for 24 h at 37°C. CTF-free DHL plates served as controls. Samples were subcultured on nutrient agar (Nissui) at a maximum of 10 colonies per agar plate. The biochemical properties of these colonies were examined using triple sugar iron medium (Nissui), lysine indole motility medium (Nissui), and oxidase tests. Final identification of E. coli was performed by API20E (bioMérieux, Tokyo, Japan).

Susceptibility Testing

β-Lactam resistance was screened using CFZ KB-disks (Eiken, Tokyo, Japan) according to the manufacturer's instructions. Isolates showing resistance to CFZ in the KB-disk method were assessed to determine the minimum inhibitory concentration (MIC) by using the microdilution method according to the recommendations of the Clinical and Laboratory Standards Institute (CLSI; 2008) [18]. MICs were determined for eight β-lactam antimicrobials: AMP, CFZ, LEX, CXM, CTF, CPD, CAZ, FEP, and two mixtures of clavulanic acid (CVA) (CVA/AMP and CVA/CTF). Breakpoint values were defined according to 2008 CLSI recommendations, except in the case of LEX, CXM, CAZ, and FEP, which were defined according to 2011 CLSI recommendations [19], because the break points for these agents have not been defined for veterinary pathogens. Antimicrobial plates for microdilution testing were purchased from Eiken.

Detection of β-lactamase Genes

β-Lactamase genes were identified by PCR and direct DNA sequencing. bla_{CTX-M} was detected as described by Xu et al. [20], and plasmid-mediated ampC was detected as described by Pérez-Pérez et al. [21]. The presence of bla_{TEM}, bla_{SHV}, and mutations in the chromosomal ampC promoter region was detected according to Kojima et al. [11]. Nucleotide sequences were determined with a BigDye Terminator v3.1 Cycle Sequencing Kit and a 3130 Genetic Analyzer (Applied Biosystems, Foster City, CA).

Pulsed-field Gel Electrophoresis (PFGE)

PFGE was performed according to the method outlined by PulseNet USA [22] by using XbaI (Takara-Bio, Tokyo, Japan). The CHEF-DR III system (Bio-Rad Laboratories, Hercules, CA, USA) was used with the following running conditions: 19 h at 11.3°C, voltage of 6 V, ramped with an initial forward time of 2.2 s, and a final forward time of 54.2 s. After electrophoresis, gels were stained with ethidium bromide and photographed. The banding patterns were visually interpreted using published guidelines, and Dice similarity indices were calculated by cluster analysis.

Transferability Test of β-lactamase Genes

Broth-mating experiments were performed using rifampicin-resistant ML4909 (F⁻ galK2 galT22 hsdR metB1 relA supE44 rifampicin-resistant) as a recipient strain [21]. Donors and recipients were grown in tryptic soy broth (TSB, Nissui) to the logarithmic phase; they were then mixed in a total volume of 2 mL at a 1:9 (v/v) ratio, and 2 mL fresh TSB was added. The mating cultures were incubated overnight at 37°C. Transconjugants were selected on CTF (final concentration, 4 μg/mL)- and rifampicin (final concentration, 64 μg/mL)-containing MH agar.

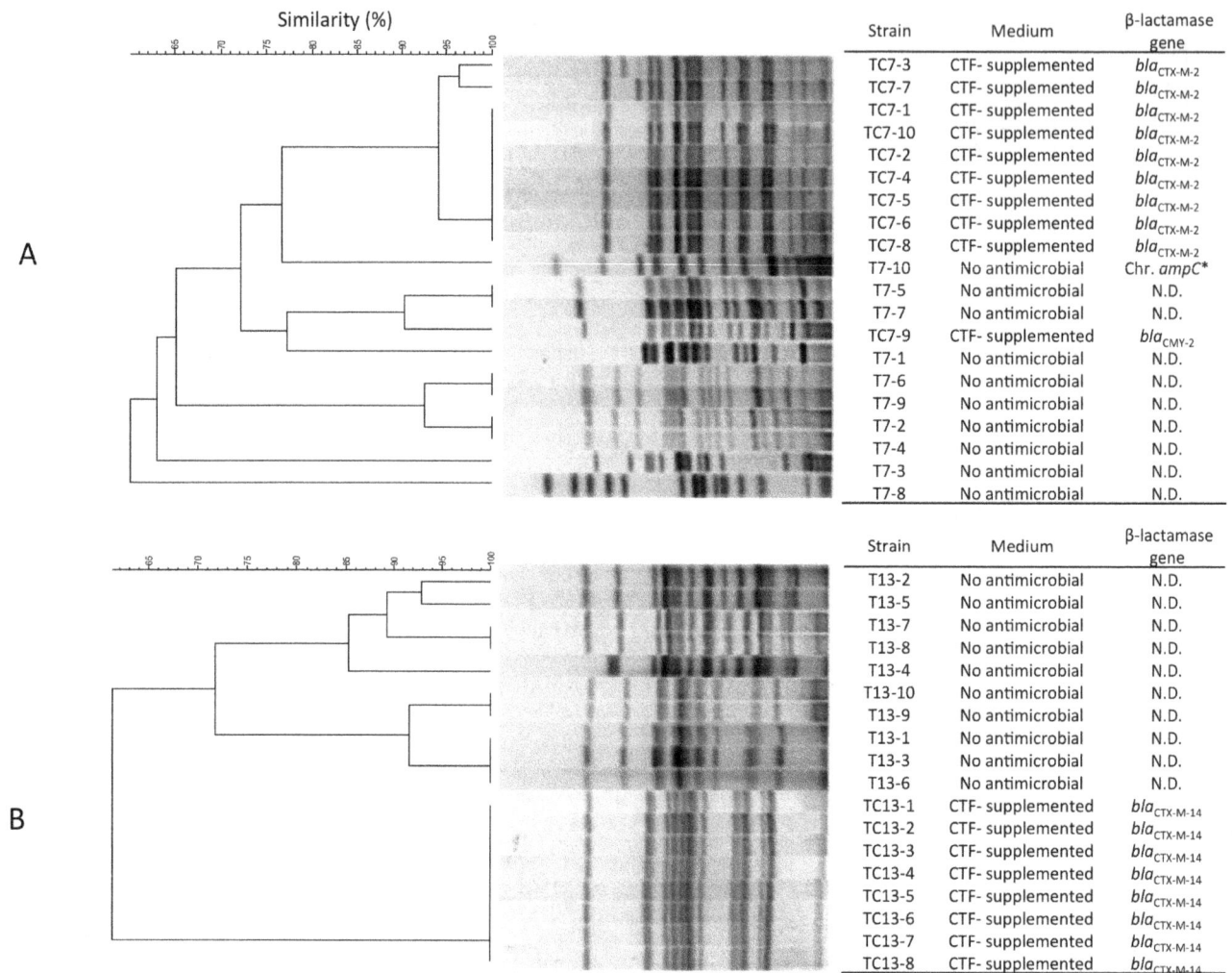

Strain	Medium	β-lactamase gene
TC7-3	CTF- supplemented	bla$_{CTX-M-2}$
TC7-7	CTF- supplemented	bla$_{CTX-M-2}$
TC7-1	CTF- supplemented	bla$_{CTX-M-2}$
TC7-10	CTF- supplemented	bla$_{CTX-M-2}$
TC7-2	CTF- supplemented	bla$_{CTX-M-2}$
TC7-4	CTF- supplemented	bla$_{CTX-M-2}$
TC7-5	CTF- supplemented	bla$_{CTX-M-2}$
TC7-6	CTF- supplemented	bla$_{CTX-M-2}$
TC7-8	CTF- supplemented	bla$_{CTX-M-2}$
T7-10	No antimicrobial	Chr. ampC*
T7-5	No antimicrobial	N.D.
T7-7	No antimicrobial	N.D.
TC7-9	CTF- supplemented	bla$_{CMY-2}$
T7-1	No antimicrobial	N.D.
T7-6	No antimicrobial	N.D.
T7-9	No antimicrobial	N.D.
T7-2	No antimicrobial	N.D.
T7-4	No antimicrobial	N.D.
T7-3	No antimicrobial	N.D.
T7-8	No antimicrobial	N.D.

Strain	Medium	β-lactamase gene
T13-2	No antimicrobial	N.D.
T13-5	No antimicrobial	N.D.
T13-7	No antimicrobial	N.D.
T13-8	No antimicrobial	N.D.
T13-4	No antimicrobial	N.D.
T13-10	No antimicrobial	N.D.
T13-9	No antimicrobial	N.D.
T13-1	No antimicrobial	N.D.
T13-3	No antimicrobial	N.D.
T13-6	No antimicrobial	N.D.
TC13-1	CTF- supplemented	bla$_{CTX-M-14}$
TC13-2	CTF- supplemented	bla$_{CTX-M-14}$
TC13-3	CTF- supplemented	bla$_{CTX-M-14}$
TC13-4	CTF- supplemented	bla$_{CTX-M-14}$
TC13-5	CTF- supplemented	bla$_{CTX-M-14}$
TC13-6	CTF- supplemented	bla$_{CTX-M-14}$
TC13-7	CTF- supplemented	bla$_{CTX-M-14}$
TC13-8	CTF- supplemented	bla$_{CTX-M-14}$

Figure 1. Pulsed-field gel electrophoresis of CTF-resistant *E. coli* isolates from two CTF-treated cattle. A, PFGE analysis of 20 isolates obtained from cow No. 7. Strains T7 and TC7 were isolated in the absence or presence of CTF, respectively. B, PFGE analysis of 18 isolates obtained from cow No. 13. Strains T13 and TC13 were isolated in the absence or presence of CTF, respectively.

Plasmid Profiling and Southern Hybridization Analysis

Plasmid profiling was performed according to previously described methods [24]. Plasmid incompatibility (Inc) groups were determined by PCR with the following primers: HI1, HI2, I1-Iγ, X, L/M, N, FIA, FIB, W, Y, P, FIC, A/C, T, FIIAs, F, K, and B/O [25].

Southern hybridization was performed as follows. Probes were prepared by PCR. Probes for bla$_{CTX-M-2}$ and bla$_{CTX-M-14}$ were prepared using a CTX-M consensus primer set [26]. The probe for bla$_{CMY-2}$ was prepared using primers described by Pérez-Pérez and Hanson [21]. These PCR products were labeled using a PCR DIG Labeling Mix (Roche Diagnostic, Tokyo, Japan) according to the manufacturer's instructions. Plasmid DNA was separated by 0.8% (w/v) agarose gel electrophoresis at 100 V for 70 min. The DNA in the gel was transferred to a positive membrane (Roche Diagnostics) by the capillary method. Pre-hybridization (>30 min) and hybridization (>16 h) were performed using Easy Hyb solution (Roche Diagnostics) under high-stringency conditions, and digoxigenin (DIG) in the hybrids was detected using a DIG Luminescent Detection Kit (Roche Diagnostics) according to the manufacturer's instructions. A hyper MP film (GE Healthcare

Japan, Tokyo, Japan) was exposed to the membranes for 2 min at room temperature and developed in a Kodak X-Omat processor.

Statistical Analysis

Statistical significance was determined using chi-square test and Fisher's exact tests. Significance was set at $p < 0.05$.

Results

Isolation and Antimicrobial Resistance of *E. coli*

Using non-supplemented agar. In this study, 193 and 182 *E. coli* isolates were obtained from CTF-treated and untreated cattle, respectively. We screened for CFZ resistance by the disk diffusion method. From the 193 strains isolated from CTF-treated cattle, 11 isolates resistant to CFZ were obtained; however, no CFZ-resistant *E. coli* was obtained from untreated cattle ($p < 0.05$). The 11 CFZ-resistant isolates (from cow No. 5 [10 strains] and cow No. 7 [1 strain]) were also resistant to AMP and CXM, but not CTF; CVA did not affect the MICs of AMP or CTF (Table 1). All 11 isolates carried mutations in the chromosomal *ampC* promoter region.

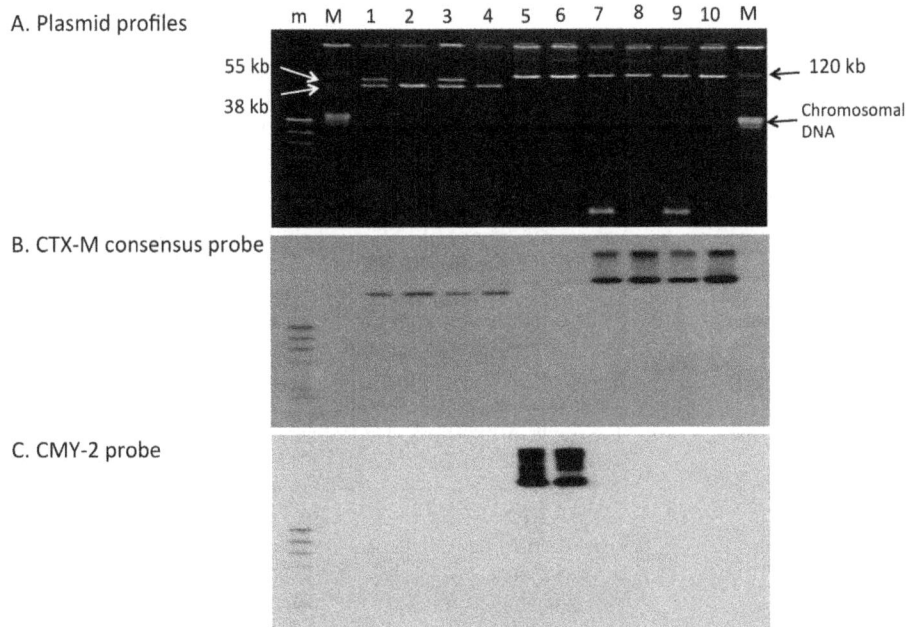

Figure 2. Plasmid profiling and Southern hybridization of β-lactamase genes in *E. coli* isolates from CTF-treated cattle. A, Plasmid profiling. B, Southern hybridization of the bla_{CTX-M} consensus probe. C, Southern hybridization of the bla_{CMY-2} probe. Lane1, ML4909 (recipient); lane 2, TC7-1 (possesses $bla_{CTX-M-2}$); lane 3, TcTC7-1; lane 4, TC7-2 (possesses $bla_{CTX-M-2}$); lane 5, TcTC7-2; lane 6, TC7-9 (possesses bla_{CMY-2}); lane 7, TcTC7-9; lane 8, TC13-1 (possesses $bla_{CTX-M-14}$); lane 9, TcTC13-1; lane 10, TC13-2 (possesses $bla_{CTX-M-14}$); lane 11, TcTC13-2; m, DNA Molecular Weight Marker II, DIG-labeled; M, BAC-Tracker Supercoiled DNA Ladder. $bla_{CTX-M-2}$ and $bla_{CTX-M-14}$ were detected using a CTX-M consensus probe.

Using CTF-supplemented agar. Eighteen *E. coli* isolates were obtained on CTF-supplemented agar (from CTF-treated cow No. 7 [10 strains] and cow No. 13 [8 strains]); no resistant strains were isolated from the untreated group ($p<0.05$). Seventeen isolates were resistant to AMP, CFZ, LEX, CXM, CPD, and CTF, and CVA influenced the MICs of AMP and CTF (Table 2). The *E. coli* isolates showed CTF resistance from cow nos. 7 and 13 possessed $bla_{CTX-M-2}$ and $bla_{CTX-M-14}$, respectively. The last strain from CTF-treated cow No. 7 showed resistance to AMP, CFZ, LEX, CXM, CPD, CAZ, and CTF; however, CVA did not affect the MICs of AMP and CTF in this isolate. This strain possessed bla_{CMY-2}. None of the isolates exceeded the breakpoint of FEP (Tables 1 and 2).

PFGE Analysis and Plasmid Analysis

To determine the clonal relationship of isolates exhibiting differential CTF selection properties, we performed PFGE of isolates derived from non-supplemented and CTF-supplemented agar after collection from two CTF-treated cattle (Nos. 7 and 13; Figure 1). The PFGE pattern showed that these isolates were clearly different clones. Isolates harboring $bla_{CTX-M-2}$ and $bla_{CTX-M-14}$, which were isolated from CTF-supplemented agar, exhibited mostly identical PFGE patterns. Plasmid profiling also showed that strains isolated from CTF-supplemented agar possessed identically sized plasmid(s) harboring their respective β-lactamase gene types (Figure 2). These results indicated that resistant strains carrying $bla_{CTX-M-2}$ from cow No. 7 and those carrying $bla_{CTX-M-14}$ from cow no. 13 originated from a single clone in each cow.

Transferability Test and Southern Hybridization of β-lactamase Genes

We investigated the transferability of β-lactamase genes using recipient ML4909 cells. The donors were TC7-1 and TC7-2,

which possessed $bla_{CTX-M-2}$ (isolated from cow No. 7); TC7-9, which possessed bla_{CMY-2} (isolated from cow No. 7); and TC13-1 and TC13-2, which possessed $bla_{CTX-M-14}$ (isolated from cow No. 13). All detected β-lactamase genes could be transferred to the recipient, and the MICs of the transconjugants increased at a level similar to that of the donor (Table 3). Replicon typing and Southern hybridization showed that $bla_{CTX-M-2}$ was located in an IncN plasmid (about 40 kb), bla_{CMY-2} was located in I1-Iγ and/or FIB plasmids (more than 100 kb), and $bla_{CTX-M-14}$ was located in an I1-Iγ plasmid (more than 100 kb; Table 3 and Figure 2).

Discussion

The occurrence of antimicrobial-resistant bacteria, including cephalosporin-resistant bacteria, is thought to be related to selection pressures resulting from antimicrobial consumption [27–29]. Previous studies have suggested an association between CTF use and the occurrence of ESC-resistant *E. coli* in cattle [2,13–15]. Although it has not reported an association between CTF use and the occurrence of ESC-resistant *E. coli* in cattle in Japan, a previous study showed that 6 (1.5%) of 396 *E. coli* isolates obtained from bovine fecal samples in Japan showed ESC resistance [30]. These data indicate an association between the isolation of ESC-resistant *E. coli* and ESC use in Japan. However, evidence supporting this association is lacking because the histories of clinical CTF use and compliance with clinical criteria were unknown and a cohort study on veterinary CTF use has never been performed. Thus, the estimation of emergence of ESC-resistant *E. coli* due to suitable clinical ESC use could help re-evaluate antimicrobial therapy to avoid the spread of ESC-resistant bacteria.

CTF was used to treat refractory pneumonia and other serious infectious diseases such as puerperal fever and hoof disease in dairy cattle, according to our inquiry survey. In this study, cephalospo-

Table 3. β-Lactam susceptibilities and detection of β-lactamase genes in transconjugants from CTF-resistant isolates.

Strain	Characteristic	MIC (µg/mL)						Inc. group	β-lactamase gene
		AMP	AMP/CVA	CFZ	CXM	CTF	CTF/CVA		
ML4909	Recipient	4	2/1	2	<1	<0.5	<0.5/0.25	ND	ND[a]
TC7-1	Donor	>128	8/4	>128	>128	>32	1/0.5	N, FIA, FIB	$bla_{CTX-M-2}$
TcTC7-1	Transconjugant	>128	8/4	>128	>128	>32	1/0.5	N	$bla_{CTX-M-2}$
TC7-2	Donor	>128	8/4	>128	>128	>32	1/0.5	N, FIA, FIB	$bla_{CTX-M-2}$
TcTC7-2	Transconjugant	>128	8/4	>128	>128	>32	1/0.5	N	$bla_{CTX-M-2}$
TC7-9	Donor	128	64/32	>128	32	8	8/4	I1-Iγ, FIB	bla_{CMY-2}
TcTC7-9	Transconjugant	64	64/32	128	8	8	4/2	I1-Iγ, FIB	bla_{CMY-2}
TC13-1	Donor	>128	8/4	>128	>128	>32	1/0.5	I1-Iγ	$bla_{CTX-M-14}$
TcTC13-1	Transconjugant	>128	8/4	>128	>128	>32	<0.5/0.25	I1-Iγ	$bla_{CTX-M-14}$
TC13-2	Donor	>128	8/4	>128	>128	>32	1/0.5	I1-Iγ	$bla_{CTX-M-14}$
TcTC13-2	Transconjugant	>128	4/2	>128	>128	>32	<0.5/0.25	I1-Iγ	$bla_{CTX-M-14}$

[a]ND, not detected.

rin-resistant isolates were found only in CTF-treated animals. All of these isolates possessed mutations in chromosomal *ampC* and were resistant to AMP and first- and second-generation cephalosporins (CFZ and CXM), but not CTF. Thus, we conclude that if CTF is used appropriately ($1–2 \text{ mg·kg}^{-1}\text{·day}^{-1}$ for 3 days) in Japanese veterinary practice, washout periods will increase the frequency of naturally occurring first- and second-generation cephalosporin resistance in *E. coli*, but will not influence the natural occurrence of ESC-resistant *E. coli* in dairy cattle.

A previous study reported the isolation of ESC-resistant *E. coli* (possessing bla_{CMY-2}) from fecal samples of calves on 8 µg/mL CTF-supplemented agar, but not on non-supplemented agar [14]. This finding suggests that ESC-resistant *E. coli* are present in the bovine rectal flora at low frequency, and additional CTF exposure selects for these ESC-resistant *E. coli*. However, the applicability of this result to real-world CTF treatment in dairying is unknown, because the histories of clinical CTF use (or other β-lactams) in these calves were unknown. In this study, all CTF-resistant isolates were obtained from treated cattle and after culture on CTF-supplemented agar; these isolates possessed a plasmid-encoded β-lactamase gene, $bla_{CTX-M-2}$, $bla_{CTX-M-14}$, or bla_{CMY-2}. Importantly, PFGE analysis showed that although ESC-resistant clones were not yet predominant in the rectal flora at the end of the washout period after CTF treatment, *in vitro* CTF exposure led to the selection of specific ESC-resistant clones in CTF-treated cattle. However, we could not determine which CTF dose (1 or 2 mg/kg of CTF) was high risk in terms of selection of ECS-resistant *E. coli* by *in vitro* testing because these dose were scattered regardless of whether ECS-resistant *E. coli* were isolated or not. Therefore, these results suggest that although appropriate CTF use ($1–2 \text{ mg·kg}^{-1}\text{·day}^{-1}$ for 3 days) in Japanese veterinary practice dose not influence the natural occurrence of ESC-resistant *E. coli* in cattle, if CTF is used inappropriately, such as by overuse and/or subcutaneous use, it might encourage the selection and spread of broad-spectrum cephalosporin-resistant *E. coli* clones in bovine flora as suggested by *in vitro* CTF selection.

β-Lactamase genes in ESC-resistant isolates were located on Inc-type plasmids, i.e., $bla_{CTX-M-2}$ (Inc-N), $bla_{CTX-M-14}$ (Inc-I1-Iγ), and bla_{CMY-2} (Inc I1-Iγ and/or FIB), and all were capable of self-transmission. bla_{CTX-M2} was found in *E. coli* from cattle in Japan from 2000 to 2001 [30]. bla_{CMY-2} was found in I1-Iγ and A/C plasmids in *Salmonella enterica* serovar Typhimurium isolated from cattle in Japan in 2007 [31]. $bla_{CTX-M-14}$ was found in *S. enterica* serovar Enteritidis from chicken meat imported from China and sold by a retailer in Japan in 2004 [32]. The presence of these genes suggests β-lactamase genes producing ESC resistance are already widespread in Japanese livestock and their products. Although these data do not show an association between veterinary ESC use and the presence of β-lactamase genes in ESC-resistant *E. coli*, the presence of these genes might be selected for by cephalosporin use or co-selected by other antimicrobials used in veterinary medicine.

Furthermore, the ESC-resistant *E. coli* isolated in current study showed resistance to both ESCs used in veterinary medicine and to ESCs used in human medicine, and their transferable β-lactamase genes have been detected in humans in a variety of clinical settings worldwide [33]. Remarkably, $bla_{CTX-M-2}$ and $bla_{CTX-M-14}$ have also been found in *E. coli* isolates from humans in Japan ($bla_{CTX-M-2}$ in Inc-N and $bla_{CTX-M-14}$ in Inc-I1 plasmids [4,34], similar to the pattern observed in our study). In particular, *E. coli* O25 (undetermined H-antigen)-ST131, which frequently possesses $bla_{CTX-M-14}$, is the most common strain that spreads to humans [34]. Our study and other studies suggest that human health may be at increased risk from the overuse of cephalosporins in livestock and that further genetic and epidemiological investigations are required to determine whether there is direct transmission of ESC-resistant *E. coli* and their β-lactamase genes from livestock to humans.

In conclusion, although appropriate veterinary use of a third-generation cephalosporin, CTF, increased the occurrence of first- and second-generation cephalosporin-resistant *E. coli*, it did not influence the natural occurrence of ECS-resistant *E. coli* in dairy cattle. However, *in vitro* CTF selection suggested that inappropriate CTF use in veterinary practice might increase the risk of selection of ESC-resistant *E. coli* possessing $bla_{CTX-M-2}$, bla_{CMY-2}, or $bla_{CTX-M-14}$. Therefore, veterinary use of ESCs should be

carefully monitored and used appropriately as described by the Joint FAO/WHO/OIE Expert Meeting on Critically Important Antimicrobials [6] to prevent the spread of ESC-resistant bacteria in veterinary medicine.

Author Contributions

Performed the experiments: TS TO. Analyzed the data: TS TO. Contributed reagents/materials/analysis tools: TS TO MU SY SI YT. Wrote the paper: TS. Contributed to, prepared and approved the manuscript: MU SY YT.

References

1. World Health Organization (WHO): Critically Important Antimicrobials for Human Medicine: Categorization for the Development of Risk Management Strategies to contain Antimicrobial Resistance due to Non-Human Antimicrobial Use Report of the Second WHO Expert Meeting, Copenhagen, 2007, 29–31.

2. Chantziaras I, Boyen F, Callens B, Dewulf J (2014) Correlation between veterinary antimicrobial use and antimicrobial resistance in food-producing animals: a report on seven countries J Antimicrob Chemother 69: 827–834.

3. Chong Y, Yakushiji H, Ito Y, Kamimura T (2011) Clinical and molecular epidemiology of extended-spectrum β-lactamase-producing Escherichia coli and Klebsiella pneumoniae in a long-term study from Japan. European Eur J Clin Microbiol Infect Dis 30: 83–87.

4. Suzuki S, Shibata N, Yamane K, Wachino J, Ito K, et al (2009) Change in the prevalence of extended-spectrum-beta-lactamase-producing Escherichia coli in Japan by clonal spread. J Antimicrob Chemother 63: 72–79.

5. Collignon P, Powers JH, Chiller TM, Aidara-Kane A, Aarestrup FM (2009) World Health Organization ranking of antimicrobials according to their importance in human medicine: A critical step for developing risk management strategies for the use of antimicrobials in food production animals. Clin Infect Dis 49: 132–141.

6. FAO/WHO/OIE: Report of the Joint FAO/WHO/OIE Expert Meeting on Critically Important Antimicrobials (2007) FAO, Rome, Italy.

7. Bertrand S, Weill FX, Cloeckaert A, Vrints M, Mairiaux E, et al. (2006) Clonal emergence of extended-spectrum β-lactamase (CTX-M-2)-producing Salmonella enterica serovar Virchow isolates with reduced susceptibilities to ciprofloxacin among poultry and humans in Belgium and France (2000 to 2003). J Clin Microbiol 44: 2897–2903.

8. Winokur PL, Vonstein DL, Hoffman LJ, Uhlenhopp EK, Doern GV (2001) Evidence for transfer of CMY-2 AmpC beta-lactamase plasmids between Escherichia coli and Salmonella isolates from food animals and humans. Antimicrob Agents Chemother 45: 2716–2722.

9. Cavaco LM, Abatih E, Aarestrup FM, Guardabassi L (2008) Selection and persistence of CTX-M-producing Escherichia coli in the intestinal flora of pigs treated with amoxicillin, ceftiofur, or cefquinome. Antimicrob Agents and Chemother 52: 3612–3616.

10. Jouini A, Vinue L, Ben Slama K, Saenz Y, Klibi N, et al. (2007) Characterization of CTX-M and SHV extended-spectrum beta-lactamases and associated resistance genes in Escherichia coli strains of food samples in Tunisia. J Antimicrob Chemother 60: 1137–1141.

11. Kojima A, Ishii Y, Ishihara K, Esaki H, Asai T, et al. (2005) Extended-spectrum-beta-lactamase-producing Escherichia coli strains isolated from farm animals from 1999 to 2002: Report from the Japanese Veterinary Antimicrobial Resistance Monitoring program. Antimicrob Agents Chemother 49: 3533–3537.

12. Liebana E, Batchelor M, Hopkins KL, Clifton-Hadley FA, Teale CJ, et al. (2006) Longitudinal farm study of extended-spectrum β-lactamase-mediated resistance. J Clin Microbiol 44: 1630–1634.

13. Daniels JB, Call DR, Hancock D, Sischo WM, Baker K, et al. (2009) Role of ceftiofur in selection and dissemination of bla(CMY-2)-mediated cephalosporin resistance in Salmonella enterica and commensal Escherichia coli isolates from cattle. Appl Environ Microbiol 2009, 75: 3648–3655.

14. Donaldson SC, Straley BA, Hegde NV, Sawant AA, DebRoy C, et al. (2006) Molecular epidemiology of ceftiofur-resistant Escherichia coli isolates from dairy calves. Appl Environ Microbiol 72: 3940–3948.

15. Singer RS, Patterson SK, Wallace RL (2008) Effects of therapeutic ceftiofur administration to dairy cattle on Escherichia coli dynamics in the intestinal tract. Appl Environ Microbiol 74: 6956–6962.

16. Nuru S, Osbaldiston GW, Stowe EC, Walker D (1972) Fecal microflora of healthy cattle and pigs. Cornell Vet 62: 242–253.

17. Clermont O, Olier M, Hoede C, Diancourt L, Brisse S, et al. (2011) Animal and human pathogenic Escherichia coli strains share common genetic backgrounds. Infect Genet Evol 11: 654–662.

18. Clinical and Laboratory Standards Institute: Performance standards for antimicrobial disk and dilution antimicrobial susceptibility tests for bacteria isolated from animals. Approved standard, 3rd ed. CLSI document 2008, M31-A3. CLSI, Wayne, PA.

19. Clinical and Laboratory Standards Institute: Performance standards for antimicrobial susceptibility testing standards 2011, M100-S21. CLSI, Wayne, PA.

20. Xu L, Ensor V, Gossain S, Nye K, Hawkey P (2005) Rapid and simple detection of bla(CTX-M) genes by multiplex PCR assay. J Med Microbiol 54: 1183–1187.

21. Pérez-Pérez FJ, Hanson ND (2002) Detection of plasmid-mediated AmpC β-lactamase genes in clinical isolates by using multiplex PCR. J Clin Microbiol 40: 2153–2162.

22. The National Molecular Subtyping Network for Foodborne Disease Surveillance: One-day (24–28 h) standardized laboratory protocol for molecular subtyping of Escherichia coli O157:H7, non-typhoidal Salmonella serotypes, and Shigella sonnei by pulsed field gel electrophoresis (PFGE) (2004) MAF, 1–12.

23. Ma L, Ishii Y, Ishiguro M, Matsuzawa H, Yamaguchi K (1998) Cloning and sequencing of the gene encoding Toho-2, a class A beta-lactamase preferentially inhibited by tazobactam. Antimicrob Agents Chemother 42: 1181–1186.

24. Kado CI, Liu ST (1981) Rapid procedure for detection and isolation of large and small plasmids. J Bact 145: 1365–1373.

25. Carattoli A, Bertini A, Villa L, Falbo V, Hopkins KL, et al. (2005) Identification of plasmids by PCR-based replicon typing. J Microbiol Methods 63: 219–228.

26. Saladin M, Cao VT, Lambert T, Donay JL, Herrmann JL, et al. (2002) Diversity of CTX-M beta-lactamases and their promoter regions from Enterobacteriaceae isolated in three Parisian hospitals. FEMS Microbiol Lett 209: 161–168.

27. Alexander TW, Inglis GD, Yanke LJ, Topp E, Read RR, et al. (2010) Farm-to-fork characterization of Escherichia coli associated with feedlot cattle with a known history of antimicrobial use. Int J Food Microbiol 137: 40–48.

28. Asai T, Kojima A, Harada K, Ishihara K, Takahashi T, et al. (2005) Correlation between the usage volume of veterinary therapeutic antimicrobials and resistance in Escherichia coli isolated from the feces of food-producing animals in Japan. Japan J Infect Dis 58: 369–372.

29. Bergman M, Nyberg ST, Huovinen P, Paakkari P, Hakanen AJ (2009) Association between antimicrobial consumption and resistance in Escherichia coli. Antimicrob Agents Chemother 53: 912–917.

30. Shiraki Y, Shibata N, Doi Y, Arakawa Y (2004) Escherichia coli producing CTX-M-2 beta-lactamase in cattle, Japan. Emerg Infect Dis 10: 69–75.

31. Sugawara M, Komori J, Kawakami M, Izumiya H, Watanabe H, et al. (2011) Molecular and phenotypic characteristics of CMY-2 beta-lactamase-producing Salmonella enterica serovar Typhimurium isolated from cattle in Japan. J Vet Med Sci 73: 345–349.

32. Matsumoto Y, Kitazume H, Yamada M, Ishiguro Y, Muto T, et al. (2007) CTX-M-14 type beta-lactamase producing Salmonella enterica serovar Enteritidis isolated from imported chicken meat. Japan J Infectious Dis 60: 236–238.

33. Bonnet R (2004) Growing group of extended-spectrum beta-lactamases: The CTX-M enzymes. Antimicrob Agents Chemother 48: 1–14.

34. Uchida Y, Mochimaru T, Morokuma Y, Kiyosuke M, Fujise M, et al. (2010) Clonal spread in Eastern Asia of ciprofloxacin-resistant Escherichia coli serogroup O25 strains, and associated virulence factors. Int J Antimicrob Agents 35: 444–450.

PERMISSIONS

LIST OF CONTRIBUTORS

Lisai Zhu, Zeli Xing, Xiaochun Gai, Sujing Li, Zhihao San and Xinping Wang
College of Veterinary Medicine, Jilin University, Changchun, Jilin, China

Álvaro Menin, Renata Fleith, Paula Fernandes and André Báfica
Laboratory of Immunobiology, Universidade Federal de Santa Catarina, Floriano´ spolis, Santa Catarina, Brazil

Carolina Reck and Célso Pilati
Laboratory of Histology and Immunohistochemistry, Universidade do Estado de Santa Catarina, Lages, Santa Catarina, Brazil

Mariel Marlow
Laboratory of Protozoology, Universidade Federal de Santa Catarina, Floriano´ spolis, Santa Catarina, Brazil

Ylva Telldahl and Jan Storå
Osteoarchaeological Research Laboratory, Department of Archaeology and Classical Studies, Stockholm University, Stockholm, Sweden

Emma Svensson and Anders Götherstrom
Department of Evolutionary Biology, Uppsala Universitet, Uppsala, Sweden

Kristina M. Adams Waldorf
Department of Obstetrics & Gynecology, University of Washington, Seattle, Washington, United States of America

Ryan M. McAdams
Department of Pediatrics, University of Washington, Seattle, Washington, United States of America

Louis J. Paolella
Global Alliance to Prevent Prematurity & Stillbirth, Seattle, Washington, United States of America

G. Michael Gough
Washington National Primate Research Center, Seattle, Washington, United States of America

David J. Carl
Ross University School of Medicine, Dominica, West Indies

H. Denny Liggitt
Department of Comparative Medicine, University of Washington, Seattle, Washington, United States of America

Raj P. Kapur
Department of Laboratories, Seattle Children's, Seattle, Washington, United States of America

Frederick B. Reitz
Center on Human Development and Disability, University of Washington, Seattle, Washington, United States of America

Michael G. Gravett
Department of Obstetrics & Gynecology, University of Washington, Seattle, Washington, United States of America
Global Alliance to Prevent Prematurity & Stillbirth, Seattle, Washington, United States of America

Craig E. Rubens
Global Alliance to Prevent Prematurity & Stillbirth, Seattle, Washington, United States of America
Division of Infectious Disease, Seattle Children's, Seattle, Washington, United States of America

Christopher Simpson and Henk R. Braig
School of Biological Sciences, Bangor University, Bangor, Wales, United Kingdom

M. Alejandra Perotti
School of Biological Sciences, University of Reading, Reading, United Kingdom

Peter Masan
School of Biological Sciences, Bangor University, Bangor, Wales, United Kingdom
Institute of Zoology, Slovak Academy of Sciences, Bratislava, Slovakia

Pascal Monestiez
INRA, UR 546, Biostatistics and Spatial Processes, Avignon, France

Simon Nusinovici, Henri Seegers, Franc¸ois Beaudeau and Christine Fourichon
INRA, UMR1300 Biology, Epidemiology and Risk Analysis in animal health, Nantes, France
LUNAM Université, Oniris, Ecole nationale vétérinaire, agroalimentaire et de l'alimentation Nantes-Atlantique, Nantes, France

Helen M. Higgins and Martic J. Green
Population Health and Welfare Group, School of Veterinary Medicine and Science, University of Nottingham, Sutton Bonington, United Kingdom

Eamonn Ferguson
Personality, Social Psychology, and Health Research Group, School of Psychology, University of Nottingham, Nottingham, United Kingdom

Robert F. Smith
Division of Livestock Health and Welfare, School of Veterinary Science, University of Liverpool, Neston, United Kingdom

Henrike C. Jäger, Trevelyan J. McKinley, James L. N. Wood, Gareth P. Pearce and Alexander W. Tucker
Department of Veterinary Medicine, University of Cambridge, Cambridge, United Kingdom

Susanna Williamson
Veterinary Laboratories Agency (AHVLA), Bury St Edmunds, Suffolk, United Kingdom

Benjamin Strugnell and Stanley Done
Veterinary Laboratories Agency (AHVLA), West House, Thirsk, North Yorkshire, United Kingdom

Henrike Habernoll
BQP Ltd, Stradbroke Business Centre, Stradbroke, Suffolk, United Kingdom

Andreas Palzer
Ludwig-Maximilians-Universität München, Clinic for Swine, Sonnenstrasse, Oberschleissheim Germany

Samuel M. Thumbi and Mark E. J. Woolhouse
Centre for Immunology, Infection and Evolution, University of Edinburgh, Edinburgh, United Kingdom

Barend Mark de Clare Bronsvoort, Amy Jennings and Ian Graham Handel
The Roslin Institute and Royal (Dick) School of Veterinary Studies, University of Edinburgh, Roslin, United Kingdom

Elizabeth Jane Poole, Henry Kiara, Philip G. Toye and Mary Ndila Mbole-Kariuki
International Livestock Research Institute, Nairobi, Kenya

Olivier Hanotte
School of Life Science, University of Nottingham, University Park, Nottingham, United Kingdom

Ilana Conradie and Jacobus Andries Wynand Coetzer
Department of Veterinary Tropical Diseases, Faculty of Veterinary Science, University of Pretoria, Onderstepoort, South Africa

Johan C. A. Steyl
Department of Paraclinical Sciences, Faculty of Veterinary Science, University of Pretoria, Onderstepoort, South Africa

Charles L. Nunn
Department of Human Evolutionary Biology, Harvard University, Cambridge, Massachusetts, United States of America

Peter H. Thrall
CSIRO Plant Industry, Canberra, Australia

Fabian H. Leendertz
Research Group Emerging Zoonoses, Robert Koch-Institute, Berlin, Germany

Christophe Boesch
Max Planck Institute for Evolutionary Anthropology, Leipzig, Germany

Katie Nightingale, Claire S. Levy, John Hopkins, Finn Grey, Suzanne Esper and Robert G. Dalziel
The Roslin Institute & R(D)SVS, University of Edinburgh, Edinburgh, Midlothian, United Kingdom

Emilie Gay
ANSES, Laboratoire de Lyon, Unité Epidémiologie, Lyon, France

Anne V. Gautier-Bouchardon and Séverine Ferré
ANSES, Laboratoire de Ploufragan/Plouzané, Unité Mycoplasmologie-Bactériologie, Ploufragan, France
Universié Européenne de Bretagne, Rennes, France

Dominique Le Grand, Agnès Paoli and François Poumarat
ANSES, Laboratoire de Lyon, UMR Mycoplasmoses des Ruminants, Lyon, France
Université de Lyon, VetAgro Sup, UMR Mycoplasmoses des Ruminants, Marcy L'Etoile, France

Scott D. Reed
Neurosignaling Laboratory, Pennington Biomedical Research Center, Louisiana State University System, Baton Rouge, Louisiana, United States of America

Nithya Mariappan and Joseph Francis
Comparative Biomedical Sciences, Louisiana State University School of Veterinary Medicine, Baton Rouge, Louisiana, United States of America

Barbara Shukitt-Hale and James A. Joseph
United States Department of Agriculture-Agriculture Research Services, Human Nutrition Research Center on Aging, Tufts University, Boston, Massachusetts, United States of America

Donald K. Ingram
Nutritional Neuroscience and Aging Laboratory, Pennington Biomedical Research Center, Louisiana State University System, Baton Rouge, Louisiana, United States of America

Carrie M. Elks
Comparative Biomedical Sciences, Louisiana State University School of Veterinary Medicine, Baton Rouge, Louisiana, United States of America
Nutritional Neuroscience and Aging Laboratory, Pennington Biomedical Research Center, Louisiana State University System, Baton Rouge, Louisiana, United States of America

Jonathon M. Tinsley, Richard Storer, Fraser J. Wilkes, Adam Lambert, Francis X. Wilson and Stephen P. Wren
Summit plc, Abingdon, United Kingdom

Rebecca J. Fairclough, Allyson C. Potter, Sarah E. Squire, Dave S. Powell and Kay E. Davies
MRC Functional Genomics Unit, Department of Physiology Anatomy and Genetics, University of Oxford, Oxford, United Kingdom

Anna Cozzoli, Roberta F. Capogrosso and Annamaria De Luca
Unit of Pharmacology, Department of Pharmaco-biology, University of Bari "A. Moro", Bari, Italy

Louis S. Kidder and Yan Zhang
Masonic Cancer Center, University of Minnesota, Minneapolis, Minnesota, United States of America

Greg Fairchild and Kayti Coghill
Department of Therapeutic Radiology, Medical School, University of Minnesota, Minneapolis, Minnesota, United States of America

Cory J. Xian
Sansom Institute, School of Pharmacy and Medical Sciences, University of South Australia, Adelaide, South Australia, Australia

Susanta K. Hui
Department of Therapeutic Radiology, Medical School, University of Minnesota, Minneapolis, Minnesota, United States of America
Masonic Cancer Center, University of Minnesota, Minneapolis, Minnesota, United States of America

Leslie Sharkey
Department of Veterinary Clinical Sciences, College of Veterinary Medicine, University of Minnesota, St. Paul, Minnesota, United States of America
Masonic Cancer Center, University of Minnesota, Minneapolis, Minnesota, United States of America

Douglas Yee
Masonic Cancer Center, University of Minnesota, Minneapolis, Minnesota, United States of America
Department of Medicine, Medical School, University of Minnesota, Minneapolis, Minnesota, United States of America

Reda E. Khalafalla
Department of Parasitology, Faculty of Veterinary Medicine, Kafrelsheikh University, Kafrelsheikh, Egypt

Renduo Zhang
School of Environmental Science and Engineering, Guangdong Provincial Key Laboratory of Environmental Pollution Control and Remediation Technology, Sun Yat-sen University, Guangzhou, China

Jinhua Zhang
Guizhou Normal University, Guiyang, China
Guizhou Institute of Pratacultural, Guiyang, China

Xiaoyun Shen
Chongqing University of Science and Technology, Chongqing, China
Office of Poverty Alleviation of Guizhou Province, Guiyang, China
Pratacultural Ecology Institute, Bijie University, Bijie, China

Mukhtar Salihu Anka, Latiffah Hassan, Siti Khairani-Bejo and Annas Salleh
Department of Veterinary Pathology and Microbiology, Faculty of Veterinary Medicine, Universiti Putra Malaysia, Serdang, Selangor, Malaysia

Mohamed Abidin Zainal
Department of Agribusiness and information system, Faculty of Agriculture, Universiti Putra Malaysia, Serdang, Selangor, Malaysia

Ramlan bin Mohamad
Veterinary Research Institute, Ipoh Perak, Malaysia

Azri Adzhar
Epidemiology and Surveillance Unit, Department of Veterinary Services, Putrajaya, Malaysia

Jean-Noël Arsac and Thierry Baron
Agence nationale de sécurité sanitaire de l'alimentation, de l'environnement et du travail (Anses), Unité Maladies Neuro-dégnératives, Lyon, France

Rowena M. A. Packer and Holger A. Volk
Department of Clinical Science and Services, Royal Veterinary College, Hatfield, Hertfordshire, United Kingdom

Bruno B. J. Torres
Department of Veterinary Medicine and Surgery, Federal University of Minas Gerais, Belo Horizonte, Minas Gerais, Brazil

Nadia K. Shihab
Department of Clinical Science and Services, Royal Veterinary College, Hatfield, Hertfordshire, United Kingdom
Department of Neurology/Neurosurgery, Southern Counties Veterinary Specialists, Ringwood, Hampshire, United Kingdom

Raul J. Cano
Center for Applications in Biotechnology, California Polytechnic State University, San Luis Obispo, California, United States of America

Jessica Rivera-Perez, Gary A. Toranzos, Erileen García-Roldán and Steven E. Massey
Department of Biology, University of Puerto Rico, San Juan, Puerto Rico

Tasha M. Santiago-Rodriguez
Department of Pathology, University of California San Diego, San Diego, California, United States of America

Yvonne M. Narganes-Storde and Luis Chanlatte-Baik
Center for Archaeological Research, University of Puerto Rico, Rio Piedras Campus, San Juan, Puerto Rico

Lucy Bunkley-Williams
Department of Biology, University of Puerto Rico, Mayaguez Campus, San Juan, Puerto Rico

Toyotaka Sato, Torahiko Okubo, Masaru Usui and Yutaka Tamura
Laboratory of Food Microbiology and Food Safety, Department of Health and Environmental Sciences, School of Veterinary Medicine, Rakuno Gakuen University, Ebetsu, Japan

Shin-ichi Yokota
Department of Microbiology, Sapporo Medical University School of Medicine, Sapporo, Japan

Satoshi Izumiyama
Nemuro District Agriculture Mutual Aid Association, Nakashibetsu, Japan

Index